Rhinitis

Editor

JONATHAN A. BERNSTEIN

IMMUNOLOGY AND ALLERGY CLINICS OF NORTH AMERICA

www.immunology.theclinics.com

Consulting Editor
STEPHEN A. TILLES

May 2016 • Volume 36 • Number 2

ELSEVIER

1600 John F. Kennedy Boulevard • Suite 1800 • Philadelphia, Pennsylvania, 19103-2899

http://www.theclinics.com

IMMUNOLOGY AND ALLERGY CLINICS OF NORTH AMERICA Volume 36, Number 2

May 2016 ISSN 0889-8561, ISBN-13: 978-0-323-44467-5

Editor: Jessica McCool

Developmental Editor: Kristen Helm

Immunology and Allergy Clinics of North America (ISSN 0889–8561) is published quarterly by Elsevier Inc., 360 Park Avenue South, New York, NY 10010-1710. Months of issue are February, May, August, and November. Periodicals postage paid at New York, NY and additional mailing offices. Subscription prices are $320.00 per year for US individuals, $508.00 per year for US institutions, $100.00 per year for US students and residents, $395.00 per year for Canadian individuals, $220.00 per year for Canadian students, $644.00 per year for Canadian institutions, $445.00 per year for international individuals, $644.00 per year for international institutions, $220.00 per year for international students. To receive student/resident rate, orders must be accompanied by name of affiliated institution, date of term, and the *signature* of program/residency coordinator on institution letterhead. Orders will be billed at individual rate until proof of status is received. Foreign air speed delivery is included in all *Clinics* subscription prices. All prices are subject to change without notice. **POSTMASTER**: Send address changes to *Immunology and Allergy Clinics of North America,* Elsevier Health Sciences Division, Subscription Customer Service, 3251 Riverport Lane, Maryland Heights, MO 63043. **Customer Service: 1-800-654-2452 (U.S. and Canada); 314-447-8871 (outside U.S. and Canada). Fax: 314-447-8029. E-mail: journalscustomerservice-usa@elsevier.com** (for print support); **journalsonlinesupport-usa@elsevier.com** (for online support).

Reprints. For copies of 100 or more, of articles in this publication, please contact the Commercial Reprints Department, Elsevier Inc., 360 Park Avenue South, New York, New York 10010-1710. Tel. 212-633-3874, Fax: 212-633-3820, E-mail: reprints@elsevier.com.

Immunology and Allergy Clinics of North America is covered in MEDLINE/PubMed (Index Medicus), Current Contents/Life Sciences, Science Citation Index, ISI/BIOMED, Chemical Abstracts, and EMBASE/Excerpta Medica.

Contributors

CONSULTING EDITOR

STEPHEN A. TILLES, MD
Executive Director, ASTHMA Inc. Clinical Research Center; Partner, Northwest Asthma and Allergy Center; Clinical Professor of Medicine, University of Washington, Seattle, Washington

EDITOR

JONATHAN A. BERNSTEIN, MD
Bernstein Allergy Group; Professor of Medicine, Division of Immunology, Rheumatology and Allergy, Department of Internal Medicine, Director of the VAH Clinical Research Unit, University of Cincinnati College of Medicine, Cincinnati, Ohio

AUTHORS

ALAN P. BAPTIST, MD, MPH
Division of Allergy and Clinical Immunology, University of Michigan, Ann Arbor, Michigan

FUAD M. BAROODY, MD, FACS, FAAAI
Professor, Section of Otolaryngology-Head and Neck Surgery, Departments of Surgery and Pediatrics, The University of Chicago Medicine and Biological Sciences, Chicago, Illinois

DAVID I. BERNSTEIN, MD
Professor of Medicine, Division of Immunology Allergy Section, Department of Internal Medicine, University of Cincinnati College of Medicine, Cincinnati, Ohio

JONATHAN A. BERNSTEIN, MD
Bernstein Allergy Group; Professor of Medicine, Division of Immunology, Rheumatology and Allergy, Department of Internal Medicine, Director of the VAH Clinical Research Unit, University of Cincinnati College of Medicine, Cincinnati, Ohio

NATALIA BLANCA-LÓPEZ, MD, PhD
Allergy Service, Hospital Infanta Leonor, Madrid, Spain

PALOMA CAMPO, MD, PhD
Allergy Unit, IBIMA-Regional University Hospital of Málaga, UMA, Málaga, Spain

JOAN DUNLOP, MD
Clinical Associate, Division of Emergency Medicine, Children's National Health System, Washington, DC

WYTSKE J. FOKKENS, MD, PhD
Head, Department of Otorhinolaryngology, Academic Medical Centre, Amsterdam, The Netherlands

LESLIE C. GRAMMER III, MD
Professor, Division of Allergy-Immunology, Department of Medicine, Northwestern University Feinberg School of Medicine, Chicago, Illinois

JUSTIN GREIWE, MD
Bernstein Allergy Group; Division of Immunology Allergy Section, Department of Internal Medicine, University of Cincinnati College of Medicine, Cincinnati, Ohio

GEORGE V. GUIBAS, MD, PhD
Centre of Paediatrics and Child Health, Institute of Human Development, University of Manchester; Royal Manchester Children's Hospital, Central Manchester University Hospitals Trust, Manchester, United Kingdom

ANJENI KESWANI, MD, MS
Clinical Instructor, Division of Pulmonary, Allergy, and Critical Care, Department of Medicine, Duke University Medical Center, Durham, North Carolina

PHILLIP L. LIEBERMAN, MD
Clinical Professor of Medicine and Pediatrics, Division of Allergy and Immunology, Department of Medicine, University of Tennessee; Department of Pediatrics, University of Tennessee, Memphis, Tennessee

ELIZABETH MATSUI, MD, MHS
Professor of Pediatrics, Division of Pediatric Allergy and Immunology, Johns Hopkins School of Medicine, Baltimore, Maryland

ELI O. MELTZER, MD
Senior Associate, Allergy and Asthma Medical Group and Research Center; Clinical Professor of Pediatrics, Division of Allergy and Immunology, University of California, San Diego, California

SHARMILEE NYENHUIS, MD
Division of Pulmonary, Critical Care, Sleep and Allergy, University of Illinois at Chicago, Chicago, Illinois

NIKOLAOS G. PAPADOPOULOS, MD, PhD
Centre of Paediatrics and Child Health, Institute of Human Development, University of Manchester; Royal Manchester Children's Hospital, Central Manchester University Hospitals Trust, Manchester, United Kingdom; Allergy Department, 2nd University Pediatrics Clinic, University of Athens, Athens, Greece

ANJU T. PETERS, MD
Professor, Division of Allergy-Immunology, Department of Medicine, Northwestern University Feinberg School of Medicine, Chicago, Illinois

CARMEN RONDÓN, MD, PhD
Allergy Unit, IBIMA-Regional University Hospital of Málaga, UMA, Málaga, Spain

MARÍA SALAS, MD, PhD
Allergy Unit, IBIMA-Regional University Hospital of Málaga, UMA, Málaga, Spain

GLENIS K. SCADDING, MD, FRCP
Honorary Consultant Allergist and Rhinologist, Royal National Throat, Nose and Ear Hospital, London, United Kingdom

GUY W. SCADDING, MBBS, MRCP
Specialist Registrar in Allergy, Royal Brompton Hospital, London, United Kingdom

GENE SCHWARTZ, MD
Fellow, Division of Immunology Allergy Section, Department of Internal Medicine, University of Cincinnati College of Medicine, Cincinnati, Ohio

HEMANT P. SHARMA, MD, MHS
Attending Physician, Division of Allergy and Immunology, Children's National Health System; Assistant Professor of Pediatrics, George Washington University School of Medicine and Health Sciences, Washington, DC

DENNIS SHUSTERMAN, MD, MPH
Professor of Clinical Medicine, Emeritus, Division of Occupational and Environmental Medicine, University of California, San Francisco, San Francisco, California

PETER SMITH, MD
Qld Allergy Services, Clinical School of Medicine, Griffith University, Southport, Queensland, Australia

PAVOL SURDA, MD
Department of Otorhinolaryngology, Academic Medical Centre, Amsterdam, The Netherlands

Contents

control, rescue medication requirements, and quality-of-life measures. A comprehensive multiple modality treatment plan customized to the individual patient can optimize outcomes.

Nonallergic rhinitis is a common disease that affects many Americans. It is characterized by nasal symptoms of congestion and rhinorrhea without evidence of allergic sensitization. The pathophysiology of the disease has not been studied extensively. In the following article, the author concentrates on summarizing the available information related to cellular inflammation and neurogenic mechanisms in patients with nonallergic rhinitis. The author also explores nasal reactivity to various stimuli in these patients.

Nonallergic rhinitis (NAR) is one of the most common conditions in medicine, affecting the quality of life of millions of patients throughout the United States. Despite its ubiquitous nature, NAR remains a poorly managed and often difficult to treat condition. NAR is often suboptimally managed by clinicians with poor clinical outcomes. Establishing the correct diagnosis requires a keen understanding of the unique underlying mechanisms involved in NAR, which is still evolving. Ultimately epidemiologic studies that better define NAR prevalence and its economic burden on society are needed to convince funding agencies of the need for research to elucidate mechanisms and specific treatment approaches for this condition.

Chronic nonallergic rhinitis (NAR) is a syndrome rather than a specific disease. A lack of understanding of the pathogenesis of this condition has led to imprecise terminology with several alternate names for the condition, including vasomotor rhinitis, nonallergic rhinopathy, and idiopathic rhinitis. The therapy for NAR is best based on the underlying pathology, which typically exists in a form whereby an abnormality of the autonomic nervous system is dominant or a form in which inflammation seems to be the cause of symptoms. In general the most effective therapy is the combination of an intranasal antihistamine and an intranasal corticosteroid.

This review focuses on local allergic rhinitis, a new phenotype of allergic rhinitis, commonly misdiagnosed as nonallergic rhinitis. It has gained attention over last decade and can affect patients from all countries, ethnic groups and ages, impairing their quality of life, and is frequently associated with conjunctivitis and asthma. Diagnosis is based on clinical history, the demonstration of a positive response to nasal allergen provocation test and/or the detection of nasal sIgE. A positive basophil activation test may support the diagnosis. Recent studies have demonstrated that allergen immunotherapy is an effective immune-modifying treatment, highlighting the importance of early diagnosis.

association with disease prevalence. Exposure to a variety of aeroallergens is strongly implicated in the pathogenesis and progression of AR. Other environmental exposures have been suggested to play potential roles in the risk of AR, including bacterial exposure, air pollution, and environmental toxicants.

Dennis Shusterman

"Nonallergic rhinitis" (NAR) is defined by intermittent or persistent nasal symptoms without evidence of immunoglobulin E-mediated sensitization to relevant aeroallergens. The largest subgroup is idiopathic, and is characterized by nasal hyperreactivity to nonspecific environmental triggers, including temperature, humidity, and chemical exposures. As nonspecific nasal hyperreactivity is often found in the absence of mucosal inflammation, some clinicians refer to this condition as "nonallergic rhinopathy." Irritant rhinitis can arise de novo after high-level and/or prolonged exposure to airborne irritant chemicals. We review the range of environmentally induced nonallergic nasal symptoms and signs, and explore issues of pathophysiology unique to environmental chemical exposures.

Pavol Surda and Wytske J. Fokkens

Rhinitis is a multifactorial disease characterized by sneezing, rhinorrhea, postnasal drip, and nasal congestion. This condition affects 10% to 40% of the population and is responsible for billions of spent health care dollars and impairment in quality of life for those affected. Currently available medical and vaccine therapies are effective for a large segment of this population; however, a subset of patients still has difficult-to-control rhinitis. This article reviews the current progress being made in novel drug and vaccine development and delves into alternative medical, surgical, and homeopathic strategies that may be promising adjunctive treatments for the difficult-to-treat rhinitis patient.

IMMUNOLOGY AND ALLERGY CLINICS OF NORTH AMERICA

THE CLINICS ARE AVAILABLE ONLINE!
Access your subscription at:
www.theclinics.com

Foreword

Rhinitis: The Great Enigma

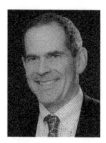

Stephen A. Tilles, MD
Consulting Editor

Since the nose is the doorway through which we continuously sample the airborne environment, and since the lifetime prevalence rates of infectious rhinitis and allergic rhinitis are 100% and 20%, respectively, it should come as no surprise that rhinitis is the indisputable "backbone" of the Allergy/Immunology specialty. And thanks to decades of painstaking research addressing the unmet needs of patients with allergic rhinitis—the most common form of chronic rhinitis—we are able to offer remarkably effective and affordable pharmacotherapies as well as safe and effective immunotherapies for our patients. However, as impressive as recent innovations have been, there are more chronic rhinitis patients than ever; we have yet to find a cure for allergic rhinitis, and the pace of progress in our understanding of the pathophysiology of nonallergic rhinitis has been sluggish. Indeed, despite more than a century of innovation, there are still far too many patients who continue to suffer greatly, and in fact, we still do not know how to help some rhinitis patients.

In this issue of *Immunology and Allergy Clinics of North America*, Editor Jonathan Bernstein has done a masterful job of assembling an international team of authors to address cutting-edge topics of interest to clinicians who take care of rhinitis patients. In addition to describing the classification, pathophysiology, diagnosis, and treatment of both allergic and nonallergic rhinitis, there are separate articles focusing on local allergic rhinitis, occupational rhinitis, rhinitis in the elderly, and complications of rhinitis. I highly recommend this *Immunology and Allergy Clinics of North America* issue as an

Immunol Allergy Clin N Am 36 (2016) xiii–xiv
http://dx.doi.org/10.1016/j.iac.2016.01.002
0889-8561/16/$ – see front matter

authoritative state-of-the-art reference for any care provider who routinely evaluates patients with this ubiquitous and enigmatic disorder.

Stephen A. Tilles, MD
ASTHMA Inc. Clinical Research Center
Northwest Asthma and Allergy Center
University of Washington School of Medicine
9725 Third Avenue NE, Suite 500
Seattle, WA 98115, USA

E-mail address:
stilles@nwasthma.com

Preface

Rhinitis

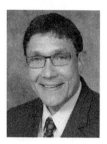

Jonathan A. Bernstein, MD
Editor

Rhinitis is an important clinical condition that affects a broad sector of the population. Our understanding of clinical phenotypes and endotypes for chronic rhinitis subtypes is still evolving as are investigations into novel and more effective treatment approaches for more difficult to treat rhinitis patients. Unfortunately, chronic rhinitis is still trivialized by many clinicians, who often treat patients as "one size fits all," and by patients who accept living daily with uncontrolled symptoms and a poor quality of life. The compendium of articles in this issue addresses the spectrum of issues pertaining to chronic rhinitis and is replete with useful information for both the primary care physician and the specialist alike. There is intentional overlap between articles to emphasize important concepts. The contributing authors are from different countries and have different specialty backgrounds. What is reassuring is that all of the authors have similar impressions regarding the current state-of-the-art for chronic rhinitis, indicating that the emerging literature in conjunction with international practice guidelines has been impactful for developing consensus opinions regarding diagnosis, management, and treatment of chronic rhinitis subtypes. However, much is still to be investigated and learned about this chronic condition, which is associated with a significant number of other comorbidities, including chronic sinusitis, sleep disturbances, and asthma. Topics included in this series include discussion on endotypes and phenotypes; burden of illness and quality of life; mechanisms, diagnosis, and treatment for allergic and nonallergic rhinitis; special populations including local allergic rhinitis, the elderly, and rhinitis in the workplace; the impact of allergic and nonallergic environmental determinants; comorbidities and emerging as well as novel potentially adjunctive medical and surgical therapies. The authors are to be congratulated for their thorough comprehensive review of these important topics. It is hoped that this issue will help stimulate the reader to pursue clinical, translational, or basic research initiatives that will fill the unmet knowledge gaps still quite apparent for chronic rhinitis.

I would like to dedicate this book in memory of my beloved Father, Leonard, Mother, Miriam, and sisters, Susan and Ellen. I was blessed to have a father who was a great

Immunol Allergy Clin N Am 36 (2016) xv–xvi
http://dx.doi.org/10.1016/j.iac.2016.01.001
0889-8561/16/$ – see front matter © 2016 Published by Elsevier Inc.
immunology.theclinics.com

mentor but also my colleague and friend, a mother whose inner strength and optimism was inspirational and a guiding light to our entire family and two beautiful, unique sisters who cared deeply about family and always faced problems head on with courage and determination. I also want to thank my older brother, David, for his support and advice throughout my career and life. Finally, last but not least, I am grateful to my wife, Lisa, and four amazing kids, Alison, Joshua, Rebecca and Caren, for their unconditional love and support. They make it all worthwhile.

Jonathan A. Bernstein, MD
University of Cincinnati College of Medicine
Division of Immunology, Rheumatology and Allergy
231 Albert Sabin Way, ML#563
Cincinnati, OH 45267-0563, USA

E-mail address:
Jonathan.Bernstein@uc.edu

Rhinitis Subtypes, Endotypes, and Definitions

Nikolaos G. Papadopoulos, MD, PhD[a,b,c,]*, George V. Guibas, MD, PhD[a,b]

KEYWORDS

- Rhinitis • Endotypes • Phenotypes • Pathophysiology • Symptoms

KEY POINTS

- Rhinitis endotypes are as numerous and diverse as the disease's phenotypes and are largely overlapping, making a clear demarcation challenging.
- Some rhinitis phenotypes previously considered important are now thought to be less relevant because of advances that have been made in understanding rhinitis subtypes.
- Consensus classification of rhinitis subsets is still an unmet need.
- Chronic rhinitis is a far more complex and burdensome condition than is generally acknowledged, and there is considerable need for research to better understand the pathobiology of nonallergic rhinitis and its interaction with allergic rhinitis.

INTRODUCTION

Chronic rhinitis (CR) is defined as an inflammation of the nasal mucosa, characterized by 2 or more symptoms of nasal congestion/obstruction, anterior or posterior rhinorrhea, and sneezing and itching for at least 1 hour daily and for more than 2 weeks.[1] CR is a prevalent pathologic condition with widespread morbidity associated with a considerable financial burden on health care systems.[2,3] Its economic impact is further magnified because it is a risk factor for other comorbidities in adults, such as sinusitis and asthma, and also a precursor to serious conditions in children, such as learning disabilities, behavioral deviation, and psychological impairment.[3,4] Nevertheless, it is an underestimated and often trivialized disease,

Conflicts of interest: Dr N.G. Papadopoulos has received grants from GSK, Nestle, and Merck, fees for development of educational presentations from AbbVie, Sanofi, Menarini, Meda, consultancy fees from GSK, AbbVie, Novartis, Menarini, ALK-Abello, and Meda, and fees for lectures by Novartis, Allergopharma, Uriach, GSK, Stallergenes, and MSD; Dr G.V. Guibas declares no relevant conflict of interest.
[a] Centre of Paediatrics and Child Health, Institute of Human Development, University of Manchester, Oxford Road, Manchester M13 9WL, UK; [b] Department of Pediatric Immunology, Royal Manchester Children's Hospital, Central Manchester University Hospitals Trust, Oxford Road, Manchester M13 9WL, UK; [c] Allergy Department, 2nd University Pediatrics Clinic, University of Athens, Aglaia Kyriakou Childrens Hospital, Thivon & Livadeias, Athens 11527, Greece
* Corresponding author. St Mary's Hospital, 5th Floor, Research, Oxford Road, Manchester M13 9WL, UK.
E-mail address: ngp@allergy.gr

Immunol Allergy Clin N Am 36 (2016) 215–233
http://dx.doi.org/10.1016/j.iac.2015.12.001
0889-8561/16/$ – see front matter © 2016 Elsevier Inc. All rights reserved.

often viewed as no more than a mere annoyance. Furthermore, the high variability in both underlying pathophysiologic mechanisms (endotypes) and clinical presentations (phenotypes) of CR has hindered efforts to develop clear guidelines for its diagnosis and treatment. Even the term rhinitis has been criticized because it connotes inflammation, whereas certain rhinitis endotypes seem to be devoid of an inflammatory component.[5]

The 3 most widely accepted rhinitis subgroups thus far are allergic rhinitis (AR), infectious rhinitis, and nonallergic noninfectious rhinitis (NAR).[1] However, this classification may be an oversimplification, because a combined (mixed) phenotype exists in many patients.[3,6] In addition, there are numerous, mostly overlapping classification systems based on independent criteria such as age of onset, disease severity, symptoms, symptom pattern/frequency, causative agents, and underlying pathophysiology. For instance, from a clinical perspective, patients are classified as blockers, with nasal congestion as the prominent symptom, and runners, with rhinorrhea being predominant. Also, rhinitis caused by mechanical/structural abnormalities is included in the NAR subgroup by some investigators[7,8] and excluded by others.[9] Furthermore, occupational rhinitis can be either allergic or nonallergic, blurring the boundaries between the 3 widely accepted categories.[10] Characterization of rhinitis phenotypes is further hampered by the scarcity of distinct biomarkers. Even for allergic rhinitis, for which the immunopathogenesis is more clearly delineated, clinical classification as proposed by Allergic Rhinitis and its Impact on Asthma (ARIA) guidelines are frequently not adhered to by treating physicians who still do not prescribe or modify treatment based on phenotypic characteristics (eg, frequency or disease severity), contrary to the ARIA guidelines.[11–14] These studies underscore the difficulty of using only the phenotype concept to classify CR and highlight the importance of developing a classification system that focuses on rhinitis endotypes.[15]

SUBTYPES, ENDOTYPES, AND DEFINITIONS
Rhinosinusitis and Overlapping Subtypes

Rhinitis frequently coexists with sinusitis because the nose and sinuses share vascular, neuronal, and anatomic pathways. Therefore, the term rhinosinusitis is preferred in patients with symptomatic sinus inflammation.[16] Rhinosinusitis can be acute or chronic.[1]

The acute form of rhinosinusitis is infectious and predominantly of viral origin (around 90% of cases[17,18]), with the usual causes being rhinovirus (common cold), coronavirus, adenovirus, parainfluenza virus, respiratory syncytial virus, or enterovirus. It is common that an acute viral rhinosinusitis is complicated by secondary bacterial superinfection that establishes a bacterial rhinosinusitis endotype (eg, Streptococcus pneumoniae, Haemophilus influenzae, Moraxella catarrhalis).

The chronic rhinosinusitis phenotype is more complicated for establishing a defined endotype because infection has a minor, if any, role. Chronic rhinosinusitis is characterized by nasal and sinus symptoms, such as nasal congestion, purulent discharge, facial pain, and impaired olfaction, which last longer than 12 weeks. Specifically, diagnosis requires:

1. The existence of 2 or more symptoms, one of which must be either nasal blockage or discharge and the other facial pain/pressure or impaired olfaction
2. Either endoscopic signs (polyps, mucopurulent discharge, and/or edema/mucosal obstruction primarily in the middle meatus) and/or computed tomography findings (sinus mucosal changes)[19]

Importantly, chronic rhinosinusitis is further classified into chronic rhinosinusitis without nasal polyps and chronic rhinosinusitis with nasal polyps.[16] Both conditions are discrete phenotypes defined by the presence or absence of nasal polyps. However, this characteristic can also be endotype defining, because the presence of polyps indicates a different underlying pathophysiologic mechanism compared with when they are absent. Chronic rhinosinusitis without polyps seems to mechanistically involve Th_1 mucosal inflammation resulting in tissue remodeling caused by overexpression of transforming growth factor beta.[20–22] The role of infection in this endotype, if any, is not clear.[21,23] In contrast, the endotype for chronic rhinosinusitis with polyps seems to be Th_2 skewed and characterized by increased levels of interleukin (IL)-4, IL-5, and IL-13 manifested as significant mucosal eosinophilia.[24] A different endotype for chronic rhinosinusitis with polyps characterized by preponderance of neutrophils may be seen in patients with cystic fibrosis,[25] or in Asian populations, in which TH_{17} cytokines and interferon gamma may be predominant.[26]

The eosinophilic endotype (chronic rhinosinusitis with polyps) may be further associated with increased levels of total and specific immunoglobulin E (IgE).[27] In addition, a role for *Staphylococcus aureus* toxins and other microbial superantigens has been suggested[28] through various pathways, including mediation of basophil degranulation, interaction with the T-cell receptor, and antienterotoxin IgE.[27,29,30] Defective epithelial barrier caused by disruption of tight junctions could also play a role in this endotype.[31] One particular phenotype/endotype that is important is aspirin-exacerbated respiratory disease, characterized by concomitant asthma and aspirin hypersensitivity and present in up to 40% of patients with nasal polyps.[32,33] This condition is also encompassed in the local inflammatory drug-induced rhinitis endotype, because it is defined by hypersensitivity to aspirin that leads to upper and lower airway inflammation, resulting in severe rhinitis and asthma symptoms.[34] Additional chronic rhinosinusitis endotypes could be characterized based on their variable responsiveness to different treatments. For example, there exist good responders, weak responders, and nonresponders to any given therapeutic agent (eg, anti–IL-5–responsive and anti-IgE–responsive endotypes).[16] However, it should be emphasized that poor treatment response may simply reflect an incorrect phenotypic/endotypic diagnosis, further emphasizing the need for better understanding of the pathogenesis of CR and chronic rhinosinusitis subtypes.

Allergic Rhinitis

Allergic rhinitis, as defined by ARIA, is a well-defined endotype. It is an inflammatory condition caused by an IgE-mediated response to a spectrum of environmental allergens, including pollens, dust mite, cockroach frass, animal dander, rodents, and molds.[35] Therefore, the diagnosis is established by skin-prick testing or specific IgE serologic testing to show IgE-mediated sensitization that corresponds with the patient's medical history of symptoms induced by exposure to 1 or more specific sensitizing allergens (**Fig. 1**). Nasally inhaled sensitizing allergens are processed by antigen-presenting cells in the nasal mucosa and presented to $CD4^+$ T lymphocytes.[36] During this sensitization phase, T lymphocytes produce cytokines (eg, IL-3, II-4, IL-5, IL-13, granulocyte-macrophage colony-stimulating factor), which lead to differentiation of B lymphocytes to plasma cells, which in turn produce antigen-specific IgE, which binds to high-affinity IgE receptors (Fc epsilon receptor I [FcERI]) on the surface of mast cells and basophils. On allergen reexposure, specific allergenic peptides are recognized by antigen-binding sites of specific IgE bound to these mast cells or basophils, resulting in cross-linking of IgE molecules and activation of signaling cascades that lead to granule exocytosis (also called degranulation) of preformed and newly

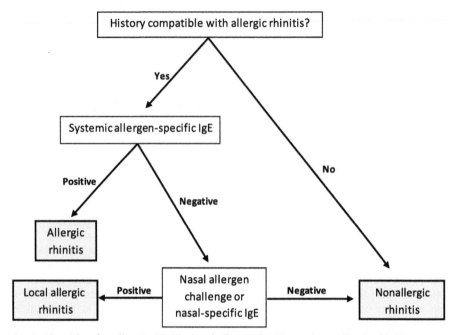

Fig. 1. Algorithm for allergic rhinitis, local allergic rhinitis, and nonallergic rhinitis.

formed bioactive mediators (eg, histamine, leukotrienes, prostaglandins, platelet-activating factor).[35,37] A late-phase reaction typically follows up to 4 to 12 hours later, as a result of the release of chemokines and other chemoattractants that cause Th_2 cells, activated eosinophils, and mast cells to migrate into the nasal epithelium where they release additional cytokines, enzymes, and mediators that perpetuate allergic inflammation,[38,39] causing delayed or persistent AR symptoms.

Although AR as an endotype seems to be fairly straightforward, the variety of AR phenotypes is much more complicated. Clinically, AR has traditionally been character-ized as seasonal, attributed to seasonal allergens (pollens); perennial, associated with year-round allergens (dust mites, mold spores, and animal dander)[3,9]; or episodic, caused by sporadic exposures. However, this phenotyping approach is often inconsis-tent and overlapping.[9] Therefore, ARIA guidelines[11,12] have categorized AR by dura-tion, either as intermittent (<4 days per week or <4 weeks) or persistent (>4 days per week and >4 weeks) and by severity as mild, characterized by normal sleep, no impair-ment of daily activities/work/leisure/sport/school, and no troublesome symptoms; and moderate/severe, associated with any of the characteristics listed earlier. Further AR phenotyping may include pattern of sensitization (monosensitized vs polysensitized). It was recently suggested in a Practical Allergy (PRACTALL) document that more atten-tion should be paid to the underlying mechanisms related to aeroallergen sensitization even if such sensitization does not seem to drive symptoms, because this patient pro-file could potentially define a novel phenotype and/or endotype.[40]

Nonallergic Rhinitis

Noninfectious nonallergic rhinitis (NAR) is a heterogeneous group of nasal conditions in which the diagnosis requires negative systemic IgE testing (see **Fig. 1**).[7,41] The NAR subtypes are common, affecting as many as 200 million individuals worldwide,[42,43] with a prevalence of 20% to 70% among adult patients.[44] However, their heterogeneity, the different criteria used for classification, and the often conflicting terminology across studies impedes uncovering of the exact prevalence of this disorder.

For instance, from nasal mucosal eosinophilia (endotype-wise), NAR variants have historically been divided into 2 groups: NAR with eosinophilia syndrome (NARES) (which was long thought to be a distinct phenotype/endotype[45]) and all the other non-eosinophilic subtypes (non-NARES); NARES was originally defined by the presence of more than 20% eosinophils in nasal smears.[46,47] However, there is currently no consensus on the eosinophilic threshold required for diagnosis, because any amount from greater than 5% to greater than 20% has been reported to indicate this condition.[2,8,48] However, recent research scrutinizing NARES mechanics has raised questions regarding whether this is a distinct condition or whether it mostly overlaps with other conditions.[40] The value of this histologic-based classification is further reduced because the methodologies used to obtain nasal cytology by swabbing or scraping the inferior turbinate or nasal lavage are variable and burdensome, making it impractical to routinely perform in the clinical setting.[10] Furthermore, because NARES pathophysiology is obscure it has often been equated to idiopathic rhinitis (IR),[45,49] local AR,[40] a local inflammatory response induced by irritants,[50] or as a precursor to aspirin triad because NARES patients frequently have eosinophilic nasal polyps, bronchial hyperreactivity, and nonallergic asthma.[2,51,52] Regardless of whether any or all of these different endotypes are relevant, it is clear that eosinophilia contributes to direct mucosal damage, protracted mucociliary clearance, and nasal hyperresponsiveness.[50] Other studies have reported different inflammatory profiles in the nasal mucosa in patients with NAR, including mast cells and neutrophils, further complicating the utility of nasal histology as a biomarker for establishing reliable NAR endotypes.[53]

In addition to NARES, at least 6 other clinical entities are included in the NAR classification: drug-induced rhinitis, gustatory rhinitis, hormone-induced rhinitis, atrophic rhinitis, rhinitis of the elderly, and IR (**Fig. 2, Table 1**).[10]

Idiopathic rhinitis

IR is the most prevalent subtype of the NAR group,[54] and is also a diagnosis requiring exclusion of AR.[44,54,55] Its terminology has been variable across studies,[7,10] including intrinsic rhinitis, IR, vasomotor rhinitis,[55,56] and nonallergic rhinopathy.[6] Its pathophysiologic mechanism is unrelated to allergy, structural defects, or underlying systemic disease, and it is typically not associated with nasal eosinophilia.[51,57]

Idiotypic rhinitis endotypes are not well elucidated. However, it is likely that the underlying mechanism is neurogenically mediated. The absence of a distinct consistent cellular inflammatory pattern in the nasal mucosa provides further indirect support for a neurogenic mechanism. Triggers for this form of NAR typically include noxious odorants or chemical irritants like tobacco smoke, perfumes/fragrance, and cleaning agents, but also changes in temperature, humidity, and barometric pressure. Other triggers may include positional changes, alcohol, or the act of eating.

Nonspecific irritants and alcohol[9,54,58] were thought to induce tachykinin release and inhibition of sympathetic mediators, enhancing the parasympathetic response and culminating in nasal congestion and/or rhinorrhea.[59] However, such a neural/vascular pathophysiologic mechanism has not been clearly documented,[3] and it is now thought that some forms of IR may be disorders of the nonadrenergic noncholinergic (NANC) or peptidergic neural system.[60,61] Nasal peptidergic neurons (mainly sensory C fibers) are activated by these nonspecific stimuli, resulting in antidromic and orthodromic release of inflammatory neuropeptides, which can exert effects on

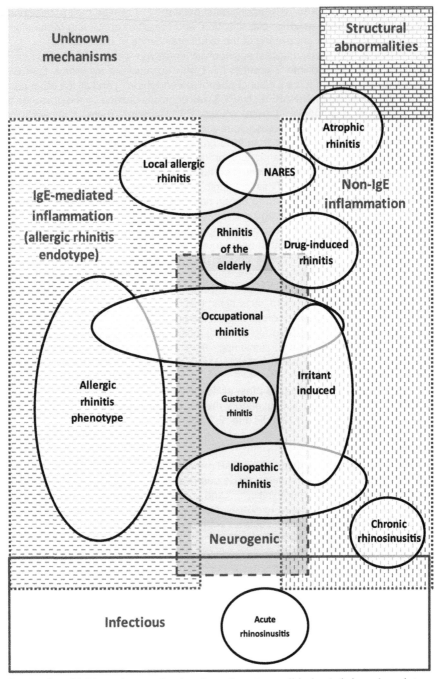

Fig. 2. The rhinitis universe. Overlapping phenotypes (*black circles*) and endotypes (*background*).

Table 1
Rhinitis phenotypes and characteristics

Phenotype	Characteristic
Rhinitis by structural/systemic causes	Systematic disease/structural causes
Acute infectious rhinosinusitis	Infection
Chronic Rhinosinusitis	Duration >12 wk and paranasal sinuses involvement/polyps
Allergic rhinitis	IgE-mediated inflammation
Nonallergic rhinitis	—
Local allergic rhinitis	Topical IgE mechanism
NARES	Nasal smear with >5%–20% of eosinophils
Gustatory rhinitis	Symptoms elicited by ingestion of foods
Rhinitis of pregnancy	Pregnancy >36 wk
Drug-induced rhinitis	Symptoms elicited by medication intake
Rhinitis medicamentosa	Prolonged use of nasal decongestants
Occupational rhinitis	Symptoms only at workplace
Many surgeries/granulomatous disease	Atrophic rhinitis
Rhinitis of the elderly	Old-age onset
Idiopathic rhinitis	All other phenotypes excluded

the blood vasculature and mucus-secreting glands, leading to symptoms of IR. These fibers are thought to be primarily activated by transient response potential (TRP) calcium ion channels whose ligands have been shown to be affected by temperature, mechanical or osmotic stimuli, or a spectrum of chemical irritants. For example, TPRV1, for which capsaicin has been shown to be a specific ligand, is activated by hot temperatures. An acute exposure to capsaicin can activate TRPV1, whereas continuous exposure to capsaicin can desensitize this receptor[40] (for a discussion of the mechanisms for NAR, see Baroody FM: Non-Allergic Rhinitis: Mechanism of Action, in this issue).

However, these pathways could define a novel umbrella endotype, the neurogenic rhinitis endotype, which can be distinguished from healthy controls by provocation to stimuli like cold dry air,[62] a challenge that stimulates TRPA1 and TRPM8 channels, which are attenuated by capsaicin.[63] Similar TRP pathways could explain gustatory rhinitis, which is another subtype with a strong neurologic basis,[64] as well as other rhinitis subtypes to a variable degree (ie, acute viral rhinosinusitis, which is known to be responsive to cold air provocation[65,66]; rhinitis of the elderly; or even AR, which may have a neural hypersensitivity facet[63]). Further support for a neurologic mechanism is that these conditions seem to be responsive to treatment with capsaicin or anticholinergic drugs.[3,67,68]

Further endotypes of IR could be defined by the trigger type; for example, irritant-sensitive IR.[8] An irritant-induced umbrella phenotype that includes not only IR but other entities such as occupational rhinitis subphenotypes has been proposed (see **Fig. 2**).[40] These novel groupings warrant further research.

Hormonal rhinitis

Hormonal rhinitis subtypes include rhinitis of pregnancy and menstrual cycle–related rhinitis.[6,69] Rhinitis of pregnancy is a common condition that affects up to 20% to 30% of pregnant women. Rhinitis of pregnancy typically begins in the last 6 weeks of pregnancy (after 34 weeks of gestation) and resolves spontaneously within 2 weeks postpartum,[70] whereas menstrual cycle–related rhinitis consists of premenstrual symptoms on a cyclical basis. These phenotypes are probably based on similar pathophysiologic mechanisms primarily mediated through increased levels of estrogen, which cause nasal congestion through vascular engorgement.[71] This assumption was based mainly on reports from women taking contraceptive pills containing high estrogen levels, which caused rhinitis as a side effect. Assuming that estrogen does cause nasal obstruction, increased congestion would be expected during the preovulatory phase of the menstrual cycle, when the levels of estrogen are highest, but this is not always the case.[71] Therefore, other mechanisms have also been suggested, including increased circulating blood volume caused by a vasodilating effect of progesterone, increased production of human growth hormone (which is also the basis of a proposed acromegaly-related rhinitis subtype), as well as enhanced production of a placental growth hormone variant, of an insulinlike growth factor-I, or of prolactin. Other key players could include beta-estradiol, which has been shown to increase the expression of histamine H1 receptors on mucosal epithelial and microvascular endothelial cells[72] and to induce eosinophil migration and/or degranulation.[71,73] Other suggested forms of hormonal rhinitis, such as those linked with thyroid disorders, are not currently supported by a high level of scientific evidence.[2,33]

Gustatory rhinitis

Gustatory rhinitis is defined by the acute onset of profuse watery rhinorrhea immediately after ingestion of certain spicy foods but can occur after the act of eating in general.[74,75] Recent studies suggest that it is a direct neurogenic event, thought to be associated with overstimulation of the parasympathetic system. Regulation of vascular and glandular processes in the nose includes complex interactions between sensory, sympathetic, and parasympathetic nerves.[76] Ingestion of the food could act as a mechanical stimulus that activates nociceptive sensory nerves, resulting in overactivation of parasympathetic fibers, as shown by the blunting of this effect by intranasal atropine.[74,77] However, the role of a hyperactive, NANC, or peptidergic neural system is still not well elucidated and remains under debate.[64] Gustatory rhinitis has various endotypes/subtypes, including idiopathic gustatory rhinitis and posttraumatic, postsurgical, and cranial nerve neuropathy–associated endotypes.[64,78] Idiopathic gustatory rhinitis, the most common of these entities, is prevalent in the general population.[64] However, up to 45% of patients consider it no more than an annoyance, probably leading to an underestimation of its prevalence.[75]

Drug-induced rhinitis

Systemic drug-induced rhinitis may be classified into 3 subtypes: local inflammatory type, neurogenic type, and idiopathic (unknown) type (**Fig. 3**).

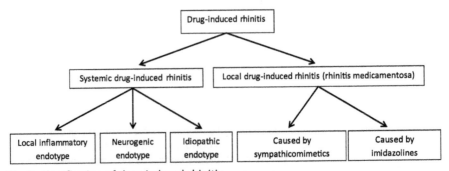

Fig. 3. Classification of drug-induced rhinitis.

The local inflammatory endotype commonly occurs after ingestion of aspirin and other nonsteroidal antiinflammatory drugs.[8,79] Although various pathogenic mechanisms have been proposed, it is thought that the inhibition of cyclooxygenase-1 shifts the metabolism of arachidonic acid to the lipooxygenase pathway, resulting in decreased production of prostaglandin E2 and increased cysteinyl leukotriene release (ie, leucotriene C4) precipitating local inflammation.[79]

The neurogenic endotype of drug-induced rhinitis can occur with sympatholytic drugs such as alpha-adrenergic and beta-adrenergic antagonists, including clonidine, guanethidine, doxazocin, and methyldopa.[8,79] Downregulation of the sympathetic tone leads to vascular engorgement, nasal congestion, and rhinorrhea. Other drug classes that could cause neurogenic-type rhinitis are phosphodiesterase-5 selective inhibitors such as sildenafil, tadalafil, and vardenafil, which act through their vasodilating properties. This group of medications is thought to affect the erectile tissue of the nasal turbinates (capacitance venous vessels) causing nasal congestion.[51,79,80] This concept is the same as that underlying the so-called honeymoon rhinitis subtype, in which sexual activities are thought to cause nasal blockade.

The idiopathic endotype of drug-induced rhinitis is caused by several different drug classes, some of which seem to have no pathophysiologic similarities (eg, β-blockers, angiotensin-converting enzyme inhibitors,[81] calcium channel blockers, antipsychotics[8,79]). Although some assumptions can be made related to underlying mechanisms causing rhinitis for some of these agents (eg, ACE inhibitors resulting in increased release of bradykinin, which is a potent vasodilator), the pathophysiologic basis of the idiopathic endotype is largely obscure[79] and no specific subendotypes have yet been defined.

Rhinitis medicamentosa is a distinct drug-induced rhinitis subtype.[79] It is defined as rebound nasal congestion following excessive local (rather than systemic) use of decongestant sprays. Physical examination in patients with rhinitis medicamentosa often reveals swollen, red nasal mucous membranes with minimal discharge. Two different endotypes can be discerned depending on the classes of nasal decongestants used that can cause this condition: sympathomimetics and imidazolines (**Box 1**).

Box 1
Classes of drugs that cause rhinitis medicamentosa

Sympathomimetics

Pseudoephedrine

Amphetamine

Benzedrine

Mescaline

Phenylephrine

Ephedrine

Phenylpropanolamine

Imidazolines

Xylometazoline

Naphazoline

Clonidine

Oxymetazoline

Sympathomimetic amines activate sympathetic nerves and cause vasoconstriction. Imidazolines cause vasoconstriction primarily through alpha2-adrenoreceptors. Cocaine (which is a potent vasoconstrictor) can also cause rhinitis medicamentosa, although usually symptoms are significantly more severe.[82] Histologic changes consistent with rhinitis medicamentosa include ciliary loss, squamous cell metaplasia, epithelial edema, goblet cell hyperplasia, and inflammatory cell accumulation.[83] When used briefly (<3–5 days consecutively), these medications provide significant relief of nasal congestion; however, prolonged use may lead to rhinitis medicamentosa. The mechanisms underlying this condition are variable and could be secondary to decreased production of endogenous norepinephrine through negative feedback[84]; the result of sympathomimetic amines with activity at both alpha and beta sites but a beta effect that outlasts the alpha effect causing rebound swelling[84]; or edema formation by altering vasomotor tone and vascular permeability through increased parasympathetic activity. Alongside rebound congestion, tachyphylaxis[85] and, rarely, nasal septal perforation[86] may also occur, although recent findings suggest that long-term use of these medications may be much safer when coadministered with intranasal steroids.[87,88]

Rhinitis of the elderly

Rhinitis of the elderly is possibly underpinned by nasal hyperresponsiveness of the parasympathetic system and exemplifies the neurogenic rhinitis endotype, because it commonly presents with profuse rhinorrhea and is responsive to anticholinergic treatment. A causal role of other age-related factors, such as changes in nasal physiology or body water content, decrease in nasal blood flow, degeneration of mucous glands, collagen atrophy, and weakening of the septal cartilage, is still under debate.[3,51,67,89] It is likely that such issues can result in drying and increased nasal congestion regardless of the underlying pathophysiology of rhinitis, and hence may magnify or bring about a more complicated endotype of rhinitis of the elderly.[51]

Atrophic rhinitis

Atrophic rhinitis is characterized by symptoms of crusting, purulent discharge, nasal obstruction, and halitosis.[90] It has a primary and secondary endotype that, symptom-wise, are fairly similar. A thorough medical history coupled with typical endoscopic findings are sufficient to diagnose both entities. Signs of sequelae (eg, atrophic pharyngitis) and of complications (eg, septal perforation and saddle nose deformity) may be seen in long-standing cases of both subtypes.[91]

The primary (idiopathic) subtype of atrophic rhinitis is defined by nasal mucosal and glandular atrophy.[6] It primarily affects people from areas with warm climates who present with nasal inflammation, dryness, crusting, a sense of severe congestion, and epistaxis.[8,91] The underlying pathophysiology is unclear but it is either caused by a lack of mucus, thereby facilitating bacterial growth, leading to mucosal colonization (usually with *Klebsiella ozaenae*, *S aureus*, *Proteus mirabilis*, and *Escherichia coli*[92]) or, vice versa, microbial colonization may be the primary cause of this condition. In any case, characteristic findings include crusting of nasal mucosa, a foul-smelling nasal discharge, and a reported sense of severe congestion, paradoxically in spite of considerably wide and unobstructed nasal cavities.[8]

The secondary subtype has a similar presentation, with the triad of fetor, crusting, and spacious nasal cavities with perceived congestion.[93] However, because this form of atrophic rhinitis is caused by extensive surgical removal of mucus-secreting tissue, trauma, or chronic granulomatous disorders,[6] signs of these underlying causes may be evident on physical examination. Aggressive resection of the turbinates often causes the empty nose syndrome, in which the patient exhibits severe nasal obstruction and inability to sense airflow despite complete nasal patency.[94]

Local allergic rhinitis

Local AR (also called entopic rhinitis) cannot easily fit into the 3-arm classification of rhinitis by formal criteria (see Campo P, Salas M, Blanca-López N, et al: Local Allergic Rhinitis, in this issue). Resent research has been scrutinizing this phenotype, which is a form of CR with symptoms similar to AR without systemic but with localized antigen-specific IgE (see **Fig. 1**).[41,95,96] Local IgE to common aeroallergens such as house dust mite and grass/olive pollen confirmed by specific provocation has previously been reported.[49,95,96] The mechanism for LAR seems to be similar to that of AR, in which allergen exposure causes nasal mucosal production of specific IgE, which gives rise to a localized Th_2 inflammatory response.[41,95–98] The localized allergic response observed with this endotype has led some clinicians to term this condition "entopy."[99] Studies have uncovered leukocyte-lymphocyte similarities in the nasal lavage of patients with AR and LAR, with increased numbers of eosinophils, basophils, mast cells, CD3+, and CD4+ T cells.[95,96] It has also been suggested that LAR could be an early AR condition rather than a distinct phenotype,[41,57] although this has been contested by more recent findings.[100] It has also been suggested that LAR could overlap with NARES.[40] However, more research is needed to further define this entity.

Occupational rhinitis

Classification of occupational rhinitis (see Grammer LC: Occupational Rhinitis, in this issue) is complex and there is currently no complete consensus (**Fig. 4**). Work-related-rhinitis is essentially an umbrella phenotype including occupational rhinitis, caused by factors in the work environment, and work-exacerbated rhinitis, in which a preexisting or concurrent rhinitis is worsened by occupational factors. Occupational rhinitis has been defined as "an inflammatory disease of the nose, which is characterized by intermittent or persistent symptoms (i.e., nasal congestion, sneezing, rhinorrhea, itching), and/or variable nasal airflow limitation and/or hypersecretion due to causes and

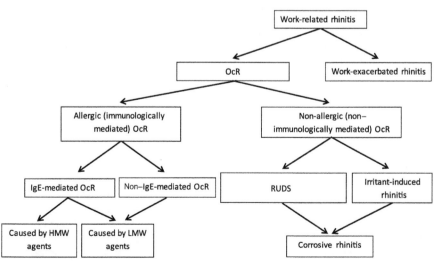

Fig. 4. Work-related rhinitis classification. OcR, occupational rhinitis; RUDS, reactive upper airways dysfunction syndrome. HMW, High molecular weight; LMW, Low molecular weight.

conditions attributable to a particular work environment and not to stimuli encountered outside the workplace."[101] Occupational rhinitis includes conditions with similar characteristics to allergic, nonallergic,[51] and irritant-induced phenotypes and to the neurogenic endotype. The nature of the workplace airborne agent exposures further defines the classification of occupational rhinitis into subvariants[50]:

- Sensitizer-induced (allergic) occupational rhinitis is an IgE immunologically mediated condition that can be induced by high-molecular-weight and low-molecular-weight antigens. High-molecular-weight agents such as plant/animal proteins and some low-molecular-weight agents like platinum salts act as complete antigens to elicit a specific IgE-mediated response, whereas low-molecular-weight agents such as some diisocyanates (hexamethylene diisocyanate) and acid anhydrides (trimellitic acid) act as haptens to bind endogenous proteins to form new allergenic peptides capable of eliciting a specific IgE-mediated response.
- The non–IgE-mediated immunologic-mediated endotype is primarily caused by low-molecular-weight agents, including reactive chemicals, transition metals, and wood dusts, and is less common.[50,102,103]
- Nonallergic occupational rhinitis, also termed reactive upper airways dysfunction syndrome, is caused by a single exposure to high chemical irritant concentrations or multiple exposures to lower chemical irritant concentrations over time, the latter form also being termed irritant-induced rhinitis.[50,104] Both of these subforms can lead to significant inflammatory and even structural damage, resulting in so-called corrosive rhinitis, which is the severe end-stage form of the irritant-induced endotype, and is most often caused by potent toxic irritants such as chlorine, sulfur dioxide, and ammonia.[105]

RHINITIS BY STRUCTURAL/MECHANICAL ABNORMALITIES

There are several structural abnormalities that predispose to and cause rhinitis. Different investigators have different views of whether these phenotypes are part of the NAR category or a stand-alone category. The most common symptom of these phenotypes is a sense of congestion either because of true blockage of the air passages or because of perceived congestion caused by a disturbance of normal airflow resistance and the development of a turbulent flow pattern.[51] Septal deviation, commonly accompanied by contralateral compensatory turbinate hypertrophy, may cause nasal obstruction. Severe septal deviations may occur and impair nasal breathing, often unilaterally.[1] Adenoidal hypertrophy typically manifests with nasal congestion, mouth breathing, nasal speech, and sleep apneic episodes/snoring.[33] It is the most common acquired anatomic cause of nasal obstruction in infants and children,[51] and is often associated with chronic allergic inflammation,[1] which causes lymphoid hypertrophy leading to prominence of the adenoidal tissue and could therefore be postulated to represent a mechanical abnormality endotype, given its association with this defined mechanism. Choanal atresia, a rare congenital disorder involving blockage of the nose–lower airways passage can go unnoticed for years if unilateral,[106] but when bilateral presents with conspicuous symptoms caused by difficulty in breathing.[107] Nasal tumors are comparably uncommon,[108] whereas nasal trauma/foreign objects are fairly common and may lead to nasal obstruction easily discernable by history or endoscopy.[109] Cerebrospinal fluid rhinorrhea, which is drainage of cerebrospinal fluid from an abnormal subarachnoid space–nasal cavity pathway, is mainly a complication of surgery or trauma[110] but can also be caused by benign intracranial hypertension or pseudotumor cerebri.[51] It is characterized by clear watery secretion occasionally accompanied by headaches and olfactory impairment.[16,111]

RHINITIS AS A SIGN OF SYSTEMIC DISEASE

Ciliary dysfunction impairs mucus clearance and can be primary or secondary (caused by viral infections and/or pollutants).[112,113] Primary ciliary dysfunction is a rare autosomal disorder that commonly manifests with recurrent respiratory infections that may manifest as Kartagener syndrome, characterized by the triad of situs inversus, chronic rhinosinusitis, and bronchiectasis. Cystic fibrosis causes recurrent nasal infections because of impaired microbial clearance and blocking of the sinus passages. Eosinophilic granulomatosis with polyangiitis (Churg-Strauss syndrome) and granulomatosis with polyangiitis (formerly known as Wegener granulomatosis) are vasculitis conditions characterized by nasal symptoms. Granulomatous inflammation causes rhinitis in sarcoidosis, a chronic syndrome that may manifest with obstruction, nasal crusting, anosmia, and epistaxis.[114,115] Amyloid deposition can occur in the sinonasal cavities in amyloidosis, causing obstruction, nasal discharge, epistaxis, and postnasal drainage.[116,117]

SUMMARY

It is likely that rhinitis phenotypes will continue to be identified clinically until the underlying mechanisms of CR subtypes are better understood, which will lead to well-defined endotypes. In view of the clinical spectrum and complexity of these conditions, this will be a major undertaking. However, it is likely that better definition of CR endotypes will greatly improve treatment and reduce symptoms, and will also reduce associated comorbidities and health care costs related to these highly prevalent and burdensome conditions.

REFERENCES

1. Roberts G, Xatzipsalti M, Borrego LM, et al. Paediatric rhinitis: position paper of the European Academy of Allergy and Clinical Immunology. Allergy 2013;68(9): 1102–16.

2. Bachert C. Persistent rhinitis - allergic or nonallergic? Allergy 2004;59:11–5.

3. Tran NP, Vickery J, Blaiss MS. Management of rhinitis: allergic and non-allergic. Allergy Asthma Immunol Res 2011;3:148–56.

4. Ledford D. Inadequate diagnosis of nonallergic rhinitis: assessing the damage. Allergy Asthma Proc 2003;24:155–62.

5. Mastin T. Recognizing and treating non-infectious rhinitis. J Am Acad Nurse Pract 2003;15:398–409.

6. Kaliner M. Classification of nonallergic rhinitis syndromes with a focus on vasomotor rhinitis, proposed to be known henceforth as nonallergic rhinopathy. World Allergy Organ J 2009;2:98–101.

7. Burns P, Powe DG, Jones NS. Idiopathic rhinitis. Curr Opin Otolaryngol Head Neck Surg 2012;20:1–8.

8. Schroer B, Pien LC. Nonallergic rhinitis: common problem, chronic symptoms. Cleve Clin J Med 2012;79:285–93.

9. Greiner AN, Meltzer EO. Overview of the treatment of allergic rhinitis and nonallergic rhinopathy. Proc Am Thorac Soc 2011;8:121–31.

10. Scarupa MD, Kaliner MA. Nonallergic rhinitis, with a focus on vasomotor rhinitis: clinical importance, differential diagnosis, and effective treatment recommendations. World Allergy Organ J 2009;2:20–5.

11. Brozek JL, Bousquet J, Baena-Cagnani CE, et al. Allergic Rhinitis and its Impact on Asthma (ARIA) guidelines: 2010 revision. J Allergy Clin Immunol 2010;126: 466–76.
12. Bousquet J, Van Cauwenberge P, Khaltaev N, et al, Aria Workshop Group, World Health Organization. Allergic rhinitis and its impact on asthma. J Allergy Clin Immunol 2001;108:S147–334.
13. Demoly P, Concas V, Urbinelli R, et al. Spreading and impact of the World Health Organization's Allergic Rhinitis and its Impact on Asthma guidelines in everyday medical practice in France. Ernani survey. Clin Exp Allergy 2008;38:1803–7.
14. Ramirez LF, Urbinelli R, Allaert FA, et al. Combining H1-antihistamines and nasal corticosteroids to treat allergic rhinitis in general practice. Allergy 2011;66: 1501–2.
15. Demoly P, Calderon MA, Casale T, et al. Assessment of disease control in allergic rhinitis. Clin Transl Allergy 2013;3:7.
16. Akdis CA, Bachert C, Cingi C, et al. Endotypes and phenotypes of chronic rhinosinusitis: a PRACTALL document of the European Academy of Allergy and Clinical Immunology and the American Academy of Allergy, Asthma & Immunology. J Allergy Clin Immunol 2013;131:1479–90.
17. Fendrick AM, Saint S, Brook I, et al. Diagnosis and treatment of upper respiratory tract infections in the primary care setting. Clin Ther 2001;23:1683–706.
18. Gwaltney JM Jr. Acute community-acquired sinusitis. Clin Infect Dis 1996;23: 1209–23.
19. Fokkens WJ, Lund VJ, Mullol J, et al. European position paper on rhinosinusitis and nasal polyps 2012. Rhinol Suppl 2012;(23). 3 p preceding table of contents, 1–298.
20. Hekiert AM, Kofonow JM, Doghramji L, et al. Biofilms correlate with TH1 inflammation in the sinonasal tissue of patients with chronic rhinosinusitis. Otolaryngol Head Neck Surg 2009;141:448–53.
21. Van Bruaene N, Derycke L, Perez-Novo CA, et al. TGF-beta signaling and collagen deposition in chronic rhinosinusitis. J Allergy Clin Immunol 2009;124: 253–9.
22. Li X, Meng J, Qiao X, et al. Expression of TGF, matrix metalloproteinases, and tissue inhibitors in Chinese chronic rhinosinusitis. J Allergy Clin Immunol 2010;125:1061–8.
23. Tatar EC, Tatar I, Ocal B, et al. Prevalence of biofilms and their response to medical treatment in chronic rhinosinusitis without polyps. Otolaryngol Head Neck Surg 2012;146:669–75.
24. Patadia M, Dixon J, Conley D, et al. Evaluation of the presence of B-cell attractant chemokines in chronic rhinosinusitis. Am J Rhinol Allergy 2010;24:11–6.
25. Van Zele T, Claeys S, Gevaert P, et al. Differentiation of chronic sinus diseases by measurement of inflammatory mediators. Allergy 2006;61:1280–9.
26. Zhang N, Liu S, Lin P, et al. Remodeling and inflammation in Chinese versus white patients with chronic rhinosinusitis. J Allergy Clin Immunol 2010;125:8.
27. Bachert C, Gevaert P, Holtappels G, et al. Total and specific IgE in nasal polyps is related to local eosinophilic inflammation. J Allergy Clin Immunol 2001;107: 607–14.
28. Van Zele T, Gevaert P, Watelet JB, et al. Staphylococcus aureus colonization and IgE antibody formation to enterotoxins is increased in nasal polyposis. J Allergy Clin Immunol 2004;114:981–3.
29. Penn R, Mikula S. The role of anti-IgE immunoglobulin therapy in nasal polyposis: a pilot study. Am J Rhinol 2007;21:428–32.

30. Bachert C, Zhang N. Chronic rhinosinusitis and asthma: novel understanding of the role of IgE 'above atopy'. J Intern Med 2012;272:133–43.
31. Soyka MB, Wawrzyniak P, Eiwegger T, et al. Defective epithelial barrier in chronic rhinosinusitis: the regulation of tight junctions by IFN-gamma and IL-4. J Allergy Clin Immunol 2012;130(5):1087–96.e10.
32. Meltzer EO, Hamilos DL, Hadley JA, et al. Rhinosinusitis: establishing definitions for clinical research and patient care. J Allergy Clin Immunol 2004;114:155–212.
33. Bernstein IL, Li JT, Bernstein DI, et al. Allergy diagnostic testing: an updated practice parameter. Ann Allergy Asthma Immunol 2008;100:S1–148.
34. Szczeklik A, Nizankowska E. Clinical features and diagnosis of aspirin induced asthma. Thorax 2000;55:42–4.
35. Sin B, Togias A. Pathophysiology of allergic and nonallergic rhinitis. Proc Am Thorac Soc 2011;8:106–14.
36. KleinJan A, Willart M, van Rijt LS, et al. An essential role for dendritic cells in human and experimental allergic rhinitis. J Allergy Clin Immunol 2006;118: 1117–25.
37. Creticos PS, Peters SP, Adkinson NF Jr, et al. Peptide leukotriene release after antigen challenge in patients sensitive to ragweed. N Engl J Med 1984;310: 1626–30.
38. Bentley AM, Jacobson MR, Cumberworth V, et al. Immunohistology of the nasal mucosa in seasonal allergic rhinitis: increases in activated eosinophils and epithelial mast cells. J Allergy Clin Immunol 1992;89:877–83.
39. Varney VA, Jacobson MR, Sudderick RM, et al. Immunohistology of the nasal mucosa following allergen-induced rhinitis. Identification of activated T lymphocytes, eosinophils, and neutrophils. Am Rev Respir Dis 1992;146:170–6.
40. Papadopoulos NG, Bernstein JA, Demoly P, et al. Phenotypes and endotypes of rhinitis and their impact on management: a PRACTALL report. Allergy 2015;70: 474–94.
41. Rondon C, Dona I, Torres MJ, et al. Evolution of patients with nonallergic rhinitis supports conversion to allergic rhinitis. J Allergy Clin Immunol 2009;123: 1098–102.
42. Settipane RA, Charnock DR. Epidemiology of rhinitis: allergic and nonallergic. Clin Allergy Immunol 2007;19:23–34.
43. Bousquet J, Fokkeins W, Burney P, et al. Important research questions in allergy and related diseases: nonallergic rhinitis: a GA2LEN paper. Allergy 2008;63: 842–53.
44. Molgaard E, Thomsen SF, Lund T, et al. Differences between allergic and nonallergic rhinitis in a large sample of adolescents and adults. Allergy 2007;62: 1033–7.
45. Settipane RA. Rhinitis: a dose of epidemiological reality. Allergy Asthma Proc 2003;24:147–54.
46. Settipane RA, Lieberman P. Update on nonallergic rhinitis. Ann Allergy Asthma Immunol 2001;86:494–507.
47. Bachert C, Van Bruaene N, Toskala E, et al. Important research questions in allergy and related diseases: 3-chronic rhinosinusitis and nasal polyposis - a GALEN study. Allergy 2009;64:520–33.
48. Ellis AK, Keith PK. Nonallergic rhinitis with eosinophilia syndrome. Curr Allergy Asthma Rep 2006;6:215–20.
49. Rondon C, Fernandez J, Lopez S, et al. Nasal inflammatory mediators and specific IgE production after nasal challenge with grass pollen in local allergic rhinitis. J Allergy Clin Immunol 2009;124:1005–11.e1.

50. Nozad CH, Michael LM, Betty Lew D, et al. Non-allergic rhinitis: a case report and review. Clin Mol Allergy 2010;8:1.
51. Wallace DV, Dykewicz MS, Bernstein DI, et al. The diagnosis and management of rhinitis: an updated practice parameter. J Allergy Clin Immunol 2008;122: S1–84.
52. Moneret-Vautrin DA, Hsieh V, Wayoff M, et al. Nonallergic rhinitis with eosinophilia syndrome a precursor of the triad: nasal polyposis, intrinsic asthma, and intolerance to aspirin. Ann Allergy 1990;64:513–8.
53. Gelardi M, Iannuzzi L, Tafuri S, et al. Allergic and non-allergic rhinitis: relationship with nasal polyposis, asthma and family history. Acta Otorhinolaryngol Ital 2014;34:36–41.
54. Settipane G. Epidemiology of vasomotor rhinitis. World Allergy Organ J 2009;2: 115–8.
55. Rondon C, Canto G, Blanca M. Local allergic rhinitis: a new entity, characterization and further studies. Curr Opin Allergy Clin Immunol 2010;10:1–7.
56. Salib RJ, Harries PG, Nair SB, et al. Mechanisms and mediators of nasal symptoms in non-allergic rhinitis. Clin Exp Allergy 2008;38:393–404.
57. Rondon C, Campo P, Togias A, et al. Local allergic rhinitis: concept, pathophysiology, and management. J Allergy Clin Immunol 2008;129:1460–7.
58. Shusterman D, Balmes J, Murphy MA, et al. Chlorine inhalation produces nasal airflow limitation in allergic rhinitic subjects without evidence of neuropeptide release. Neuropeptides 2004;38:351–8.
59. Jaradeh SS, Smith TL, Torrico L, et al. Autonomic nervous system evaluation of patients with vasomotor rhinitis. Laryngoscope 2000;110:1828–31.
60. van Rijswijk JB, Blom HM, Fokkens WJ. Idiopathic rhinitis, the ongoing quest. Allergy 2005;60:1471–81.
61. Van Gerven L, Boeckxstaens G, Hellings P. Up-date on neuro-immune mechanisms involved in allergic and non-allergic rhinitis. Rhinology 2012;50:227–35.
62. Braat JP, Mulder PG, Fokkens WJ, et al. Intranasal cold dry air is superior to histamine challenge in determining the presence and degree of nasal hyperreactivity in nonallergic noninfectious perennial rhinitis. Am J Respir Crit Care Med 1998;157:1748–55.
63. Sarin S, Undem B, Sanico A, et al. The role of the nervous system in rhinitis. J Allergy Clin Immunol 2006;118:999–1016.
64. Georgalas C, Jovancevic L. Gustatory rhinitis. Curr Opin Otolaryngol Head Neck Surg 2012;20:9–14.
65. Piedimonte G. Pathophysiological mechanisms for the respiratory syncytial virus-reactive airway disease link. Respir Res 2002;3:S21–5.
66. Doyle WJ, Skoner DP, Seroky JT, et al. Effect of experimental rhinovirus 39 infection on the nasal response to histamine and cold air challenges in allergic and nonallergic subjects. J Allergy Clin Immunol 1994;93:534–42.
67. Tan R, Corren J. Optimum treatment of rhinitis in the elderly. Drugs Aging 1995; 7:168–75.
68. Platt M. Pharmacotherapy for allergic rhinitis. Int Forum Allergy Rhinol 2014;4: S35–40.
69. Kaliner M. Recognizing and treating nonallergic rhinitis. Female Patient 2002;27: 20–32.
70. Ellegard E, Karlsson G. Nasal congestion during pregnancy. Clin Otolaryngol Allied Sci 1999;24:307–11.
71. Ellegard EK. Clinical and pathogenetic characteristics of pregnancy rhinitis. Clin Rev Allergy Immunol 2004;26:149–59.

72. Hamano N, Terada N, Maesako K, et al. Expression of histamine receptors in nasal epithelial cells and endothelial cells – the effects of sex hormones. Int Arch Allergy Immunol 2008;115:220–7.
73. Hamano N, Terada N, Maesako K, et al. Effect of sex hormones on eosinophilic inflammation in nasal mucosa. Allergy Asthma Proc 1998;19:263–9.
74. Raphael GD, Raphael MH, Kaliner MA. Gustatory rhinitis: a syndrome of food-induced rhinorrhea. J Allergy Clin Immunol 1989;13:110–5.
75. Waibel KH, Chang C. Prevalence and food avoidance behaviors for gustatory rhinitis. Ann Allergy Asthma Immunol 2008;100:200–5.
76. Lacroix JS, Landis BN. Neurogenic inflammation of the upper airway mucosa. Rhinology 2008;46:163–5.
77. Malik V, Ghosh S, Woolford TJ. Rhinitis due to food allergies: fact or fiction? J Laryngol Otol 2007;121:526–9.
78. Jovancevic L, Georgalas C, Savovic S, et al. Gustatory rhinitis. Rhinology 2010; 48:7–10.
79. Varghese M, Glaum MC, Lockey RF. Drug-induced rhinitis. Clin Exp Allergy 2010;40:381–4.
80. Vitezic D, Pelcic JM. Erectile dysfunction: oral pharmacotherapy options. Int J Clin Pharmacol Ther 2002;40:393–403.
81. Materson BJ. Adverse effects of angiotensin-converting enzyme inhibitors in antihypertensive therapy with focus on quinapril. Am J Cardiol 1992;69:46–53.
82. Goodger NM, Wang J, Pogrel MA. Palatal and nasal necrosis resulting from cocaine misuse. Br Dent J 2005;198:333–4.
83. Lin CY, Cheng PH, Fang SY. Mucosal changes in rhinitis medicamentosa. Ann Otol Rhinol Laryngol 2004;113:147–51.
84. Graf P. Rhinitis medicamentosa: a review of causes and treatment. Treat Respir Med 2005;4:21–9.
85. Knipping S, Holzhausen HJ, Goetze G, et al. Rhinitis medicamentosa: electron microscopic changes of human nasal mucosa. Otolaryngol Head Neck Surg 2007;136:57–61.
86. Keyserling HF, Grimme JD, Camacho DL, et al. Nasal septal perforation secondary to rhinitis medicamentosa. Ear Nose Throat J 2006;85:8–9.
87. Baroody FM, Brown D, Gavanescu L, et al. Oxymetazoline adds to the effectiveness of fluticasone furoate in the treatment of perennial allergic rhinitis. J Allergy Clin Immunol 2011;127(4):927–34.
88. Vaidyanathan S, Williamson P, Clearie K, et al. Fluticasone reverses oxymetazoline-induced tachyphylaxis of response and rebound congestion. Am J Respir Crit Care Med 2010;182:19–24.
89. Edelstein DR. Aging of the normal nose in adults. Laryngoscope 1996;106:1–25.
90. Chhabra N, Houser SM. The diagnosis and management of empty nose syndrome. Otolaryngol Clin North Am 2009;42:311–30.
91. Dutt SN, Kameswaran M. The aetiology and management of atrophic rhinitis. J Laryngol Otol 2005;119:843–52.
92. Moore EJ, Kern EB. Atrophic rhinitis: a review of 242 cases. Am J Rhinol 2001; 15:355–61.
93. deShazo RD, Stringer SP. Atrophic rhinosinusitis: progress toward explanation of an unsolved medical mystery. Curr Opin Allergy Clin Immunol 2011;11:1–7.
94. Houser SM. Empty nose syndrome associated with middle turbinate resection. Otolaryngol Head Neck Surg 2006;135:972–3.

95. Rondon C, Romero JJ, Lopez S, et al. Local IgE production and positive nasal provocation test in patients with persistent nonallergic rhinitis. J Allergy Clin Immunol 2007;119:899–905.

96. Rondon C, Dona I, Lopez S, et al. Seasonal idiopathic rhinitis with local inflammatory response and specific IgE in absence of systemic response. Allergy 2008;63:1352–8.

97. Powe DG, Huskisson RS, Carney AS, et al. Evidence for an inflammatory pathophysiology in idiopathic rhinitis. Clin Exp Allergy 2001;31:864–72.

98. Powe DG, Huskisson RS, Carney AS, et al. Mucosal T-cell phenotypes in persistent atopic and nonatopic rhinitis show an association with mast cells. Allergy 2004;59:204–12.

99. Powe DG, Jagger C, Kleinjan A, et al. 'Entopy': localized mucosal allergic disease in the absence of systemic responses for atopy. Clin Exp Allergy 2003; 33:1374–9.

100. Rondon C, Campo P, Zambonino MA, et al. Follow-up study in local allergic rhinitis shows a consistent entity not evolving to systemic allergic rhinitis. J Allergy Clin Immunol 2014;133:1026–31.

101. Moscato G, Vandenplas O, Gerth Van Wijk R, et al. Occupational rhinitis. Allergy 2008;63:969–80.

102. Palczynski C, Walusiak J, Ruta U, et al. Nasal provocation test in the diagnosis of natural rubber latex allergy. Allergy 2000;55:34–41.

103. Archambault S, Malo JL, Infante-Rivard C, et al. Incidence of sensitization, symptoms, and probable occupational rhinoconjunctivitis and asthma in apprentices starting exposure to latex. J Allergy Clin Immunol 2001;107:921–3.

104. Meggs WJ. RADS and RUDS–the toxic induction of asthma and rhinitis. J Toxicol Clin Toxicol 1994;32:487–501.

105. Graham D, Henderson F, House D. Neutrophil influx measured in nasal lavages of humans exposed to ozone. Arch Environ Health 1988;43:228–33.

106. Assanasen P, Metheetrairut C. Choanal atresia. J Med Assoc Thai 2009;92: 699–706.

107. Sadek SA. Congenital bilateral choanal atresia. Int J Pediatr Otorhinolaryngol 1998;42:247–56.

108. Baumgartner BJ, Ladd T, Esquivel C. Low-grade adenocarcinoma of the nasal cavity–an unusual presentation: case report and review of the literature. Ear Nose Throat J 2007;86:97–100.

109. Alvi A, Doherty T, Lewen G. Facial fractures and concomitant injuries in trauma patients. Laryngoscope 2003;113:102–6.

110. Clark D, Bullock P, Hui T, et al. Benign intracranial hypertension: a cause of CSF rhinorrhoea. J Neurol Neurosurg Psychiatry 1994;57:847–9.

111. Ryall RG, Peacock MK, Simpson DA. Usefulness of beta 2-transferrin assay in the detection of cerebrospinal fluid leaks following head injury. J Neurosurg 1992;77:737–9.

112. Carson JL, Collier AM, Hu SS. Acquired ciliary defects in nasal epithelium of children with acute viral upper respiratory infections. N Engl J Med 1985;312: 463–8.

113. Pedersen M. Ciliary activity and pollution. Lung 1990;168:368–76.

114. Reed J, deShazo RD, Houle TT, et al. Clinical features of sarcoid rhinosinusitis. Am J Med 2010;123:856–62.

115. Qazi FA, Thorne JE, Jabs DA. Scleral nodule associated with sarcoidosis. Am J Ophthalmol 2003;136:752–4.

116. Panda NK, Saravanan K, Purushotaman GP, et al. Localized amyloidosis masquerading as nasopharyngeal tumor: a review. Am J Otolaryngol 2007;28: 208–11.
117. Tsikoudas A, Martin-Hirsch DP, Woodhead CJ. Primary sinonasal amyloidosis. J Laryngol Otol 2001;115:55–6.

Allergic Rhinitis
Burden of Illness, Quality of Life, Comorbidities, and Control

 CrossMark

Eli O. Meltzer, MD

KEYWORDS

- Allergic rhinitis • Qualify of life • Comorbidities • Control • Burden of illness • RCAT

KEY POINTS

- Allergic rhinitis is a highly prevalent and costly condition.
- The disease burden suffered by patients includes the morbidity of the nasal symptoms, the impairment of multiple domains of quality of life (QOL), and numerous comorbidities.
- The goal of therapy is long-term good control.

INTRODUCTION

The World Health Organization in 1948[1] provided the following definition: health is a state of complete physical, mental, emotional, and social well-being and not merely the absence of disease or infirmity. In this context, most patients with allergic rhinitis are not healthy. This article describes the burden of this disease, which manifests itself as disease in terms of high prevalence, uncontrolled symptoms, impaired QOL, and unpleasant comorbidities. It also suggests that the goal of therapy is control of this disease.

PREVALENCE OF ALLERGIC RHINITIS

Allergic rhinitis is a common condition. It affects up to 60 million people in the United States annually, including self-reported rates of 10% to 30% of adults and as many as 40% of children. Recent surveys that required a physician-confirmed diagnosis of allergic rhinitis published prevalence rates of US adults, 14%; US children, 13%; Latin America adults, 7%; and Asia-Pacific adults, 9%.[2] Another survey from a representative Belgian population (n = approximately 5000) found a self-declared overall prevalence of approximately 39% for recent rhinitis symptoms. Detailed information from a

Conflict of Interest Statement: There are no commercial conflicts of interest, financial conflicts of interest, or funding sources associated with this article.
Allergy & Asthma Medical Group and Research Center, 5776 Ruffin Road, San Diego, CA 92123, USA
E-mail address: eliomeltzer@gmail.com

sample of approximately 750 respondents determined a prevalence of allergic rhinitis of approximately 30% and of nonallergic rhinitis of approximately 10%. Compared with the nonallergic rhinitis patients, statistically significantly more patients with allergic rhinitis had persistent symptomatology (41% vs 24%) and moderate/severe symptom intensity (75% vs 53%). A greater number of symptoms and comorbidities were also significantly more commonly reported in the allergic rhinitis patients.[3]

There are risk factors for the development of allergic rhinitis. These include (1) a family history of atopy, (2) a serum IgE greater than 100 IU/mL before age 6 years, (3) a higher socioeconomic class, and (4) the presence of a positive allergy skin prick test.[4–7] The influence of early childhood exposure to infections (the hygiene hypothesis), animals, and secondary tobacco smoke on the development of atopy and allergic rhinitis is still unclear.[8–13]

The presentation of allergic rhinitis in childhood is more frequent in boys, but in adults, it is more common in women. Children with a bilateral family history of atopy may develop symptoms more frequently and at a younger age than those with a unilateral family history.[14,15] Aeroallergen sensitization rarely begins before 6 months of age[16] but may start between 6 months and 2 years of life.[17] Infants born to atopic families are sensitized to pollen aeroallergens more frequently than to indoor aeroallergens in the first year of life.[17] The frequency of sensitization to inhalant allergens is increasing and is more than 40% in many populations in the United States and Europe.[18]

Seasonal allergic rhinitis symptoms generally do not develop until 2 to 7 years of age.[19,20] Food ingestion rarely causes allergic rhinitis in infants, children, or adults unless there are associated gastrointestinal, dermatologic, or systemic manifestations. The prevalence of seasonal allergic rhinitis is higher in children and adolescents, whereas perennial allergic rhinitis has a higher prevalence in adults.[21]

QUALITY OF LIFE IN ALLERGIC RHINITIS

"Quality of life" has been defined as the subjective value a person places on satisfaction with his or her life.[22] Health-related QOL focuses on patients' perceptions of their disease and measures impairments that have a significant impact on a patient. The burden of disease, as a patient perceives it, forms the basic motivation to seek medical aid and undergo therapy. The burden is usually described by patients in terms of symptoms and impact on QOL.

The 4 major symptoms of allergic rhinitis are nasal congestion, rhinorrhea, sneezing, and nasal itch. Nasal congestion is the most frequent and generally the most bothersome symptom in both adults and children. In adults, 60% report it the most common symptom during the worst time of the year, and in the pediatric population aged 4 to 17 years it is noted every day or most days by 52%.[2,23] Postnasal drip, runny nose, and sneezing are similarly common and more so than nasal itch. Postnasal drip and runny nose, however, are generally more bothersome than either sneezing or nasal itch.

The impact of nasal allergies on patient-perceived health status is substantial. Although a majority of patients with allergic rhinitis have reported a good overall sense of their health (excellent, 11%; very good, 29%; and good, 34%), when compared with adults without nasal allergies, it was evident that allergic rhinitis patients rated their overall heath significantly lower. Nearly twice as many adults without nasal allergies described their health as excellent (23%) and at the other extreme, nearly twice as many allergic rhinitis patients rated their health as only fair/poor/very poor (27%) compared with adults without nasal allergies (15%).[24] According to physicians' assessments, nearly half of patients (47%) have persistent disease and almost two-thirds (63%) have moderate or severe disease. Comparison of the physicians' and patients' evaluations of disease severity found that patients rated their disease as more severe than did the physicians[25] (**Fig. 1**).

Adverse consequences on patients' QOL have included impairment of physical and social functioning, disturbed sleep, daytime somnolence and fatigue, irritability, depression, and attention, learning, and memory deficits. In the US, Latin America and Asia-Pacific surveys, between 35% and 50% of adults reported that nasal allergies have at least a moderate effect on daily life[2] (**Fig. 2**). In the physical domain of QOL, sleep disturbances are one of these impaired matters and include difficulty falling asleep, staying asleep, and awakening refreshed. Approximately 1 in 4 (22%) of adult US respondents report they are unable to sleep or are awakened most days or every day and 26% to 45% of children experience sleep disruption because of nasal allergy symptoms.[2,23]

Almost twice as many patients with allergic rhinitis compared with adults without nasal allergies say that their health limited them in daytime physical indoor activities (20% vs 11%) and outdoor activities (44% vs 21%).[24] In a Spanish study, the negative impact on daily activities for patients with allergic rhinitis was greater (27%) than for patients with type 2 diabetes mellitus (17%) and hypertension (9%); it was less than for symptomatic depression (59%).[26] In athletes with rhinitis, factors with a potential negative effect on sports performance include outdoor exposure to pollen and pollutants (ozone and particulate matter) and sports-specific environmental conditions (eg, cold temperatures, dry air, and indoor chlorine).[27] Nasal inflammation and obstruction also interfere with the conditioning of inspired air by nasal turbinates and this may potentiate exercise-induced asthma symptoms.[28]

In a US survey of adults in response to questions regarding the worst month of allergy symptoms, the percentage of patients who reported adverse effects in their emotional domain regarding their mood and feelings, sometimes or frequently, was

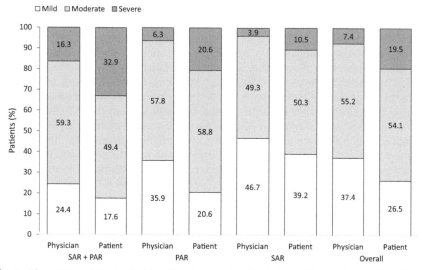

Fig. 1. Disease severity reported by physicians and patients in the United States. PAR, Perennial allergic rhinitis; SAR, Seasonal allergic rhinitis. (*From* Schatz M. A survey of the burden of allergic rhinitis in the USA. Allergy 2007;62:11; with permission.)

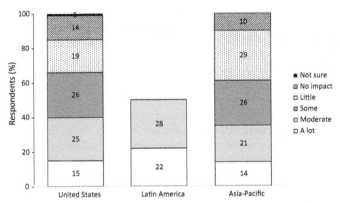

Fig. 2. Patient perceptions of effect of nasal allergy symptoms on daily life. (*From* Meltzer EO, Blaiss MS, Naclerio RM, et al. Burden of allergic rhinitis: allergies in America, Latin America, and Asia-Pacific adult surveys. Allergy Asthma Proc 2012;33:S123; with permission.)

85% fatigue, 67% irritable, 60% miserable, 28% depressed or blue, 25% anxious, and 15% embarrassed.[24] In a review of relevant articles, a majority of studies indicate associations between nasal allergies and anxiety/mood syndromes. There are several mechanisms that might mediate this relationship: allergic reactions triggering the immune system and cytokines, allergies impairing sleep through nasal obstruction, and allergies negatively affecting cognitive function.[29]

In the US, Latin America, and Asia-Pacific surveys, 10%, 4%, and 4%, respectively, of the workers reported absenteeism because of their nasal allergies; 22%, 17%, and 25%, respectively, reported work interference (presenteeism); and 20%, 16%, and 21%, respectively, experienced both. These different surveys noted between a 23% and 33% estimate of loss of productivity on days when allergies were at their worst compared with days when the respondent experienced no symptoms.[2] A study from the Netherlands of more than 2000 patients concluded that symptom severity, sleep, QOL, and certain antihistamines were significantly related to work productivity.[30] Regarding the mental domain, allergic rhinitis can, by itself, introduce significant inattention, impairment of cognition, and decreased daytime school performance. In addition, by impeding restorative sleep, learning during the school years and beyond can be compromised.[31] Furthermore, the first-generation antihistamines have unacceptable central and anticholinergic effects that can worsen this situation.[32] In a Swedish study of approximately 1000 adolescents, nasal symptoms severe enough to affect daily activity were associated with lower grades.[33] Successful management requires communication and collaboration among parents, educators, and health care professionals to ensure good QOL and maximal school performance in this population.[34] Moreover, allergic rhinitis has a negative impact on the QOL of the whole family because, it can cause interference with social relationships and increase financial costs. Few data are available on the health-related QOL of patients with nonallergic rhinitis.[35]

A variety of validated and standardized questionnaires have been developed to quantify the effect of allergic rhinitis on the physical, social, emotional, and mental domains of an individual's life.[36] In a French study of 990 adult patients, both severity and duration of symptoms had an impact on the visual analog scale (VAS) and the QOL as measured by the Rhinoconjunctivitis Quality of Life Questionnaire (RQLQ). Nasal congestion and ocular symptoms had the greatest impact on QOL.[37] A cutoff variation of a VAS of 23/100 discriminated significant changes in symptoms and was associated with a cutoff variation of 0.5 units for the QOL measurement (RQLQ).[38] In meta-analyses, calculations for the minimal important differences (the smallest changes in an outcome important to a patient) were for total nasal symptom score, 0.55 units; peak nasal inspiratory flow, 5 L/min; and Mini RQLQ: 0.4 units.[39] Although the disease-specific RQLQ instrument reflects an allergic rhinitis patient's QOL, when multiple organs are involved, such as when there are comorbidities, for example, asthma, a generic instrument seems to generate a more comprehensive view of the impact of the allergen exposure on a patient's QOL.[40] Better allergic rhinitis control, as reflected by the Rhinitis Control Assessment Test (RCAT), is associated with improved QOL as reflected by scores on the RQLQ.[41]

A decreased sense of smell can lead to a significant decrease in QOL, including disturbing a patient's ability to taste, losing the pleasures of eating, and increasing health risks, such as not appreciating spoiled food or leaking gas and adding larger quantities of sugar and salt to highlight flavors, thus worsening general health.[42] The mechanism underlying olfactory impairment in nasal and sinonasal disease relates to either obstruction of the olfactory cleft due to congestion of the nasal mucosa or dysfunction of the olfactory bulb from local inflammation.[43] In a prospective controlled study in Spain, most patients with persistent allergic rhinitis, in particular those with moderate to severe persistent allergic rhinitis and in those with self-reported hyposmia, have significant reduction in smell detection and smell identification compared with healthy controls. This finding seems to depend on both nasal congestion and inflammation.[44]

The economic burden of allergic rhinitis is substantial; the total direct medical cost is approximately $3.4 billion, with almost half attributable to prescription medications.[45] Compared with matched controls, patients with allergic rhinitis have an approximately 2-fold increase in medication costs and a 1.8-fold increase in the number of visits to health care practitioners.[46] Indirect cost ranges were higher in studies estimating only indirect costs ($5.5–$9.7 billion) than in those estimating both direct and indirect costs ($1.7–$4.3 billion).[47] In Europe, the total societal cost of persistent allergic rhinitis and its comorbidities in 2002 was estimated at 355.06 Euros per patient per month.[48] Appropriate therapy can substantially reduce both societal and employer costs. Few of the economic evaluations have formal cost assessments that compare the incremental costs and benefits of alternative treatment strategies. Lack of treatment, undertreatment, and nonadherence to treatment have all been seen to increase direct and indirect costs.[49]

COMORBIDITIES OF ALLERGIC RHINITIS
Associated Headaches

In a US national sample of adults with allergic rhinitis, more than a third (37%) were at least somewhat bothered by headaches and in multiple surveys headaches ranked as one of the most bothersome symptoms for adults and children with allergic rhinitis.[2,23,24] In 1 US survey, 17% of the nasal allergy population identified themselves as having migraine headaches compared with 9% of the nonallergy adults.[50] In a similar survey of the Latin American population, 41% of the allergic adults claimed they had migraine headaches.[2] If a thorough evaluation is performed, a majority of patients presenting with a "sinus headache" (a headache of rhinogenic origin) in the absence of significant acute inflammatory findings are diagnosed with migraine.[51]

Associated Allergic Conjunctivitis

In a recent French study, 52% of allergic rhinitis patients (women more often than men) described ocular symptoms. The troublesome symptoms were itchy eyes, 51%; watery eyes, 39%; red eyes, 7%; and swollen eyelids, 4%.[52] These symptoms had a negative impact on daily activities. One mechanism is direct allergen contact with an eye. More likely causes are the cross talk between neurologic (nasal-nasal and nasal-ocular reflexes) and inflammatory pathways in the upper airways.[53,54]

Associated Otitis Media

Otitis media likely results from an increase in blood flow to and, thus, gas loss from the middle ear, in combination with a dysfunctional eustachian tube that cannot resupply that gas. These processes could be induced by viral and/or allergen driven inflammation.[55] A large body of epidemiologic and mechanistic evidence supports the role for allergic rhinitis as a risk factor for otitis media. In contrast to the general, nonallergic population without chronic rhinitis symptoms who have a rate of earaches in the prior 4 weeks of 3%, the allergic rhinitis adults reported a 16% incidence of earaches.[50] Furthermore, the observed prevalence of allergic rhinitis in patients with chronic or recurrent otitis media with effusion ranges from 24% to 89%.[56] Analysis of inflammatory mediators indicates that the mucosa of the middle ear can respond to antigen in the same way as the mucosa of the lower respiratory tract. Characterization of the mucosa and effusion from atopic patients with otitis media with effusion reveals Th2 cytokine and cellular profiles consistent with an allergic response.[57] Benefits of considering medical treatment in patients with otitis media with effusion both prior to and after surgery include the potential reduction in allergic inflammation.

Associated Rhinosinusitis

A theory has been developed suggesting that allergic rhinitis and rhinosinusitis may be manifestations of an inflammatory process within a continuous airway rather than fully separate diseases.[58] Genetic studies highlight common associations and excessive mucosal inflammation with immune dysregulation is a common feature, including a role for bacterial superantigens.[59] There are also strong epidemiologic findings. The Allergies in America surveys revealed that 50% of adults and 43% of children ages 4 to 17 years with nasal allergies reported having chronic sinus issues.[23,60] Sinus problems were identified by 33% of Latin American respondents.[61] An important role for innate immunity is now apparent and offers prospects of novel therapeutic approaches in the future.

Associated Cough Sensitivity

Chronic upper airway cough syndrome (also referred to as postnasal drip syndrome) and/or subclinical inflammatory changes within the lower airways are probably responsible for the greater afferent nerve endings reactivity (cough sensitivity) in patients with allergic rhinitis. This increased reactivity has been demonstrated in a series of studies that documented increased cough responses to capsaicin in pollen-allergic patients in season compared with allergic patients out of season, and in allergic patients out of pollen season compared with nonallergic subjects without chronic rhinitis.[62,63] The research suggests that both direct stimulatory effects on the larynx and secondary effects of mucus production and mucus trafficking can create a range of laryngeal symptoms, including cough.[64]

Associated Asthma

Rhinitis and asthma are linked by common epidemiologic, physiologic, and patho-logic mechanisms as well as common therapeutic approaches.[65,66] Epidemiologic surveys have consistently shown allergic rhinitis as an independent risk factor for developing asthma and a growing body of evidence demonstrates that patients with allergic rhinitis, in the absence of asthma, have distinct abnormalities of lower airway function, including alterations in physiology, histology, and biochemistry.[67] Nasal symptoms, nasal airflow, and markers of inflammation directly correlate with lower airway involvement. Local tissue factors, such as microbial stimuli and systemic inflammatory mechanisms, play a role in the clinical expression of the allergic airway syndrome.[68] US surveys report that 38% of patients with allergic rhinitis have asthma and up to 78% of asthma patients have allergic rhinitis,[69] and in a study of young adults in Italy, patients with allergic rhinitis had an 8-fold risk of having asthma compared with subjects without allergic rhinitis.[70] Even in pa-tients with rhinitis who do not have asthma, subclinical changes in the lower airways and inflammatory mediators can be detected. Bronchial hyper-reactivity has often been reported in patients with allergic rhinitis and a decreased forced expiratory flow at 25% and 75% of pulmonary volume has been proposed as an early marker of bronchial involvement in patients with allergic rhinitis who only perceive nasal symptoms.[71] In a large group of children, those with rhinitis showed a significant forced expiratory volume in the first second of expiration (FEV_1) increase after a bronchodilation test in comparison with basal values and to the measures in control children. Patients with reversibility had lower FEV_1 levels and longer rhinitis dura-tion.[72] Measurements of exhaled nitric oxide in nonasthmatic allergic rhinitis sub-jects were significantly higher than healthy controls both in pollen season and to a lesser degree outside of the pollen season. This study also confirms the presence of eosinophilic lower airway inflammation in allergic rhinitis patients.[73] Therefore, it has been suggested that patients with persistent allergic rhinitis be evaluated for asthma, which should include pulmonary function tests.[74] The presence of asthma may not be apparent because allergic rhinitis patients (1) may have difficulty in recognizing their symptoms, (2) may not have consistent symptoms, (3) may have a normal physical examination of the respiratory system, and (4) may present with symptoms that are atypical. There are more patients with incomplete asthma control[75] and higher medical resources use, including acute asthma exacerbations, emergency department visits, unscheduled and scheduled physician office visits, and prescription medication use among asthmatic patients with concomitant allergic rhinitis compared with those without allergic rhinitis.[76,77] The roles of various therapies for patients who are dually afflicted by upper and lower airway disease are important considerations.

Associated Gastroesophageal Reflux

Heartburn or gastroesophageal reflux disorder is often described by patients with allergic rhinitis. In the Allergies in America and Allergies in Latin America surveys, 23% and 30%, respectively, of the respondents reported this issue.[2] This is a greater frequency than the 16% noted in the general nonallergic population of adults without chronic rhinitis evaluated in the National Allergy Survey Assessing Limitations.[50] The suggested mechanism by which allergic rhinitis increases gastroesophageal reflux is through the increased negative intrathoracic pressure developed by patients as they try to inspire through their obstructed nose. There are inadequate data to support this supposed association.[78]

Associated Sexual Dysfunction

In women with symptomatic allergic rhinoconjunctivitis, the results from the Female Sexual Function Index were significantly lower than in those treated for their allergic rhinoconjunctivitis or in control women. In men, the International Index of Erectile Function results of treated allergic rhinoconjunctivitis and controls were significantly higher than for symptomatic allergic patients.[79] The mechanism of this association has not been determined.

Associated Skin Rashes

The frequency of skin rashes is higher in patients with allergic rhinitis (10%-15%) than nonallergic adults (3%) as reported in surveys.[2,50] The interrelationship between atopic dermatitis and allergic rhinitis is the best studied having a high prevalence and coincidence, with both conditions involving specific IgE responses to allergens as well as mast cell and eosinophilic inflammatory infiltrates. Genetics, epithelial barrier defects, and colonization with Staphylococcus aureus are also important issues that link these 2 conditions by complex and currently unclear mechanisms.[80]

Associated Sleep Disturbances

Sleep is fundamental for physical and mental health. Many allergic rhinitis patients suffer from sleep disorders.[81] Nasal congestion is the most common and bothersome symptom of rhinitis and is thought to be a key cause of sleep impairment in individuals with rhinitis.[82] Nasal congestion also demonstrates circadian rhythm and positional variability, worsening during nighttime hours and in the supine position.[83] The degree of sleep disturbance is directly related to the severity of the disease. In a French study of approximately 600 patients, all dimensions of sleep were impaired by allergic rhinitis, significantly more in patients with severe disease than in those with the mild type.[84] In a Spanish survey of more than 2200 patients, with 88% classified as having moderate-severe rhinitis and 12% as mild rhinitis, 53% had poor sleep quality according to the Pittsburgh sleep quality index and 21% suffered from excessive diurnal somnolence based on the Epworth sleepiness scale. In a logistic regression model, moderate-severe rhinitis and nasal obstruction were associated with a worse sleep quality.[85] Nasal obstruction is an independent risk factor for obstructive sleep apnea. Rhinitis alone is associated with mild obstructive sleep apnea but commonly causes microarousals and sleep fragmentation.[86] In a systematic review of existing literature over the past 25 years in children, a statistically significant association was found between allergic rhinitis and sleep-disordered breathing, including snoring and obstructive sleep apnea.[87] Atopy has been associated with habitual snoring in infants.[88] In children, the presence of rhinitis is a strong predictor of habitual snoring.[89] Children who are African American, have upper respiratory disease, and have a family history of sleep apnea are at enhanced risk for sleep-disordered breathing.[90] Thus, formal evaluation for obstructive sleep apnea syndrome may be considered in children as well as adults presenting with chronic rhinitis and other risk factors associated with sleep-disordered breathing.

In snoring adults with rhinitis and sleep apnea symptoms, increased nasal airway resistance has been associated with apnea and hypopnea.[91] Sleep impairment is likely a major contributor to overall disease morbidity, including impairment of QOL, daytime fatigue and somnolence, loss of work productivity, poorer cognitive abilities (difficulty concentrating, memory deficits) and school performance, and direct and indirect health care costs.[92–94] Instruments available to assess the impact that rhinitis has on sleep include subjective general and disease-specific QOL questionnaires (including rhinitis-specific and sleep-specific questionnaires, such as the Pittsburgh Sleep Quality Index and Epworth Sleepiness Scale), and objective measures of nasal patency (nasal inspiratory peak flow rhinomanometry, acoustic rhinometry, and measures of sleep, such as polysomnography, the Multiple Sleep Latency Test, the Maintenance of Wakefulness Test, and learning and performance tests).[94] Actigraphy scores are another objective tool to evaluate sleep disturbances and response to therapy.[95]

CONTROL OF ALLERGIC RHINITIS

Despite the availability of effective therapy, allergic rhinitis continues to be associated with a high clinical and economic burden. Guidelines have not been implemented effectively by many clinicians, adherence to recommendations is commonly lacking, and poor control of the disease is widespread. Accurate assessment of rhinitis control is an essential element in a strategy to simplify and improve management.

Clear therapeutic targets exist for many chronic diseases. Examples include for hypertension, a systolic blood pressure of less than 140 mm Hg and a diastolic blood pressure of less than 90 mm Hg; for diabetes, a hemoglobin A_{1c} of 7% or less; and for asthma, a control test in the normal range, for example, having a score greater than 19 on the Asthma Control Test.

With regard to allergic rhinitis, there are several options as to how to measure control using patient-based data. Symptoms of nasal itching, sneezing, rhinorrhea, and congestion reported by a patient can be added up to create a Total Nasal Symptom Score. The lower the score, the better the rhinitis control. The physical, social, emotional, and mental domains of a patient's QOL can be quantified using the RQLQ. Lower scores suggest better control. Nighttime sleep disturbances and daytime work and school performance can be assessed quantitatively and qualitatively. Patients can self-rate functional status and emotional issues, such as fatigue, irritability, anxiety, and depression. Nasal airflow can be measured using such instruments as rhinomanometry or the nasal peak flow meter. Lower scores suggest poorer control. Furthermore, the number of medications and the frequency used can reflect the degree of control.

Recently, a formal tool for evaluating allergic and nonallergic rhinitis control was developed and validated. The RCAT has 6 questions that ask about nasal and other allergy symptoms that are not related to a cold or the flu and control of these symptoms.[96] For each question patients are asked to choose a rating that describes their condition over the past week, from a range of 5, which is the best the person could be, to 1, which is the worst they could be. The maximum, optimal total score is 30 and the lowest, poorest score a 6[96] (Table 1). A cutpoint of 21 on the 6-point to 30-point range provides the best combination of specificity and sensitivity in screening for rhinitis control. Scores of 21 or less indicate uncontrolled rhinitis; a score of 17 or less suggests poor control and referral to a specialist may be appropriate. Finally, a 3 or more point change from a previous RCAT assessment indicates a clinically meaningful change, either a relevant improvement or a relevant worsening. The RCAT generates a rhinitis score that can be understood by patients as to where they are in the range of possible levels of rhinitis control. The RCAT is a simple and validated tool that can rapidly measure control at home, in a pharmacy, or in a health care provider's office. The RCAT results can be shared with a clinician to enhance further dialogue and for guiding therapeutic decisions. It can empower patients to seek a higher score and ultimately the goal of therapy, namely, better control of their rhinitis.

Table 1
Rhinitis Control Assessment Test: questionnaire

During the past week, how often did you have nasal congestion?				
Never 5	Rarely 4	Sometimes 3	Often 2	Extremely Often 1

During the past week, how often did you sneeze?				
Never 5	Rarely 4	Sometimes 3	Often 2	Extremely Often 1

During the past week, how often do you have watery eyes?				
Never 5	Rarely 4	Sometimes 3	Often 2	Extremely Often 1

During the past week, to what extent did your nasal or other allergy symptoms interfere with your sleep?				
Never 5	Rarely 4	Sometimes 3	Often 2	Extremely Often 1

During the past week, how often did avoid activities (for example, visiting a house with a dog or cat, gardening) because of your nasal or other allergy symptoms?				
Never 5	Rarely 4	Sometimes 3	Often 2	Extremely Often 1

During the past week, how well were your nasal or other allergy symptoms controlled?				
Completely (5)	Very (4)	Somewhat (3)	A little (2)	Not at all (1)

From Meltzer EO, Schatz M, Nathan R, et al. Reliability, validity and responsiveness of the Rhinitis Control Assessment Test in patients with rhinitis. J Allergy Clin Immunol 2013;131:381; with permission.

REFERENCES

1. Preamble to the Constitution of the World Health Organization as adopted by the International Health Conference, New York, 19-22 June, 1946; signed on 22 July 1946 by the representatives of 61 States (Official Records of the World Health Organization, no. 2, p. 100) and entered into force on 7 April 1948.
2. Meltzer EO, Blaiss MS, Naclerio RM, et al. Burden of allergic rhinitis: allergies in America, Latin America, and Asia-Pacific adult surveys. Allergy Asthma Proc 2012;33:S113–41.
3. Bachert C, van Cauwenberge P, Olbrecht J, et al. Prevalence, classification and perception of allergic and nonallergic rhinitis patients in Belgium. Allergy 2006; 61:693–8.
4. Settipane RJ, Hagy GW, Settipane GA. Long-term risk factors for developing asthma and allergic rhinitis: a 23-year follow-up study of college students. Allergy Proc 1994;15:21–5.
5. Hagy GW, Settipane GA. Prognosis of allergy skin tests in an asymptomatic population: a three tear follow-up of college students. J Allergy Clin Immunol 1971;48: 200–11.
6. Tang RB, Tsai LC, Hwang HM, et al. The prevalence of allergic disease and IgE antibodies to house dust mite in schoolchildren in Taiwan. Clin Exp Allergy 1990; 20:33–8.
7. Wright AL, Holberg CJ, Martinez FD, et al. Epidemiology of physician-diagnosed allergic rhinitis in childhood. Pediatrics 1994;94:895–901.

8. Hagerhed-Engman L, Bornehag CG, Sundell J, et al. Day-care attendance and increased risk for respiratory and allergic symptoms in preschool age. Allergy 2006;61:447–53.

9. Karmaus W, Botezan C. Does a higher number of siblings protect against the development of allergy and asthma? A review. J Epidemiol Community Health 2002;56:209–17.

10. Romagnani S. The increased prevalence of allergy and the hygiene hypothesis: missing immune deviation, reduced immune suppression, or both? Immunology 2004;112:352–63.

11. Balemans WA, Rovers MM, Schilder AG, et al. Recurrent childhood upper respiratory tract infections do not reduce the risk of adult atopic disease. Clin Exp Allergy 2006;36:198–203.

12. Hesselmar B, Aberg N, Aberg B, et al. Does early exposure to cat or dog protect against later allergy development? Clin Exp Allergy 1999;29:611–7.

13. Frosh AC, Sandhu G, Joyce R, et al. Prevalence of rhinitis, pillow type, and past and present ownership of furred pets. Clin Exp Allergy 1999;29:457–60.

14. Smith JM. A five-year prospective survey of rural children with asthma and hay fever. J Allergy 1971;47:23–30.

15. Fougard T. Allergy and allergy-like symptoms in 1,050 medical students. Allergy 1991;46:20–6.

16. Hill LW. Certain aspects of allergy in children: a critical review of the recent literature. N Engl J Med 1961;265:1194–2000.

17. LeMasters GK, Wilson K, Levin L, et al. High prevalence of aeroallergen sensitization among infants of atopic parents. J Pediatr 2006;149:505–11.

18. Wheatley LM, Togias A. Allergic rhinitis. N Engl J Med 2015;372:456–63.

19. Biagini JM, LeMasters GK, Ryan PH, et al. Environmental risk factors of rhinitis in early infancy. Pediatr Allergy Immunol 2006;17:278–84.

20. Kulig M, Klettke U, Wahn V, et al. Development of seasonal allergic rhinitis during the first 7 years of life. J Allergy Clin Immunol 2000;106:832–9.

21. Jessen M, Malm L. Definition, prevalence and development of nasal obstruction. Allergy 1997;52:3–6.

22. Blaiss MS, Thompson AK, Juniper E, et al. Quality of life in patients with allergic rhinitis. Ann Allergy Asthma Immunol 2000;85:338–44.

23. Meltzer EO, Blaiss MS, Derebery MJ, et al. Burden of allergic rhinitis: results from the pediatric allergies in America survey. J Allergy Clin Immunol 2009;124:S43–70.

24. Meltzer EO, Gross GN, Katial R, et al. Allergic rhinitis substantially impacts patient quality of life: findings from the nasal allergy survey assessing limitations. J Fam Pract 2012;61:S5–10.

25. Schatz M. A survey of the burden of allergic rhinitis in the USA. Allergy 2007;62:9–16.

26. de la Hoz Caballer B, Rodriguez M, Fraj J, et al. Allergic rhinitis and its impact on work productivity in primary care practice and a comparison with other common diseases: the Cross–sectional study to evaluate work productivity in allergic rhinitis compared with other common diseases (CAPRI) study. Am J Rhinol Allergy 2012;26:390–4.

27. Delgado L, Moreira A, Capao-Filipe M. Rhinitis and its impact on sports. Allergy Clin Immunol Int 2006;18:98–105.

28. Fisher LH, Davies MJ, Craig TJ. Nasal obstruction, the airway, and the athlete. Clin Rev Allergy Immunol 2005;29:151–8.

29. Sansone RA, Sansone LA. Allergic rhinitis: relationships with anxiety and mood syndromes. Innov Clin Neurosci 2011;8:12–7.
30. Szeinbach SL, Seoane-Vazquez EC, Beyer A, et al. The impact of allergic rhinitis on work productivity. Prim Care Respir J 2007;16:98–105.
31. Bender BG. Cognitive effects of allergic rhinitis and its treatment. Immunol Allergy Clin North Am 2005;25:301–12.
32. Jauregui I, Mullol J, Davila I, et al. Allergic rhinitis and school performance. J Investig Allergol Clin Immunol 2009;19:32–9.
33. Sundberg R, Toren K, Hoglund D, et al. Nasal symptoms are associated with school performance in adolescents. J Adolesc Health 2007;40:581–3.
34. Blaiss MS. Allergic rhinitis and impairment issues in schoolchildren: a consensus report. Curr Med Res Opin 2004;20:1937–52.
35. Helgren J. Quality of life in nonallergic rhinitis. Clin Allergy Immunol 2007;19:383–7.
36. Ozdoganoglu T, Songu M, Inancli HM. Quality of life in allergic rhinitis. Ther Adv Respir Dis 2012;6:25–39.
37. Bousquet PJ, Demoly P, Devillier P, et al. Impact of allergic rhinitis on quality of life in primary care. Int Arch Allergy Immunol 2013;160:393–400.
38. Demoly P, Bousquet PJ, Mesbah K, et al. Visual analogue scale in patients treated for allergic rhinitis: an observational prospective study in primary care of asthma and rhinitis. Clin Exp Allergy 2013;43:881–8.
39. Barnes ML, Vaidyanathan S, Williamson PA, et al. The minimal clinically important difference in allergic rhinitis. Clin Exp Allergy 2010;40:242–50.
40. Petersen KD, Kronborg C, Gyrd-Hansen D, et al. Quality of life in rhinoconjunctivitis assessed with generic and disease specific questionnaires. Allergy 2008;63:284–91.
41. Everhart RS, Kopel SJ, Esteban CA, et al. Allergic rhinitis quality of life in urban children with asthma. Ann Allergy Asthma Immunol 2014;112:365–70.
42. Passali GC, Ralli M, Galli J, et al. How relevant is the impairment of smell for the quality of life in allergic rhinitis? Curr Opin Allergy Clin Immunol 2008;8:238–42.
43. Hellings PW, Rombaux P. Medical therapy and smell dysfunction. B-ENT 2009;5:S71–5.
44. Guilemany JM, Garcia-Pinero A, Alobid I, et al. Persistent allergic rhinitis has a moderate impact on the sense of smell depending on both nasal congestion and inflammation. Laryngoscope 2009;119:233–8.
45. Meltzer EO, Bukstein DA. The economic impact of allergic rhinitis and current guidelines for treatment. Ann Allergy Asthma Immunol 2011;106:S12–6.
46. Nathan RA. The burden of allergic rhinitis. Allergy Asthma Proc 2007;28:3–9.
47. Reed SD, Lee TA, McCrory DC. The economic burden of allergic rhinitis: a critical evaluation of the literature. Pharmacoeconomics 2004;22:345–61.
48. Bousquet J, Demarteau N, Mullol J, et al. Costs associated with persistent allergic rhinitis are reduced by levocetirizine. Allergy 2005;60:788–94.
49. Schoenwetter WF, Dupclay L Jr, Appajosyula S, et al. Economic impact and quality of life burden of allergic rhinitis. Curr Med Res Opin 2004;20:305–17.
50. Hadley JA, Derebery MJ, Marple BF. Comorbidities and allergic rhinitis: not just a runny nose. J Fam Med 2012;61:S11–5.
51. Patel ZM, Kennedy DW, Setzen M, et al. "Sinus headache": rhinogenic headache or migraine? An evidence-based guide to diagnosis and treatment. Int Forum Allergy Rhinol 2013;3:221–30.
52. Klossek JM, Annesi-Maesano I, Pribil C, et al. The burden associated with ocular symptoms in allergic rhinitis. Int Arch Allergy Immunol 2012;158:411–7.

53. Baroody FM, Foster KA, Markaryan A, et al. Nasal ocular reflexes and eye symptoms in patients with allergic rhinitis. Ann Allergy Asthma Immunol 2008;100: 194–9.
54. Bielory L. Allergic conjunctivitis and the impact of allergic rhinitis. Curr Allergy Asthma Rep 2010;10:122–34.
55. Skoner AR, Skoner KR, Skoner DP. Allergic rhinitis, histamine and otitis media. Allergy Asthma Proc 2009;30:470–81.
56. Lack G, Caulfield H, Penagos M. The link between otitis media with effusion and allergy: a potential role for intranasal corticosteroids. Pediatr Allergy Immunol 2011;22:258–66.
57. Luong A, Roland PS. The link between allergic rhinitis and chronic otitis media with effusion in atopic patients. Otolaryngol Clin North Am 2008;41:311–23.
58. Meltzer EO, Szwarcberg J, Pill MW. Allergic rhinitis, asthma and rhinosinusitis: diseases of the integrated airway. J Manag Care Pharm 2004;10:310–7.
59. Kariyawasam HH, Rotiroti G. Allergic rhinitis, rhinosinusitis and asthma. Unravelling a complex relationship. Curr Opin Otolaryngol Head Neck Surg 2013;21: 79–86.
60. Blaiss MS, Meltzer EO, Derebery MJ, et al. Patient and health-care-provider perspectives on the burden of allergic rhinitis. Allergy Asthma Proc 2007;28(Suppl 1):S4–10.
61. Neffen H, Mello JF Jr, Sole D, et al. Nasal allergies in the Latin American population: results from the allergies in Latin America survey. Allergy Asthma Proc 2010; 31(Suppl 1):S9–27.
62. Pecova R, Vrlik M, Tatar M. Cough sensitivity in allergic rhinitis. J Physiol Pharmacol 2005;56:171–8.
63. Pecova R, Zucha J, Pec M, et al. Cough reflex sensitivity testing in seasonal allergic rhinitis patients and healthy volunteers. J Physiol Pharmacol 2008;59: 557–64.
64. Krouse JH, Altman KW. Rhinogenic laryngitis, cough, and the unified airway. Otolaryngol Clin North Am 2010;43:111–21.
65. Rowe-Jones JM. The link between the nose and lung, perennial rhinitis and asthma: is it the same disease? Allergy 1997;52:20–8.
66. Vignola AM, Chanez P, Godard P, et al. Relationships between rhinitis and asthma. Allergy 1998;53:833–9.
67. Corren J. The connection between allergic rhinitis and bronchial asthma. Curr Opin Pulm Med 2007;13:13–8.
68. Compalati E, Ridolo E, Passalacqua G, et al. The link between allergic rhinitis and asthma: the united airways disease. Expert Rev Clin Immunol 2010;6:413–23.
69. Casale TB, Dykewicz MS. Clinical implications of the allergic rhinitis-asthma link. Am J Med Sci 2004;327:127–38.
70. Bugiani M, Carosso A, Migliore E, et al. Allergic rhinitis and asthma comorbidity in a survey of young adults in Italy. Allergy 2005;60:165–70.
71. Ciprandi G, Cirillo I. The lower airway pathology of rhinitis. J Allergy Clin Immunol 2006;118:1105–9.
72. Capasso M, Varricchio A, Ciprandi G. Impact of allergic rhinitis on asthma in children: effects on bronchodilation. Allergy 2010;65:264–8.
73. Bencova A, Rozborilova E, Antosova M. Bidirectional link between upper and lower airways in patients with allergic rhinitis. Eur J Med Res 2009;14:18–20.
74. Bernstein L, Li J, Bernstein D, et al. Allergy diagnostic testing: an updated practice parameter. Ann Allergy 2008;100:S1–148.

75. de Groot EP, Nijkamp A, Duiverman EJ, et al. Allergic rhinitis is associated with poor asthma control in children with asthma. Thorax 2012;67:582–7.

76. Gaugris S, Sazonov-Kocevat V, Thomas M. Burden of concomitant allergic rhinitis in adults with asthma. J Asthma 2006;43:1–7.

77. Lasmar LM, Camargos P, Ordones AB, et al. Prevalence of allergic rhinitis and its impact on the use of emergency care services in a group of children and adolescents with moderate to severe persistent asthma. J Pediatr (Rio J) 2007;83:555–61.

78. Flook EP, Kumar BN. Is there evidence to link acid reflux with chronic sinusitis or any nasal symptoms? A review of the evidence. Rhinology 2011;49:11–6.

79. Kirmaz C, Aydemir O, Bayrak P, et al. Sexual dysfunction in patients with allergic rhinoconjunctivitis. Ann Allergy Asthma Immunol 2005;95:525–9.

80. Olze H, Zuberbier T. Comorbidities between nose and skin allergy. Curr Opin Allergy Clin Immunol 2011;11:457–63.

81. Mullol J, Maurer M, Bousquet J. Sleep and allergic rhinitis. J Investig Allergol Clin Immunol 2008;18:415–9.

82. Craig TJ, Sherkat A, Safaee S. Congestion and sleep-impairment in allergic rhinitis. Curr Allergy Asthma Rep 2010;10:113–21.

83. Gonzalez-Nunez V, Valero AL, Mullol J. Impact of sleep as a specific marker of quality of life in allergic rhinitis. Curr Allergy Asthma Rep 2013;13:131–41.

84. Leger D, Annesi-Maesano I, Carat F, et al. Allergic rhinitis and its consequences on quality of sleep: an unexplored area. Arch Intern Med 2006;166:1744–8.

85. Colas C, Galera H, Anibarro B, et al. Disease severity impairs sleep quality in allergic rhinitis. Clin Exp Allergy 2012;42:1080–7.

86. Staevska MT, Mandajieva MA, Dimitrov VD. Rhinitis and sleep apnea. Curr Allergy Asthma Rep 2004;4:193–9.

87. Lin SY, Melvin TA, Boss EF, et al. The association between allergic rhinitis and sleep-disordered breathing in children: a systematic review. Int Forum Allergy Rhinol 2013;3:504–9.

88. Kalra M, Lemasters G, Bernstein D, et al. Atopy as a risk factor for habitual snoring at age 1 year. Chest 2006;129:942–6.

89. Chng SY, Goh DY, Wang XS, et al. Snoring and atopic disease: a strong association. Pediatr Pulmonol 2004;38:210–6.

90. Redline S, Tishler PV, Schluchter M, et al. Risk factors for sleep-disordered breathing in children: associations with obesity, race, and respiratory problems. Am J Respir Crit Care Med 1999;159:1527–32.

91. Kramer MF, de la Chaux R, Fintelmann R, et al. NARES: a risk factor for obstructive sleep apnea? Am J Otolaryngol 2004;25:173–7.

92. Soose RJ. Role of allergy in sleep-disordered breathing. Otolaryngol Clin North Am 2011;44:625–35.

93. Fisher L, Ghaffari G, Davies M, et al. Effects of poor sleep in allergic rhinitis. Curr Opin Allergy Clin Immunol 2005;5:11–6.

94. Pratt EL, Craig TJ. Assessing outcomes from the sleep disturbance associated with rhinitis. Curr Opin Allergy Clin Immunol 2007;7:249–56.

95. Yuksel H, Sogut A, Yilmaz H, et al. Sleep actigraphy evidence of improved sleep after treatment of allergic rhinitis. Ann Allergy Asthma Immunol 2009;103:290–4.

96. Meltzer EO, Schatz M, Nathan R, et al. Reliability, validity and responsiveness of the Rhinitis Control Assessment Test in patients with rhinitis. J Allergy Clin Immunol 2013;131:379–86.

Diagnosing Allergic Rhinitis

Glenis K. Scadding, MD, FRCP[a],*, Guy W. Scadding, MBBS, MRCP[b]

KEYWORDS

- Allergic rhinitis (AR) • Diagnosis • History • Skin prick tests • Specific IgE
- Nasendoscopy • Nasal allergen challenge

KEY POINTS

- Typical symptoms of allergic rhinitis (AR) include nasal blockage, discharge, itching, and sneezing; eye symptoms are common.
- AR may present with comorbidities, including cough, impaired asthma control, chronic otitis media with effusion, and sleep disturbance.
- Diagnosis requires suitable history plus confirmation of allergy by skin or serum IgE testing.
- Nasal allergen challenge may be necessary if local AR is suspected.
- Differential diagnosis is wide, including nonallergic, infective, inflammatory, and structural disease.

INTRODUCTION

The need to diagnose rhinitis accurately and to treat it effectively is undeniable given its prevalence and negative impact on quality of life and productivity.[1] Nevertheless, the condition is too often ignored, underdiagnosed, or misdiagnosed and hence managed inadequately.[2] The starting point is to be aware of the many underlying causes and the many ways in which rhinitis manifests. Beyond establishing the diagnosis of AR, the physician and patient should identify the worst/most troublesome symptoms, their timing, likely exacerbating factors, and effects on quality of life.

DIAGNOSIS OF ALLERGIC RHINITIS

Patients with AR may present with classical symptoms making the diagnosis more straightforward but more challenging when patients present with atypical features,

The authors have nothing to disclose.
[a] Department of Allergy and Rhinology, Royal National Throat, Nose and Ear Hospital, 330 Gray's Inn Road, London WC1X 8DA, UK; [b] Allergy, Royal Brompton Hospital, Sydney Street, London SW3 6NP, UK
* Corresponding author.
E-mail address: g.scadding@ucl.ac.uk

Immunol Allergy Clin N Am 36 (2016) 249–260
http://dx.doi.org/10.1016/j.iac.2015.12.003
0889-8561/16/$ – see front matter © 2016 Elsevier Inc. All rights reserved.

immunology.theclinics.com

for example, chronic cough in an atopic child. Rhinitis should also be differentiated from chronic rhinosinusitis (CRS) (**Box 1**).[3]

The next step is accurately making a diagnosis of AR is to determine whether the rhinitis is allergic in origin or due to 1 of myriad alternative, nonallergic causes. In addition, efforts should be made to identify the likely causative allergens. This is generally unproblematic in cases of isolated seasonal allergy (seasonal AR/hay fever) but more complicated in polysensitized individuals with perennial disease. An accurate allergy diagnosis allows selection of appropriate pharmacotherapy, informs the possibility of allergen avoidance, and allows consideration of allergen-specific immunotherapy. Additionally, the importance for patients of understanding triggering factors should be acknowledged because that is likely to improve outcomes, including adherence to therapy.

Diagnosis is made based on patient history, clinical examination, and skin prick tests (SPTs) or serum-specific IgE tests. Additional tests may be required in cases of uncertainty and in consideration of differential, nonallergic diagnoses.[4]

HISTORY

The classic symptoms of rhinitis are nasal running, nasal congestion, sneezing, and itching. Two or more of these symptoms, for more than an hour per day, for more than 2 weeks is diagnostic,[1] but a more detailed history is necessary to identify specific triggers. Causes of rhinitis may be broadly grouped into allergic, infective, structural, or other. There may be overlap between these categories. For example, an individual with AR's condition may be complicated by the presence of nasal septal deviation. To ensure a comprehensive history, patients can be asked to complete a rhinitis questionnaire prior to consultation. They should also be notified ahead of time of the need to avoid use of antihistamines for at least 72 hours prior to the appointment, if possible, to allow for skin testing.

Manifestations of rhinitis, which are particularly suggestive of allergy, include sneezing, itchy nose, itchy palate, and eye involvement. The timing of these – perennial, seasonal, in certain locations, or during certain activities – may provide a clue to the responsible allergen(s). Recurrent seasonal symptoms suggest triggers, such as pollens or mold spores. Symptoms experienced within the home may be due to pets, infestations (cockroaches or mice) or house dust mites. Symptoms predominantly at work might indicate an occupational allergen, for example, bakers sensitized to flour or bread improvers or laboratory animal allergy.[5] Because disease progresses, chronic nasal inflammation produces generalized nasal mucosal hyper-reactivity and more persistent symptoms, potentially masking a clear correlation with allergen exposure. Periods of prolonged absence from allergen, such as holidays, may result in disease remission or attenuation, further suggesting the correlation of an allergic trigger exposure with disease.

Box 1
Symptoms of rhinitis and chronic rhinosinusitis

Rhinitis: nasal running, blocking, sneezing, and itching; eye symptoms, particularly in seasonal allergis rhinitis

CRS: nasal blockage, discharge (anterior and/or posterior), facial pain/pressure, reduced olfaction; diagnosis confirmed by endoscopic findings and/or CT scan

Data from Fokkens W, Lund V, Bachert C, et al. EAACI position paper on rhinosinusitis and nasal polyps executive summary. Allergy 2005;60(5):583–601.

Eye symptoms associated with AR, especially seasonal AR, include itching, redness, and swelling of the conjunctiva with lacrimation. This complex of symptoms is termed *rhinoconjunctivitis*. More severe allergic eye diseases – atopic keratoconjunctivitis and vernal keratoconjunctivitis – may occur in individuals with eczema and warrant a specialist ophthalmologic opinion.[6]

Rhinorrhea (nose running) can be anterior or posterior, manifesting as postnasal drip, and may or may not be due to allergy. Classically, AR causes bilateral clear secretions. Isolated, unilateral clear nasal discharge is uncommon and in this circumstance cerebrospinal fluid leak should be excluded.[7] Cerebrospinal fluid leak most commonly occurs after sinus surgery or trauma, but may be spontaneous. Discolored secretions can be associated with allergy. For example, eosinophils in secretions give a yellow coloration whereas neutrophils yield green secretions, potentially indicating infection, although this may mask underlying AR. Crusting of secretions within the nose is possible in AR but is not usually pronounced. Primary complaints of nasal crusting and nose bleeding may suggest other pathologies, such as CRS, nose picking, Wegener granulomatosis, sarcoidosis, other vasculitides, ozena/atrophic rhinitis (wasting away of the bony ridges and mucous membranes inside the nose), noninvasive ventilation, cocaine abuse, or frequent use of nasal decongestants. Crusting may also occur for a period after nasal or sinus surgery. Intranasal corticosteroids not uncommonly, particularly if applied incorrectly, cause some nasal bleeding and may, rarely, cause crusting.

Nasal obstruction may be accepted as normal by some patients with longstanding rhinitis and also by the parents of some rhinitic children because of the common tendency for them to mouth breathe for some time after the common cold, or because of adenoid hypertrophy. Obstruction may be partial or complete, with severity often correlating with systemic manifestations, for example, sleep problems. AR usually results in bilateral nasal congestion, but other common factors, such as septal deviation, may make it appear unilateral. Alternating nostril obstruction may occur due to changes in blood pooling in capacitance vessels from one side of the nose to the other, contributing to mucosal swelling, which is a normal physiologic phenomenon referred to as the nasal cycle.[8] Other causes of obstruction include nasal polyps, foreign bodies, and rarely tumors. The differential diagnosis is age dependent with consideration of encephaloceles and choanal atresia in young children. Paradoxically, the dry, spacious intranasal appearances seen in atrophic rhinitis or after aggressive inferior turbinectomy surgery (empty nose syndrome) are often associated with a subjective sensation of nasal obstruction.

The diagnosis of AR may be missed when a patient's primary complaint is 1 of its many comorbidities (**Box 2**). Allergic conjunctivitis may be the focus of attention but

---

Box 2
Comorbidities of allergic rhinitis

Conjunctivitis

Chronic otitis media with effusion; eustachian tube dysfunction

Sleep impairment; obstructive sleep apnea

Rhinosinusitis; hyposmia

Bronchial hyper-reactivity; asthma

Pollen-food cross-reactivity

Laryngeal irritation; globus phenomenon

is virtually always accompanied by rhinitis. Children with chronic otitis media with effusion often have concomitant rhinitis. Most asthmatics have rhinitis or rhinosinusitis of some kind. A diagnosis of rhinosinusitis requires symptoms of nasal obstruction and discharge together, or 1 of these symptoms plus hyposmia, facial pain, or headache, alongside confirmatory findings on endoscopy or CT scan.[3] CRS may be associated with or without nasal polyps. AR seems to be a risk factor for the development of CRS without polyps but less so in CRS with polyps.

AR can be associated with systemic manifestations, such as difficulty sleeping, snoring, fatigue, and impaired concentration, leading to reduced productivity or poor school performance.[9] Repeated sniffing or a nasal intonation of the voice can be caused or exacerbated by nasal obstruction and rhinorrhea from any cause.

Lower respiratory tract symptoms, including cough, wheeze, and exertional dyspnea, may be associated with AR even in the absence of overt asthma. Bronchial hyper-reactivity can be induced by upper airway inflammation, as evidenced by changes in histamine/methacholine bronchial provocation doses after seasonal allergen exposure in hay fever sufferers.[10] Disorders of the upper and lower respiratory tract often coexist: most asthmatics have rhinitis or rhinosinusitis of some kind,[11] whereas a significant minority of individuals with AR have coexistent asthma.[12] Importantly, rhinitis/rhinosinusitis may impair asthma control[13] and should always be considered in the assessment of patients with poorly controlled asthma. Aspirin-sensitive asthma in particular is frequently associated with CRS with polyps. Typically both upper and lower respiratory tract symptoms are more severe than in other forms of rhinitis and asthma.

AR may be associated with food allergy due to cross-reactivity between aeroallergens and allergens within foods, described as pollen-food syndrome (also oral allergy syndome). In Northern Europe, by far the most common presentation is seen in silver birch pollen–allergic patients. The major birch allergen, Bet v 1, shows structural homology with proteins in stone and seed fruits of the Rosaceae family as well as with many tree nuts.[14] Other aeroallergen sensitizations associated with cross-reactivity include grass pollens, weed pollens, and latex. Typically, symptoms on ingestion of cross-reacting foods are limited to the mouth and oropharynx but may occasionally be more generalized.

A diagnosis of AR is more likely when rhinitis is seasonal, in the presence of asthma, or with a family history of atopy. To assess exposure to possible allergens and irritants a full social history is required, including housing conditions (floor level, dampness and mildew odors, dust reservoirs like carpet and bedding, soft toys, carpeting, central forced air heating, or cockroach or rodent infestations), the presence of pets or other contact with animals, and school environment; and, in young children, feeding details should be obtained. Information regarding smoking, exposure to second-hand smoke and other pollutants, hobbies, and alcohol consumption should be considered. Occupational history may be relevant either as a direct cause of AR or because of workplace triggers that exacerbate preexisting rhinitis (work-exacerbated rhinitis).[5] It is important to recognize occupational rhinitis because it usually precedes the development of occupational asthma and, therefore, these patients should be more closely monitored to prevent the development of occupational asthma. Professions most at risk for occupational asthma that may present as occupational rhinitis include bakers, furriers, and animal laboratory workers.[15]

Drug history is important because several medications can cause or aggravate rhinitis symptoms. These include antihypertensive medications, aspirin and other nonsteroidal anti-inflammatory drugs, oral contraceptives, and, in particular, topical sympathomimetics/nasal decongestants, which can provoke a rebound nasal congestion (rhinitis medicamentosa) if used for extended periods of time without the use of a nasal corticosteroid spray. It is also important to inquire about the efficacy of previous rhinitis treatments and specifically whether they were used preventatively on a daily basis or as needed in response to acute symptoms only.[2]

EXAMINATION

Examination effectively begins during the history taking process – observation of frequent sniffing, mouth breathing, use of tissues, nasal speech, and nose rubbing (allergic salute) may all be seen. Initial inspection of the face may reveal clues to allergy, such as a horizontal nasal crease across the dorsum of nose (**Fig. 1**), the presence of red watery eyes suggestive of allergic conjunctivitis, facial eczema, and dark circles/shadowing beneath the eyes referred to as allergic shiners. Depression of the nasal bridge can be a postsurgical phenomenon or caused by Wegener granulomatosis or cocaine misuse. A widened bridge suggests nasal polyposis. Purple discoloration of the nasal tip can be due to sarcoidosis; prominent telangiectasia suggests hereditary hemorrhagic telangiectasia, which may present with epistaxis.

Chronic mouth breathing suggests complete or near-complete nasal obstruction. Nasal airflow can be simply assessed by observing for misting of a cold metal spatula held beneath the nostrils in patients of any age or by more complex methods (nasal inspiratory peak flow, acoustic rhinometry, and rhinomanometry) in older children and adults.

The nose should then be examined internally, preferably with a nasal endoscope, but if not available using a head-mounted light and nasal speculum (anterior rhinoscopy) or with an otoscope using the largest diameter end piece. Examination by nasal endoscopy is more specific than anterior rhinoscopy and alters the diagnosis in up to a

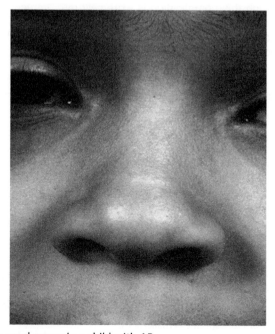

Fig. 1. Transverse nasal crease in a child with AR.

fifth of patients with nasal disease.[16] Appearances may be normal in AR (particularly if examined outside of seasonal allergen exposure) or may classically demonstrate hypertrophic, pale, boggy inferior and/or middle turbinates with clear secretions. Polyps, if visible, can be distinguished from the inferior turbinate by their insensitivity to touch, yellow/gray color, and the ability to get between them and the side wall of the nose. Yellow submucosal nodules with a cobblestone appearance suggest sarcoidosis.[17] Crusting and granulations raise the possibility of vasculitis. Septal perforation may occur after septal surgery, due to chronic vasoconstriction (cocaine or topical decongestants), Wegener granulomatosis, nose picking, or use of nasal-prong oxygen supplementation and rarely secondary to corticosteroid nasal sprays. Although septal deviation is common and rarely the main cause of symptoms, it may contribute to lateralization of symptoms and to difficulty with application of intranasal sprays. The throat, postnasal space, palate, and ears should also be inspected. All patients with persistent rhinitis should also have chest examination, including spirometry or peak flow, to assess for possible asthma.

INVESTIGATIONS

Allergen-specific IgE can be detected with SPTs or by serum immunoassay (**Boxes 3 and 4**). SPTs have the advantage of being immediate, educational for patients, and relatively cheap. SPTs should be carried out routinely in all patients to determine the presence of atopy and possible causative allergens except those patients with dermatographism or chronic eczema or when medications blocking histamine receptors cannot be discontinued (antihistamines, tricyclic antidepressants, and topical, but not oral, corticosteroids). In these circumstances, serum-specific IgE testing should be performed. Skin testing to standardized aeroallergens is extremely safe. Regardless of whether standardized or nonstandardized reagents are used, injectable adrenaline should be available given the theoretic risk of inducing a systemic allergic reaction, even though this complication is extremely rare. Intracutaneous tests are more sensitive and as a result are more likely to yield false-positive results. Furthermore, they are more painful for patients and, therefore, not routinely recommended for inhalant allergens, especially when all SPTs are negative and a patient's clinical

---

Box 3
Skin prick testing

A basic set of SPT allergens: in the United Kingdom, house dust mite, grass and tree pollens, and cat and dog danders show positivity in up to 95% of AR sufferers. Supplementation with other allergens suggested by the history may further improve diagnosis, for example, other animals, cockroach, rodents, molds, latex, and flour.

In young children, SPTs may be extended to include certain common allergenic foods for example, cow's milk, egg, soy, wheat, fish, peanut, and tree nuts.

A negative control: saline/allergen diluent, plus a positive control; histamine should be used.

Contraindications: widespread eczema, dermographism, recent antihistamines or extensive topical corticosteroid, pregnancy.

Interpret in relation to history: positive tests may be found in symptom-free patients – increased risk of developing allergic symptoms in time – and may persist even after immunotherapy. Negative testing in patients with high clinical suspicion may warrant blood analysis for serum-specific IgE to exclude a false-negative result and, if also negative, possibly nasal challenge to 1 or more specific aeroallergens.

Box 4
Serum-specific IgE testing

Typically by modified sandwich immunoassay

When skin testing not possible (eczema, use antihistamines) or allergen reagent not available

In cases of equivocal/unexpected skin test results

Allergen component diagnostics may aid differentiation between primary allergy and cross-reactivity.[18]

Data from Luengo O, Cardona V. Component resolved diagnosis: when should it be used? Clin Transl Allergy 2014;4:28.

---

history is less than convincing for AR. In circumstances where a patient gives a clear history of symptoms in response to exposure (ie, cat or dog), it is not unreasonable to place a selective intracutaneous test at a nonirritating dilution (1:1000 weight/volume) to rule out sensitization definitively. This still misses, however, local AR, and nasal provocation testing to 1 or more specific aeroallergens is the most definitive way to exclude an allergic component to chronic rhinitis. If a patient has a history of anaphylaxis or severe allergic symptoms in response to the inciting allergy, SPT administration is inadvisable outside an allergy specialist's office.

Testing total IgE alone is of limited benefit and may lead to erroneous assumption of allergy as the cause of symptoms if it is elevated. It may aid interpretation, however, of specific IgE in certain circumstances, such as severe eczema, where total IgE may be grossly elevated and modest elevations in serum-specific IgE may have a lower positive predictive value. Serum allergen–specific IgE generally correlates with the results of SPTs, showing similar sensitivity for house dust mite, but SPTs are more sensitive for other inhalant allergens, such as cat epithelium, mold, and grass pollen.[19] Regardless of which test is used, a certain degree of expertise is required to read and/or interpret the results to ensure a correct diagnosis of AR is established.

Component-based analysis, in which the actual proteins to which a patient is sensitized are revealed, is probably unnecessary for aeroallergen diagnosis in most settings where there are clearly defined allergen seasons. Confusion can arise, however, due to cross-reacting molecules, such as profilins, present in many pollens and fruits, when there is a long pollen season due to multiple trees and grasses, as in Southern Europe. For example, in this situation, testing for Bet v 1, the major birch allergen, can reveal those genuinely sensitized to birch pollen as opposed to sensitization to a minor profilin allergen only.[18] Such an approach may be advisable before embarking on treatment with allergen-specific immunotherapy.

When SPTs/serum-specific IgE tests and clinical history are concordant, then a diagnosis of AR can be made and treatment instituted. When they are discordant, further investigations may be needed (**Fig. 2**). If AR is strongly suspected from the history but not supported by these initial tests, nasal allergen challenge (**Box 5**) may be considered, but its use is generally limited to specialist centers. Challenges may also be undertaken in cases of occupational rhinitis where a high degree of diagnostic certainty is required and when considering allergen-specific immunotherapy for perennial allergens where causality of rhinitis symptoms is often more difficult to infer compared with seasonal allergens. Nasal allergen challenge typically involves administration of a defined concentration of allergen in aqueous solution by nasal spray. Outcomes include increased clinical symptoms, objective measures of decreased nasal airflow

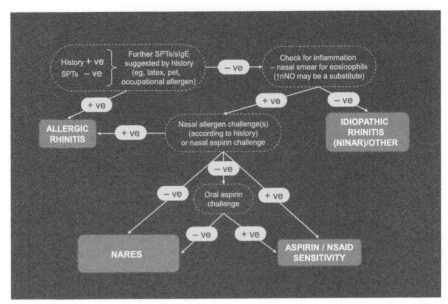

Fig. 2. Further investigations in cases of discordant history and skin/specific IgE tests. NINAR, noninfectious non-AR. NSAID, Non-steroidal anti-inflammatory drug.

or volume, and changes in cytology, local cytokines, tryptase, and other mediators as measured in nasal lavage fluid prechallenge and postchallenge. In individuals with a history of aspirin hypersensitivity, nasal lysine aspirin challenge may confirm hypersensitivity.[20] Nonspecfiic generalized nasal hyperresponsiveness, independent of allergy, can be investigated by provocation with histamine, metacholine or cold, dry air.

Objective measurements of the nasal airway (**Box 6**) are not generally made in routine clinical practice but are important measures of nasal challenge outcomes and may be helpful in assessing the nasal airway objectively if septal surgery or turbinate reduction is contemplated.

Additional laboratory investigations may be considered in cases of diagnostic uncertainty, to address differential diagnoses (**Table 1**), and may provide information to assist with treatment.[4] A complete blood cell count with differential white cell count may reveal peripheral eosinophilia in cases of CRS with nasal polyps or coexistent

---

Box 5
Uses of nasal allergen challenge

Confirmation of clinical relevance in cases of polysensitization to aeroallergens

Selection of patients for allergen immunotherapy (eg, for house dust mite)

Investigation of symptoms in the absence of evidence of systemic allergen sensitization (local AR)

Proof of symptom causation for novel and occupational allergens

Assessment of pathomechanisms of AR

Assessment of therapeutic interventions, such as antihistamines, corticosteroids, and allergen-specific immunotherapy

---

Box 6
Objective measures of the nasal airway

Peak nasal inspiratory flow is simple, inexpensive, and reproducible but effort dependent. Results correlate with rhinoscopic evidence of rhinitis but not with symptom scores. Most useful for comparing changes in airway patency within the same subject, although some normative data are now available.[21]

Acoustic rhinometry is the measure of acoustic impedance within the nasal cavity from which the cross-sectional area at different depths within the nasal cavity can be calculated. The method requires standardization and considerable experience to interpret and obtain reproducible results. Guidelines for its use are published.[22]

Rhinomanometry allows an estimation of nasal resistance from pressure-flow relationships and is difficult to perform reproducibly but still regarded by some investigators as the most accurate measure of nasal airway patency. The technique requires expensive equipment and considerable experience in interpretation.[23]

Data from Refs.[21–23]

---

asthma. C-reactive protein and erythrocyte sedimentation rate may be elevated in inflammatory conditions, such as vasculitis.

Nasal smears/mucus cytologic examination with estimation of eosinophil percentage and/or evidence of eosinophil degranulation (Charcot-Leyden crystals) may provide a diagnosis of non-AR with eosinophilia syndrome (NARES) and may be helpful in

---

Table 1
Differential diagnosis of allergic rhinitis

Type	Features
NARES	Skin tests negative; nasal smears show eosinophilia. May go on to develop nasal polyposis.
Autonomic rhinitis (vasomotor)	Physical/chemical triggers. More common in middle age with clear rhinorrhea, especially in the morning.
Drug induced	β-Adrenergic blockers, angiotensin-converting enzyme inhibitors. Rhinitis medicamentosa with chronic nasal decongestant use.
Hormonal	Pregnancy, oral contraceptives, thyroid disease.
Food	Gustatory rhinorrhea, for example, with spicy foods, sulphites.
Atrophic	Foul-smelling odor, crusting, hyposmia, nasal blockage.
Cystic fibrosis	Children with polyps must be screened for cystic fibrosis.
Primary ciliary dyskinesia	Rhinosinusitis, bronchiectasis, and reduced fertility.
Systemic/inflammatory	For example, Churg-Strauss syndrome.
Immunodeficiency	Chronic infective sinusitis secondary to antibody deficiency.
Malignancy	Bloody, purulent discharge, pain, and nasal blockage – symptoms may be unilateral.
Granulomatous diseases	Sarcoidosis. Wegener disease.
Structural abnormalities	Unilateral nasal obstruction secondary to nasal septal deviation.
Idiopathic/noninfectious non-AR	Cause unclear; may respond to topical capsaicin.
Local AR	Skin and serum IgE test negative but positive response to nasal allergen challenge.

predicting response to corticosteroids. Nasal swabs, taken from the middle meatus, may provide evidence of relevant infection; however, it should be known that asymptomatic carriage of *Staphylococcus aureus* in particular may be found in many individuals.

In cases of nasal crusting, blood-stained discharge, and/or nasal perforation, consideration should be given to the possibility of cocaine abuse – toxicology testing of urine or hair samples, with patient consent, can confirm recent use. In cases of unilateral, watery discharge, particularly after sinus surgery or head injury, a sample may be sent for assay of beta-2 transferrin, an isoform of transferrin limited to cerebrospinal fluid.

Concerning olfactory tests, the University of Pennsylvania Smell Identification Test is well validated, can identify malingerers,[24] and is accepted for legal cases.

Fractional exhaled nitric oxide (FeNO) measurement can be useful clinically in the diagnosis and monitoring of asthma. Normal levels are less than 20 parts per billion but increase in response to lower respiratory tract inflammation. FeNO levels may be elevated in AR patients, even in the absence of overt, clinical asthma. Nasal levels (nasal nitric oxide [nNO]) are widely variable in AR but in general tend to be elevated; very low FeNO levels can be a guide to the presence of primary ciliary dyskinesia or cystic fibrosis.[25]

Radiology is not routinely recommended for AR patients. Sinus CT scans are abnormal in a third of the adult population and almost half of children, probably because of the common cold and its prolonged after effects, so should only be undertaken when absolutely necessary, as advised by otorhinolaryngologists.

Referral to an otorhinolaryngologist is indicated for patients who have worrying symptoms, such as unilateral symptoms, blood-stained discharge, new-onset nasal polyp(s), and pressure effects on the orbit or orbital cellulitis (urgent referral). Cases of confirmed AR with persistent symptoms despite aggressive medical therapy require referral to an allergy specialist to confirm the diagnosis of AR versus mixed or non-AR and/or for consideration of allergen immunotherapy if appropriate.

SUMMARY

All patients presenting with upper and/or lower respiratory complaints should be questioned for symptoms of AR and asthma. Although AR can be simple to assess, it can also hide amid a variety of comorbidities and complications, thereby obfuscating its diagnosis. It can also form part of a mixed rhinitis alongside nonallergic nasal hyper-reactivity. A detailed history is the most important part of diagnosis, supported by testing for allergen-specific IgE to identify whether allergen sensitization correlates with reported symptoms on exposure. Discordance in test results and history of exposure necessitates further assessment and likely referral to an allergy or otolaryngology specialist.

REFERENCES

1. Bousquet J, Van CP, Khaltaev N. Allergic rhinitis and its impact on asthma. J Allergy Clin Immunol 2001;108(5 Suppl):S147–334.

2. Price D, Smith P, Hellings P, et al. Current controversies and challenges in allergic rhinitis management. Expert Rev Clin Immunol 2015;11(11):1205–17.

3. Fokkens W, Lund V, Bachert C, et al. EAACI position paper on rhinosinusitis and nasal polyps executive summary. Allergy 2005;60(5):583–601.

4. Hellings PW, Scadding G, Alobid I, et al. Executive summary of European task force document on diagnostic tools in rhinology. Rhinology 2012;50(4): 339–52.

5. Hox V, Steelant B, Fokkens W, et al. Occupational upper airway disease: how work affects the nose. Allergy 2014;69(3):282–91.

6. La Rosa M, Lionetti E, Reibaldi M, et al. Allergic conjunctivitis: a comprehensive review of the literature. Ital J Pediatr 2013;39:18.

7. Marshall AH, Jones NS, Robertson IJ. CSF rhinorrhoea: the place of endoscopic sinus surgery. Br J Neurosurg 2001;15(1):8–12.

8. Flanagan P, Eccles R. Spontaneous changes of unilateral nasal airflow in man. A re-examination of the 'nasal cycle'. Acta Otolaryngol 1997;117(4):590–5.

9. Blaiss MS, Allergic Rhinitis in School Children Consensus Group. Allergic rhinitis and impairment issues in schoolchildren: a consensus report. Curr Med Res Opin 2004;20(12):1937–52.

10. Corren J, Adinoff AD, Irvin CG. Changes in bronchial responsiveness following nasal provocation with allergen. J Allergy Clin Immunol 1992;89(2):611–8.

11. Corren J. The connection between allergic rhinitis and bronchial asthma. Curr Opin Pulm Med 2007;13(1):13–8.

12. Eriksson J, Bjerg A, Lotvall J, et al. Rhinitis phenotypes correlate with different symptom presentation and risk factor patterns of asthma. Respir Med 2011; 105(11):1611–21.

13. Clatworthy J, Price D, Ryan D, et al. The value of self-report assessment of adherence, rhinitis and smoking in relation to asthma control. Prim Care Respir J 2009; 18(4):300–5.

14. Skypala IJ, Bull S, Deegan K, et al. The prevalence of PFS and prevalence and characteristics of reported food allergy; a survey of UK adults aged 18-75 incorporating a validated PFS diagnostic questionnaire. Clin Exp Allergy 2013;43(8): 928–40.

15. Raulf M, Buters J, Chapman M, et al. Monitoring of occupational and environmental aeroallergens– EAACI position paper. concerted action of the EAACI IG occupational allergy and aerobiology & air pollution. Allergy 2014;69(10): 1280–99.

16. Hughes RG, Jones NS. The role of nasal endoscopy in outpatient management. Clin Otolaryngol Allied Sci 1998;23(3):224–6.

17. Fergie N, Jones NS, Havlat MF. The nasal manifestations of sarcoidosis: a review and report of eight cases. J Laryngol Otol 1999;113(10):893–8.

18. Luengo O, Cardona V. Component resolved diagnosis: when should it be used? Clin Transl Allergy 2014;4:28.

19. Gleeson M, Cripps AW, Hensley MJ, et al. A clinical evaluation in children of the Pharmacia ImmunoCAP system for inhalant allergens. Clin Exp Allergy 1996; 26(6):697–702.

20. Miller B, Mirakian R, Gane S, et al. Nasal lysine aspirin challenge in the diagnosis of aspirin - exacerbated respiratory disease: asthma and rhinitis. Clin Exp Allergy 2013;43(8):874–80.

21. Ottaviano G, Scadding GK, Coles S, et al. Peak nasal inspiratory flow; normal range in adult population. Rhinology 2006;44(1):32–5.

22. Hilberg O, Pedersen OF. Acoustic rhinometry: recommendations for technical specifications and standard operating procedures. Rhinology 2000;16(Suppl): 3–17.

23. Clement PA. Committee report on standardization of rhinomanometry. Rhinology 1984;22(3):151–5.

24. Doty RL, Shaman P, Kimmelman CP, et al. University of Pennsylvania Smell Identification Test: a rapid quantitative olfactory function test for the clinic. Laryngoscope 1984;94(2 Pt 1):176–8.

25. Scadding G, Scadding GK. Update on the use of nitric oxide as a noninvasive measure of airways inflammation. Rhinology 2009;47(2):115–20.

Allergic Rhinitis
Mechanisms and Treatment

David I. Bernstein, MD*, Gene Schwartz, MD, Jonathan A. Bernstein, MD

KEYWORDS

- Mechanisms • Allergic rhinitis treatment • Leukotrienes • Intranasal corticosteroids
- Intranasal antihistamines • Subcutaneous immunotherapy • Treatment

KEY POINTS

- Allergic rhinitis is an immunoglobulin E (IgE) -mediated inflammatory disease.
- Allergic rhinitis has a significant impact on patient morbidity and is a major economic burden to society.
- There are several effective treatment modalities available for allergic rhinitis that target receptors of bioactive mediators or inflammation.
- Subcutaneous allergen immunotherapy induces tolerance to aeroallergens and is highly effective in mitigating symptoms and preventing progression of disease and comorbidities such as asthma.
- Sublingual immunotherapy formulations offer an alternative approach to subcutaneous immunotherapy, allowing for symptomatic relief to specific seasonal allergens also likely through tolerogenic mechanisms.

INTRODUCTION

Atopic diseases, including allergic rhinitis (AR), are very prevalent, especially in developed countries. Prevalence estimates of chronic rhinitis around the world range between 10% and 40%.[1–11] The impact of AR on quality of life is very significant. Allergic rhinitis is a major contributor to the total cost of health-related absenteeism (eg, missing work) and presenteeism (ie, showing up to work but having reduced productivity). For example, costs of AR and allergic conjunctivitis in the United States have been estimated at more than $6 billion per year.[12–14] Lamb and colleagues[15] estimated the productivity loss from AR to be the highest of 15 chronic conditions among employees in the United States.

There are multiple phenotypes and endotypes of rhinitis, but in recent years, rhinitis control has been increasingly emphasized.[16] AR has been traditionally categorized as

Division of Immunology and Allergy, Department of Internal Medicine, University of Cincinnati College of Medicine, Cincinnati, OH, USA
* Corresponding author. 231 Albert Sabin Way, Cincinnati, OH 45267-0563.
E-mail address: bernstdd@ucmail.uc.edu

Immunol Allergy Clin N Am 36 (2016) 261–278
http://dx.doi.org/10.1016/j.iac.2015.12.004
0889-8561/16/$ – see front matter © 2016 Elsevier Inc. All rights reserved.

seasonal allergic rhinitis (SAR), perennial allergic rhinitis (PAR), and mixed rhinitis (ie, combined allergic and nonallergic phenotype). AR has recently been classified via the ARIA (Allergic Rhinitis and its Impact on Asthma) guideline as mild versus moderate to severe and intermittent versus persistent (**Table 1**).[17,18] Regardless of the classification system, the main goal of treatment is to achieve control of nasal and ocular symptoms of SAR and PAR.

The 3 key elements of AR management are reduction of exposure to the sensitizing allergen, which includes a spectrum of environmental avoidance recommendations specific to the inciting allergen, targeted pharmacotherapy, and either subcutaneous or sublingual immunotherapy.[19,20] Environmental control should focus on avoidance of known allergens as well as nonspecific aggravating triggers, such as noxious odorants and chemical irritants (eg, fragrances, cleaning agents, environmental tobacco smoke) identified by medical history. Broad environmental control measures aimed at reducing allergen exposure (eg, house dust mite) should not be instituted without first confirming clinical relevance, which involves demonstrating sensitization by skin prick testing or serum-specific IgE and correlation of symptoms with exposure to the specific sensitizing allergen.[17,19] Often patients may exhibit sensitization but are not able to correlate their symptoms with exposure, and in these instances, nasal provocation testing using standardized methodologies to the specific allergen may be useful to confirm or exclude the clinical relevance of sensitization.[21,22] Diagnosis of AR is discussed more extensively elsewhere in this issue. (See Scadding GK, Scadding GW: Diagnosing Allergic Rhinitis, in this issue.) The importance of environmental determinants in causing AR and eliciting related symptoms with continuous or intermittent exposures is discussed more extensively elsewhere in this issue. (See Dunlop J, Matsui E, Sharma H: Allergic Rhinitis: Environmental Determinants, in this issue.) This article focuses on providing a brief overview of the mechanisms related to AR and current treatment options for this chronic and often debilitating condition.

Allergic Rhinitis Mechanisms

AR is caused by specific immunoglobulin E (IgE) -mediated reactions against inhaled allergens driven by type 2 helper T (Th2) cells. AR results in mucosal inflammation with tissue influx of eosinophils and basophils.[23,24] IgE constitutes a very small fraction of the total antibody amount in human serum, but its biological activity is enhanced by specific cell surface receptors whose affinity can vary in strength.[24] IgE is produced as a result of complex interactions between B cells, T cells, mast cells, and basophils and involves multiple cytokines, such as interleukin (IL) -4, IL-13, and IL-18.[25] On exposure of allergen into the upper respiratory tract, the allergen is taken up by antigen-presenting cells (ie, dendritic cells, B cells) and processed to a small peptide

Table 1
Rhinitis severity grading based on joint task force rhinitis guidelines

Rhinitis Severity	Medication Requirement Example
Step 1: Episodic	—
Step 2: Mild	1 medication
Step 3: Mild to moderate	2 medications or change to another medication
Step 4: Moderate to severe	2–3 medications and/or change of 1 or more medications
Step 5: Severe	Oral corticosteroid

Data from Wallace DV, Dykewicz MS, Bernstein DI, et al. The diagnosis and management of rhinitis: an updated practice parameter. J Allergy Clin Immunol 2008;122(2 Suppl):S1–84.

that binds to specific major histocompatibility complex (MHC) class II molecules.[25] The MHC class II-peptide complex is then expressed on the cell surface, where it is recognized by Th0 receptor and other costimulatory molecules, resulting in differentiation into Th2 CD4+ lymphocytes that produce cytokines like IL-4, IL-5, and IL-13, all important in driving different components of the IgE inflammatory immune response.[25] The MHC class II-peptide complex activation of antigen-specific Th2 also can stimulate B-cell receptors, which in conjunction with B-cell costimulatory molecules cause B-cell differentiation to antibody-producing plasma cells.[25] Specific cytokines like IL-4 induce antibody class switching to IgE isotypes that specifically recognize the peptide linked to the MHC class 2 molecule. The antigen-specific IgE binds to high-affinity IgE receptors (FcER1 or CD23 + molecules) on mast cells and basophils.[25]

On re-exposure to the antigen/allergen, the relevant peptide is recognized by the FcER1 receptor, and after cross-linking these receptor molecules, a cascade of pathways is set in motion that lead to release of preformed bioactive mediators like histamine and newly formed lipid mediators derived from membrane phospholipids, such as leukotrienes, prostaglandins, and platelet-activating factor, that can cause smooth muscle contraction, increased vascular permeability, and mucus secretion (**Fig. 1**).[26] The release of these mediators leads to the early or immediate phase allergic response. These lipid mediators also have chemoattractant properties important for attracting inflammatory cells into the tissue, resulting in the late phase allergic response that can manifest approximately 4 to 8 hours after the early or immediate phase response.[25] In addition, enzymes, such as mast-cell chymase, tryptase, and serine esterases, are released that can activate matrix metalloproteinases that down tissue matrix proteins leading to tissue damage.[25] Tumor necrosis factor-α is also released by activated mast cells that can activate endothelial cells, causing increased expression of adhesion molecules that facilitates the influx of inflammatory leukocytes (ie, eosinophils) and lymphocytes influx into tissues.[25] The release of epithelial cell cytokines, such as thymic stromal lymphopoietin, IL-25, and IL-33, also bolsters the Th2 response further. Thus, the pharmacologic therapies to be discussed in later sections of this article target mediators, cytokines, or nonspecific inflammation to attenuate or ablate allergic symptoms.[25] Although these therapies block receptors or reduce inflammation, allergen immunotherapy can modify Th2-driven responses through different mechanisms, including through increased IgG4

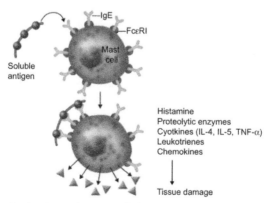

Fig. 1. Mast cell activation by antigen cross-linking of specific IgE molecules on FcER126 (Fc epsilon Receptor). TNF-α, tumor necrosis factor-α. (*From* Bernstein JA, Moellman J. Emerging concepts in the diagnosis and treatment of patients with undifferentiated angioedema. Int J Emerg Med 2012;5(1):39; with permission.)

blocking antibodies and increased production of T regulatory (CD4+ Foxp3+) cells that produce immunomodulatory cytokines (IL-10 and transforming growth factor [TGF] -β) and is the only potential curative treatment for AR.[23,24]

PHARMACOTHERAPY FOR ALLERGIC RHINITIS SUBTYPES
Seasonal Allergic Rhinitis

For the management of intermittent mild or intermittent SAR, an oral nonsedating second-generation H1 receptor antihistamine (AH) is recommended over a first-generation H1-antagonist, which is associated with more adverse effects, such as sedation, excessive drying, and impaired motor coordination. For persistent moderate or severe symptoms of seasonal rhinoconjunctivitis, daily use of an intranasal corticosteroid (INCS) or intranasal antihistamine (INAH) is the treatment of choice. Although INCS have been consistently shown to reduce associated allergic conjunctival symptoms of SAR, a topical ocular H1 AH with mast cell stabilizing properties (eg, cromolyn, pemirolast, nedocromil, olopatadine, azelastine) may be necessary to achieve better control of ocular symptoms.[27] Clinical studies have demonstrated little benefit of adding oral AHs or a leukotriene-modifying agent like montelukast to INCSs for treating moderate or severe SAR, although this approach may be beneficial in individual patients who are experiencing more nasal sneezing, itching, or conjunctival symptoms.[28] If an INCS is the first treatment of choice for treatment of SAR or PAR and is not sufficient for controlling symptoms, addition of an INAH would likely be the most appropriate next choice given the recent evidences reported in the literature regarding combination therapy.[16,20,29–31] A combination product of fluticasone proprionate plus azelastine HCl has been demonstrated to have greater efficacy in reducing nasal symptoms of SAR when compared with either drug alone.[16,31,32]

In patients with severe nasal and/or ocular symptoms of SAR or PAR refractory to nasal corticosteroids and topical AHs, especially nasal congestion, a brief course of oral corticosteroids should be considered to achieve symptomatic relief. Although still commonly used by some practitioners, long-acting depot intramuscular corticosteroid injections should not be used to treat SAR patients because of multiple systemic adverse effects, such as adrenal insufficiency as well as localized tissue atrophy at the site of the injection.[33,34] In adults with allergic or mixed rhinitis, oral decongestants such as pseudoephedrine may be added (if tolerated) in patients whose nasal symptoms (eg, nasal congestion, postnasal drainage) are not controlled with H1 blockers and nasal corticosteroids.[35] However, caution should be exercised in using these agents in patients prone to hypertension, urinary retention, and cardiac arrhythmias.[35]

Daily use of montelukast, a LTD_4 (leukotriene D) antagonist, may be considered in selected patients with SAR but is considered less effective than nasal corticosteroids. Despite good safety and tolerability in adults and children, montelukast, like oral AHs, has limited efficacy for treatment of moderate or severe SAR comparable to oral AHs.[16,17,20,29,30,36]

Perennial Allergic Rhinitis

As discussed in this issue, some environmental control measures for indoor aeroallergens can be effective in reducing allergen exposure and symptoms but are often insufficient alone. (See Dunlop J, Matsui E, Sharma H: Allergic Rhinitis: Environmental Determinants, in this issue.) Because rhinoconjunctival symptoms of PAR may not always be as pronounced as those symptoms experienced by SAR patients, pharmacologic treatment may differ. Double-blind placebo-controlled studies have demonstrated that second-generation oral AHs are more effective than placebo in patients with PAR. Both cetirizine and levocetirizine have an indication for the treatment of AR and are well tolerated.[37] In a large controlled trial, montelukast was also found to be more effective than placebo in treating adults with PAR.[38] Thus, it may be reasonable to initiate therapy of PAR with a second-generation oral AH for some patients with mild persistent PAR followed by addition of an INCS or INAH if symptoms are not well controlled. Ocular AHs and/or mast cell stabilizing agents should be initiated for allergic conjunctivitis symptoms if necessary.[27] Allergen immunotherapy is considered an alternative for any patient requiring chronic controller medications or incompletely responsive to medications and environmental control measures.[16,17,20,30]

Allergen Immunotherapy

Allergy immunotherapy (AIT) is the only potential curative therapy for SAR and/or PAR.[16,20,24,30,39] It has been reported that one-third of children and two-thirds of adults with AR experience insufficient relief with pharmacotherapy alone.[23,40,41] Allergen immunotherapy should be considered in patients uncontrolled by allergen avoidance measures and daily use of medications. Patient preference, acceptance, expected adherence, and costs are other important considerations in initiating either subcutaneous (SCIT) or sublingual immunotherapy.[16,30,42] **Fig. 2** summarizes what is known about the mechanistic responses to AIT.[43] Initially, mast cell and basophil desensitization is followed by an increase in T-regulatory cells driven by IL-10 and TGF-β cytokines, resulting in tolerance.[43] Blocking antibody and nasal mucosal tissue expression of Th1 cytokines (eg, interferon-γ), suggesting "Th1 shift," is demonstrated months after initiating SCIT.[43] SCIT has been used worldwide for more than a century and has been demonstrated to be effective in controlling symptoms of SAR and PAR.[44] Administration of high doses of allergens must be achieved to realize the full efficacy of SCIT.[45] A long-term placebo-controlled study conducted in patients with grass pollen SAR demonstrated that 3 years of SCIT with a standardized grass pollen allergen resulted in prolonged benefit for several years after discontinuation, suggesting a disease-modifying effect.[46] Although SCIT has been considered effective in the treatment of PAR due to house dust mite, the published evidence supporting this indication is relatively weak.[47] Benefits of SCIT must be weighed against the potential risks of systemic reactions known to occur with approximately 0.1% of injections.[48] Identifying and screening patients at high risk for fatal and near-fatal reactions, especially those with uncontrolled asthma, can significantly mitigate risk of severe systemic allergic reactions.[49,50] Allergen immunotherapy has many other benefits, including the prevention or progression of allergic asthma and reduction of other comorbidities, such as recurrent sinusitis.

Sublingual immunotherapy has been widely practiced in Europe for many years and has only recently been approved for use in the United States for the treatment of grass- and ragweed-induced SAR based on large placebo-controlled clinical trials.[51,52] Similar to SCIT, it too has a good safety profile. The most common side effect associated with SLIT is local oral and pharyngeal itching and swelling reactions that begin within days after initiation of therapy. In clinical trials, rare mild systemic reactions were reported, but there were no cases of severe anaphylaxis related to treatment. As with SCIT for grass pollen–induced SAR, a sustained therapeutic effect was demonstrated for 2 years following discontinuation after 3 years of continuous SLIT with grass tablets.[53] One advantage of SLIT is that there is no required buildup period and patients can self-administer the treatment at home after the first dose is given under observation in the office. At least 12 weeks of preseasonal therapy followed by coseasonal treatment with daily sublingual pollen tablets are required to see optimal clinical benefit in reducing symptoms and rescue medication.[54]

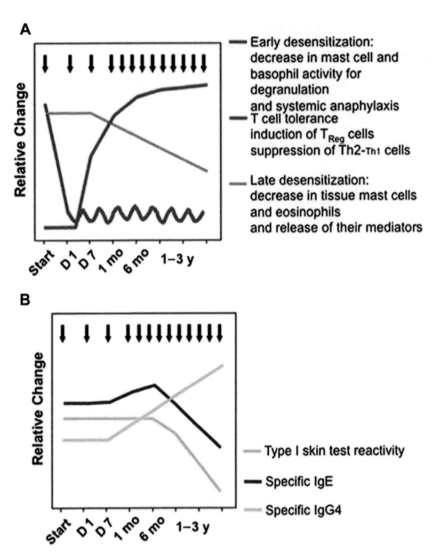

Fig. 2. Immunologic changes during allergen immunotherapy showing time course of effects on effector cells (*A*) and changes in allergy specific IgE, IgG4 and skin test reactivity (*B*). (*From* Burks AW, Calderon MA, Casale T, et al. Update on allergy immunotherapy: American Academy of Allergy, Asthma & Immunology/European Academy of Allergy and Clinical Immunology/PRACTALL Consensus Report. J Allergy Clin Immunol 2013;131(5):1290; with permission.)

PHARMACOTHERAPY, MECHANISMS OF ACTION, AND DOSING

Allergen avoidance is a very important adjunctive therapy for AR but is often hard to achieve. Nasal saline irrigation using a squeeze bottle or Neti Pot can be an important component for removing excess secretions and crusting in the nasal passages while also acting as a mild decongestant. If administered properly, it has minimal side effects. It is important to use boiled or distilled water to prepare the saline irrigation solution.[55] A recent meta-analysis of saline irrigation confirms it has a beneficial effect in the management of AR.[55]

Pharmacotherapy with AHs was a milestone in pharmacology and immunology. The Nobel Prize in Physiology and Medicine was awarded in 1957 to Daniel Bovet for the discovery of AHs (anti-H1 receptor), and in 1988 to Sir James Black for the discovery of anti-H2 receptor antagonists. Subsequently, additional H3 and H4 receptors were identified, and although research investigating the pathobiology of these receptors is ongoing, no specific receptor antagonists are currently available commercially in the United States.[56]

The pharmacologic properties and dosing regimens for first and second generation as well as INAH are summarized in **Table 2**.[20] As discussed earlier, oral AHs are considered first-line treatment recommendations for mild SAR and PAR.[16,20,30] First-generation oral AHs should be used cautiously because of side effects such as drowsiness but can be dosed relatively safely at bedtime and may be beneficial to help some patients sleep and to dry up excessive postnasal drainage.[16,20,56,57] INAHs are also recommended for mild AR and can be used more effectively as needed because of their relative quick onset of action (30 minutes). In general, oral AHs do not induce tachyphylaxis or tolerance.[16]

INCS are key to the management of moderate to severe AR and have been shown to be superior to either oral H1 AHs[58] or leukotriene receptor antagonists.[59,60] Characteristics of INCS are summarized in **Table 3**. INCSs take at least 24 hours to demonstrate a clinical effect and therefore are not as effective when used on an as-needed basis.[20,61–63] Scheduled regular administration of INCS is therefore usually superior and recommended.[64,65]

INAHs are often used to treat SAR and can be used as first-line treatment or in combination with INCS for treatment of AR according to guidelines. A recent study found that intranasal azelastine had comparable efficacy to intranasal fluticasone in the treatment of moderate to severe SAR.[32] The 2 available INAHs in the United States are olopatadine and azelastine. Olopatidine is a selective H1 receptor antagonist, whereas azelastine has multiple mechanisms of action, including H1 receptor antagonism, mast cells stabilization, and inhibition of leukotriene receptors.[30,66,67] Intranasal azelastine may also downregulate expression of adhesion molecules, regulate chemotaxis, and enhance apoptosis of inflammatory cells.[29,66–68]

Intranasal cromolyn sodium is an over-the-counter topical mast cell stabilizing agent that has been found to be effective in blocking release of allergic mediators such as histamine from sensitized mast cells.[69] Cromolyn sodium reduces both the early- and the late-phase allergic response and has been approved for use in both SAR and PAR.[70] Cromolyn sodium nasal spray has minimal systemic absorption and is very safe for chronic use without evidence of tachyphylaxis. The main disadvantage of nasal cromolyn is its rather short duration of action, necessitating administration 4 to 6 times a day for ongoing treatment effect.[16,71]

Leukotrienes are newly formed mediators that have been found to be important mediators in allergic disease. Inhibition of leukotriene C4, D4, and E4 or 5-lipoxygenase has been an important strategy for management of asthma and AR. However, the leukotriene receptor antagonist montelukast is the only agent in this class approved for the treatment of SAR and PAR. Studies have demonstrated similar efficacy of montelukast to a second-generation oral AH, and there might be an additive effect in combination with an AH.[38,72–76] In patients with AR and asthma, montelukast could potentially help treat both conditions if they are mild in severity because its effect on asthma is relatively weak.[76–79] Combination therapy with intranasal azelastine and fluticasone (Dymista) has been shown to be more effective than either

Table 2
First- and second-generation oral antihistamines and intranasal antihistamines properties, pharmacologic characteristics, and dosing

Generic Drug	Trade Name Example	Metabolites if Significant (T1/2 in Hours of Product or Metabolite)	Tmax Hours (Metabolite)	Skin Test Suppression Mean (Max) Days	% Sedation/Somnolence or Central Nervous System Impairment (Control)	Dosage Forms	Age Limit	Adult Dose
Second generation								
Acrivastine[d]	Semprex-D	(1.4–3.1)	1.15 1.4	~3, T1/2 = 1.7 h	812 (6)[PI]	8 mg	12 y	8 mg qid
Azelastine hydrogen chloride	Astelin nasal	Desmethylazelastine (22)[PI]	2.5 0.25[a]	2	11.5 (5.4)[PI]	137 µg/spray	5 y	2 sp/nostril bid
Cetirizine[d]	Zyrtec	None (7–11)	1.0 ± 0.5	3	14 (10)[PI]	5, 10 mg 5 mg/5 mL	6 mo	5–10 mg qd
Desloratadine[d]	Clarinex	3 Hydroxy desloratadine (7.8 ± 4.2)	3.17 (4.76)	~7 (T1/2 = 21–31 h)	2.1 (1.8)[PI]	5 mg 2.5 mg/5 mL	6 mo	5 mg qd
Fexofenadine[d]	Allegra	None (14.4–14.6)	2.6	2	1.3 (0.9)[PI]	30, 60, 180 mg 30 mg/5 mL	2 y	180 mg qd or 60 mg bid
Levocetirizine	Xyzal	None (7 ± 1.5)	0.9 1.25[PI]	Unknown	6 (2)[PI]	5 mg	6 y	5 mg qd
Loratadine[d]	Claritin	Descarboethoxyloratadine (7.8 ± 4.2)	1.2 ± 0.3 (1.5 ± 0.7)	7	8 (6)[PI]	10 mg 5 mg/5 mL	2 y	10 mg qd
Olopatadine hydrochloride	Patanase nasal	No major metabolites (8–12)[PI]	0.5–1.0[PI]	Unknown	0.9 (03)[PI]	665 µg/spray	12 y	2 sp/nostril bid

First generation

Drug	Trade name	Active metabolite (T1/2)					Preparations	Age	Dose
Chlorpheniramine[d]	Chlor-Trimeton	Monodesmethyl and didesmethyl chlorpheniramine (27.9 ± 8.7)	2-6	2.8	3 (6)	45%	4, 8, 12 mg 2 mg/5 mL	2 y	4 mg qid
Clemastine[d]	Tavist	(21.3 ± 11.6)		4.77 ± 2.26	5 (10)	14 (1.5)	1.34, 2.68 mg .67 mg/5 mL	6 y	1.34 mg bid to tid
Cyproheptadine	Periactin	(16)		4	9 (11)	8-50	4 mg 2 mg/5 mL	2 y	4 mg tid
Diphenhydramine	Benadryl	Nordiphenhydramine (9.2 ± 2.5)	2.6	1.7 ± 1.0	2 (5)	50%	25, 50 12.5 mg/mL	2 y	25–50 mg qid
Hydroxyzine	Atarax	(20 ± 4.1)		2.1 ± 0.4	5 (8)	80%	10, 25, 50, 100 mg 10 mg/5 mL	All ages	25 mg qid
Promethazine	Phenergan	Promethazine sulfoxide & N-desmethylpromethazine (9–16)[PI]		4.4	3 (5)	60-73	12.5, 25, 50 mg 6.25 mg/5 mL	2 y	25 mg qid
Triprolidine	Actifed	(3.2)[PI]		2.0	3 (7)	10% to 25%	—	—	—

Abbreviations: bid, 2 times a day; d, available with decongestant; PI, package insert; qd, every day; qid, 4 times a day; T1/2, half-life; tid, 3 times a day.

[a] Onset of action, not Tmax.

From Wallace DV, Dykewicz MS, Bernstein DI, et al. The diagnosis and management of rhinitis: an updated practice parameter. J Allergy Clin Immunol 2008;122:S20; with permission.

Table 3
Intranasal corticosteroids: dosing and characteristics

Spray Trade Name	Generic Drug	Type	μg/Spray	Adult Dose	Usual Child Dose	Age Limit (y)	Pregnancy/ Nursing Risk Category	Alcohol BKC Propylene Glycol
Beconase AQ	Beclometasone, monohydrate	Pump 200 spray	42	1–2 spray nos bid	1–2 sp/nos bid	6	C	Alcohol BKC
Flonase	Fluticasone propionate	Pump 120 spray	50	2 spray nos qd	1–2 sp/nos qd	4	C	Alcohol BKC
Nasarel	Flunisolide	Pump 200 spray	25	2 spray nos bid to tid	2 sp/nos bid	6	C	BKC, propylene glycol
Nasacort AQ	Triamcinolone	Pump 120 spray	55	1–2 spray nos qd	1–2 sp/nos qd	6	C	No alcohol BKC
Nasonex	Mometasone	Pump 120 spray	50	2 spray nos qd	1 sp/nos qd	2	C	No alcohol BKC
Rhinocort AQ	Budesonide	Pump 120 spray	32	1–4 spray/nos qd	1–2 sp/nos qd	6	C	No alcohol, no BKC
Veramyst	Fluticasone funoate	Pump 120 spray	50	2 spray/nos qd	1 sp/nos qd	2	C	No alcohol BKC
Omnaris	Ciclesonide	Pump 120 spray	50	2 spray/nos qd	NA	12	C	No alcohol, no BKC

Abbreviations: bid, 2 times a day; BKC, benzalkonium chloride; NA, not applicable; nos, Nostril; qd, every day; tid, 3 times a day.
From Wallace DV, Dykewicz MS, Bernstein DI, et al. The diagnosis and management of rhinitis: an updated practice parameter. J Allergy Clin Immunol 2008;122:S21; with permission.

monotherapy alone.[31] This treatment is approved for the management of SAR but is also clinically effective for PAR.[31] For many patients using Dymista, the ability to use a single spray with the INCS and INAH without having to wait in between the 2 nasal sprays is of significant convenience and prevents potential loss of medication if using the individual nose sprays separately.

Intranasal ipratropium bromide 0.03% is approved for treatment of rhinorrhea associated with perennial or SAR or non-AR and the higher concentration 0.06% is approved for rhinorrhea associated with the common cold. This medication is not effective for treatment of nasal congestion or other AR symptoms, such as nasal itching, sneezing, or nasal obstruction.[16,20,30,80,81] Intranasal ipratropium does not produce tolerance and therefore can be used on a daily basis.[16,30]

Although the chronic use of nasal decongestant spray is not currently recommended, recent studies indicate that they can be used in conjunction with INCS safely for some adult and adolescent patients not sufficiently responding to INCS alone. Specifically, oxymetazoline nasal spray has recently been shown to be effective and safe when used for an extended time period in conjunction with an INCS to treat recalcitrant nasal congestion in SAR patients.[82] Tachyphylaxis or rhinitis medicamentosa associated with daily use of an intranasal decongestant can be prevented when used with an INCS spray, which presumably prevents downregulation of the α-1 receptors.[82–85] It has also been demonstrated that INCSs are effective for treating rhinitis medicamentosa when intranasal decongestants are used inappropriately.[84,85]

MEDICATION ADMINISTRATION CAVEATS

It is essential to teach patients to administer nasal sprays away from the midline septum in order to prevent septal bleeding and ulceration. Proper administration will also help maximize the efficacy of nasal sprays by optimizing medication delivery and is especially important for INCSs, which have a greater incidence of nasal septal damage than INAH.[86] Oxymetazoline nasal spray cannot be used more than 3 to 5 days without an INCS because of rhinitis medicamentosa risk.[85] SCIT should not be administered to a patient with uncontrolled asthma or during an acute upper respiratory infection.[49,50,87] Management of local or systemic AIT reactions should include dose or concentration reduction depending on the severity of the reaction.[45]

MEDICATION SAFETY AND SIDE EFFECTS

Oral AHs, especially first-generation oral AHs, can interact with other medications and/or alcohol, causing sedation. In general, sedation is much less of a problem for second- and third-generation AHs compared with first-generation AHs. Among the second- or third-generation AHs, cetirizine is both more efficacious and also more likely to cause sedation.[88] All of the second- and third-generation H1 antagonists are pregnancy category B except fofexofenadine. Over-the-counter cromolyn sodium nasal spray is very safe and is pregnancy category B but requires administration every 4 to 6 hours because of its relatively short half-life and its decreased efficacy compared with INCS and INAH, making it less practical for use in patients with moderate to severe AR.[16,71] INCS sprays are very safe to use long term but are all pregnancy category C except budesonide nasal spray. However, long-term clinical experience indicates that INCSs are safe to use during pregnancy. INCS and to a lesser extent INAH sprays can cause nasal dryness, epistaxis, and in some cases, nasal septal ulceration and perforation. Debate is ongoing whether patients taking INCSs long term are at risk for glaucoma; however, a recent study investigating the effect of intranasal beclomethasone had no effect after 6 weeks of continuous treatment on increasing intraocular pressure.[89] Overall, INCS sprays have an excellent safety track record in both adults and children at the recommended doses.[58,60,90] Intranasal ipratropium may cause excessive nasal dryness but is otherwise very safe and is pregnancy category B.[16,20,80] The INAH sprays are generally very safe to use but are designated as pregnancy category C. Intranasal azelastine in the original phase 3 pivotal trials was associated with increased sedation, which has resulted in this warning in the package insert. However, all subsequent azelastine studies have not been associated with sedation compared with placebo.[16,20,30,67,91]

Recent meta-analyses found significant overuse of anticholinergic agents in cognitively impaired individuals, preventing them from attending memory clinic.[92,93] Many of these medications were AHs.[93] Therefore, special care should be taken when prescribing sedating AHs to elderly patients, especially if they are at risk for being cognitively impaired.[94,95]

FUTURE TREATMENT DIRECTIONS

Previously, H3 and H4 receptors have been well characterized, and work is ongoing to develop an effective H3 antagonist.[29,66] Recent studies seem to indicate that probiotics may have a beneficial effect in the management of AR, but research is ongoing.[96,97]

Other therapeutic modalities currently under investigation for treatment of AR are summarized in **Fig. 3**.[43] Other therapeutic modalities include intralymphatic injection of aqueous allergens, percutaneous administration of aqueous allergens using patch application devices, intradermal injection of allergen-specific T-cell epitopes, and

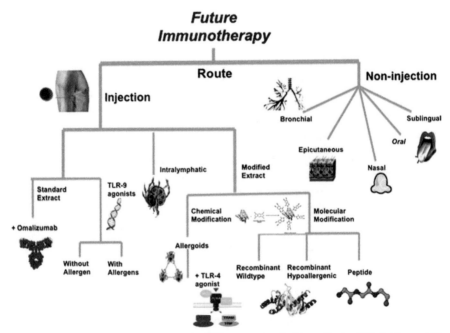

Fig. 3. Novel therapies for AIT. TLR-9, toll-like receptor-9. (*From* Burks AW, Calderon MA, Casale T, et al. Update on allergy immunotherapy: American Academy of Allergy, Asthma & Immunology/European Academy of Allergy and Clinical Immunology/PRACTALL Consensus Report. J Allergy Clin Immunol 2013;131(5):1297; with permission.)

development of tyrosine-absorbed polymerized allergens combined with lipid adjuvants among others.[43,97]

SUMMARY

Treatment of AR involves a comprehensive approach, including environmental control measures, pharmacotherapy, and if indicated, allergen immunotherapy. Treatment regimens should be tailored to the severity and duration of the patient's symptoms, taking into account their tolerance of medications, costs, and personal preferences. AR is very responsive to the spectrum of medications approved to treat this condition. When patients are not responsive to treatment, it is important to confirm that they do not have a component of non-AR, are not being adherent to medications, are not chronically exposed to allergens at home or in the workplace, or have no subclinical complications such as chronic sinusitis that is interfering with treatment responsiveness. Proper therapy can significantly improve patient quality of life and significantly impact short- and long-term clinical outcomes.[13,18]

REFERENCES

1. Gergen PJ, Turkeltaub PC. The association of allergen skin test reactivity and respiratory disease among whites in the US population. Data from the Second National Health and Nutrition Examination Survey, 1976 to 1980. Arch Intern Med 1991;151(3):487–92.
2. Sibbald B, Rink E. Epidemiology of seasonal and perennial rhinitis: clinical presentation and medical history. Thorax 1991;46(12):895–901.
3. Sibbald B, Rink E. Labelling of rhinitis and hayfever by doctors. Thorax 1991; 46(5):378–81.
4. Turkeltaub PC, Gergen PJ. Prevalence of upper and lower respiratory conditions in the US population by social and environmental factors: data from the second National Health and Nutrition Examination Survey, 1976 to 1980 (NHANES II). Ann Allergy 1991;67(2 Pt 1):147–54.
5. Ng TP, Tan WC. Epidemiology of allergic rhinitis and its associated risk factors in Singapore. Int J Epidemiol 1994;23(3):553–8.
6. Ng TP, Tan WC. Epidemiology of chronic (perennial) rhinitis in Singapore: prevalence estimates, demographic variation and clinical allergic presentation. Ann Acad Med Singapore 1994;23(1):83–8.
7. Droste JH, Kerhof M, de Monchy JG, et al. Association of skin test reactivity, specific IgE, total IgE, and eosinophils with nasal symptoms in a community-based population study. The Dutch ECRHS Group. J Allergy Clin Immunol 1996;97(4): 922–32.
8. Kerkhof M, Droste JH, de Monchy JG, et al. Distribution of total serum IgE and specific IgE to common aeroallergens by sex and age, and their relationship to each other in a random sample of the Dutch general population aged 20-70 years. Dutch ECRHS Group, European community respiratory health study. Allergy 1996;51(11):770–6.
9. Sakurai Y, Nakamura K, Teruya K, et al. Prevalence and risk factors of allergic rhinitis and cedar pollinosis among Japanese men. Prev Med 1998;27(4):617–22.
10. Dinmezel S, Ogus C, Erengin H, et al. The prevalence of asthma, allergic rhinitis, and atopy in Antalya, Turkey. Allergy Asthma Proc 2005;26(5):403–9.
11. Bachert C, van Cauwenberge P, Olbrecht J, et al. Prevalence, classification and perception of allergic and nonallergic rhinitis in Belgium. Allergy 2006;61(6): 693–8.

12. Ray NF, Baraniuk JN, Thamer M, et al. Direct expenditures for the treatment of allergic rhinoconjunctivitis in 1996, including the contributions of related airway illnesses. J Allergy Clin Immunol 1999;103(3 Pt 1):401–7.

13. Thompson AK, Juniper E, Meltzer EO. Quality of life in patients with allergic rhinitis. Ann Allergy Asthma Immunol 2000;85(5):338–47 [quiz: 347–8].

14. Blaiss MS. Allergic rhinoconjunctivitis: burden of disease. Allergy Asthma Proc 2007;28(4):393–7.

15. Lamb CE, Ratner PH, Johnson CE, et al. Economic impact of workplace productivity losses due to allergic rhinitis compared with select medical conditions in the United States from an employer perspective. Curr Med Res Opin 2006;22(6):1203–10.

16. Papadopoulos NG, Bernstein JA, Demoly P, et al. Phenotypes and endotypes of rhinitis and their impact on management: a PRACTALL report. Allergy 2015;70(5):474–94.

17. Brozek JL, Bousquet J, Baena-Cagnani CE, et al. Allergic rhinitis and its impact on asthma (ARIA) guidelines: 2010 revision. J Allergy Clin Immunol 2010;126(3):466–76.

18. Bousquet J, Schunemann HJ, Fonseca J, et al. MACVIA-ARIA Sentinel NetworK for allergic rhinitis (MASK-rhinitis): the new generation guideline implementation. Allergy 2015;70(11):1372–92.

19. Platts-Mills TA. Allergen avoidance. J Allergy Clin Immunol 2004;113(3):388–91.

20. Wallace DV, Dykewicz MS, Bernstein DI, et al. The diagnosis and management of rhinitis: an updated practice parameter. J Allergy Clin Immunol 2008;122(2 Suppl):S1–84.

21. Rondon C, Campo P, Zambonino MA, et al. Follow-up study in local allergic rhinitis shows a consistent entity not evolving to systemic allergic rhinitis. J Allergy Clin Immunol 2014;133(4):1026–31.

22. Rondon C, Romero JJ, Lopez S, et al. Local IgE production and positive nasal provocation test in patients with persistent nonallergic rhinitis. J Allergy Clin Immunol 2007;119(4):899–905.

23. Wheatley LM, Togias A. Clinical practice. Allergic rhinitis. N Engl J Med 2015;372(5):456–63.

24. Bousquet J, Khaltaev N, Cruz AA, et al. Allergic Rhinitis and its Impact on Asthma (ARIA) 2008 update (in collaboration with the World Health Organization, GA(2) LEN and AllerGen). Allergy 2008;63(Suppl 86):8–160.

25. Janeway CA Jr, Travers P, Walport M, et al. Immunobiology: the immune system in health and disease. 5th edition. New York: Garland Science; 2001.

26. Bernstein JA, Moellman JJ. Progress in the emergency management of hereditary angioedema: focus on new treatment options in the United States. Postgrad Med 2012;124(3):91–100.

27. Bielory L, Meltzer EO, Nichols KK, et al. An algorithm for the management of allergic conjunctivitis. Allergy Asthma Proc 2013;34(5):408–20.

28. Di Lorenzo G, Pacor ML, Pellitteri ME, et al. Randomized placebo-controlled trial comparing fluticasone aqueous nasal spray in mono-therapy, fluticasone plus cetirizine, fluticasone plus montelukast and cetirizine plus montelukast for seasonal allergic rhinitis. Clin Exp Allergy 2004;34(2):259–67.

29. Mygind N. Allergic rhinitis. Chem Immunol Allergy 2014;100:62–8.

30. Greiner AN, Meltzer EO. Overview of the treatment of allergic rhinitis and nonallergic rhinopathy. Proc Am Thorac Soc 2011;8(1):121–31.

31. Bousquet J, Bachert C, Bernstein J, et al. Advances in pharmacotherapy for the treatment of allergic rhinitis; MP29-02 (a novel formulation of azelastine

hydrochloride and fluticasone propionate in an advanced delivery system) fills the gaps. Expert Opin Pharmacother 2015;16(6):913–28.

32. Carr W, Bernstein J, Lieberman P, et al. A novel intranasal therapy of azelastine with fluticasone for the treatment of allergic rhinitis. J Allergy Clin Immunol 2012;129(5):1282–9.e10.

33. Mygind N, Laursen LC, Dahl M. Systemic corticosteroid treatment for seasonal allergic rhinitis: a common but poorly documented therapy. Allergy 2000;55(1): 11–5.

34. Ameratunga R. Gluteal subcutaneous atrophy after depot steroid injection for allergic rhinitis. World Allergy Organ J 2012;5(11):168–9.

35. Meltzer EO, Caballero F, Fromer LM, et al. Treatment of congestion in upper respiratory diseases. Int J Gen Med 2010;3:69–91.

36. Grainger J, Drake-Lee A. Montelukast in allergic rhinitis: a systematic review and meta-analysis. Clin Otolaryngol 2006;31(5):360–7.

37. Tzanetos DB, Fahrenholz JM, Scott T, et al. Comparison of the sedating effects of levocetirizine and cetirizine: a randomized, double-blind, placebo-controlled trial. Ann Allergy Asthma Immunol 2011;107(6):517–22.

38. Patel P, Philip G, Yang W, et al. Randomized, double-blind, placebo-controlled study of montelukast for treating perennial allergic rhinitis. Ann Allergy Asthma Immunol 2005;95(6):551–7.

39. Calderon MA, Casale T, Cox L, et al. Allergen immunotherapy: a new semantic framework from the European Academy of Allergy and Clinical Immunology/American Academy of Allergy, Asthma and Immunology/PRACTALL consensus report. Allergy 2013;68(7):825–8.

40. Meltzer EO, Blaiss MS, Derebery MJ, et al. Burden of allergic rhinitis: results from the pediatric allergies in America survey. J Allergy Clin Immunol 2009;124(3 Suppl):S43–70.

41. White P, Smith H, Baker N, et al. Symptom control in patients with hay fever in UK general practice: how well are we doing and is there a need for allergen immunotherapy? Clin Exp Allergy 1998;28(3):266–70.

42. Calderon MA, Alves B, Jacobson M, et al. Allergen injection immunotherapy for seasonal allergic rhinitis. Cochrane Database Syst Rev 2007;(1):CD001936.

43. Burks AW, Calderon MA, Casale T, et al. Update on allergy immunotherapy: American Academy of Allergy, Asthma & Immunology/European Academy of Allergy and Clinical Immunology/PRACTALL consensus report. J Allergy Clin Immunol 2013;131(5):1288–96.e3.

44. Matricardi PM, Kuna P, Panetta V, et al. Subcutaneous immunotherapy and pharmacotherapy in seasonal allergic rhinitis: a comparison based on meta-analyses. J Allergy Clin Immunol 2011;128(4):791–9.e6.

45. Cox L, Nelson H, Lockey R, et al. Allergen immunotherapy: a practice parameter third update. J Allergy Clin Immunol 2011;127(1 Suppl):S1–55.

46. Durham SR, Emminger W, Kapp A, et al. Long-term clinical efficacy in grass pollen-induced rhinoconjunctivitis after treatment with SQ-standardized grass allergy immunotherapy tablet. J Allergy Clin Immunol 2010;125(1): 131–8.e131–137.

47. Nelson HS. Update on house dust mite immunotherapy: are more studies needed? Curr Opin Allergy Clin Immunol 2014;14(6):542–8.

48. Epstein TG, Liss GM, Murphy-Berendts K, et al. AAAAI and ACAAI surveillance study of subcutaneous immunotherapy, year 3: what practices modify the risk of systemic reactions? Ann Allergy Asthma Immunol 2013;110(4):274–8, 278.e1.

49. Bernstein DI, Epstein T. Systemic reactions to subcutaneous allergen immuno-therapy. Immunol Allergy Clin N Am 2011;31(2):241–9, viii–ix.

50. Bernstein DI, Wanner M, Borish L, et al. Immunotherapy Committee AAoAA, Immunology. Twelve-year survey of fatal reactions to allergen injections and skin testing: 1990-2001. J Allergy Clin Immunol 2004;113(6):1129–36.

51. Maloney J, Bernstein DI, Nelson H, et al. Efficacy and safety of grass sublingual immunotherapy tablet, MK-7243: a large randomized controlled trial. Ann Allergy Asthma Immunol 2014;112(2):146–53.e2.

52. Creticos PS, Maloney J, Bernstein DI, et al. Randomized controlled trial of a ragweed allergy immunotherapy tablet in North American and European adults. J Allergy Clin Immunol 2013;131(5):1342–9.e6.

53. Dahl R, Kapp A, Colombo G, et al. Sublingual grass allergen tablet immuno-therapy provides sustained clinical benefit with progressive immunologic changes over 2 years. J Allergy Clin Immunol 2008;121(2):512–8.e2.

54. Li JT, Bernstein DI, Calderon MA, et al. Sublingual grass and ragweed immuno-therapy: clinical considerations—a PRACTALL consensus report. J Allergy Clin Immunol 2015. [Epub ahead of print].

55. Hermelingmeier KE, Weber RK, Hellmich M, et al. Nasal irrigation as an adjunc-tive treatment in allergic rhinitis: a systematic review and meta-analysis. Am J Rhi-nol Allergy 2012;26(5):e119–125.

56. Cataldi M, Borriello F, Granata F, et al. Histamine receptors and antihistamines: from discovery to clinical applications. Chem Immunol Allergy 2014;100:214–26.

57. Church MK, Maurer M, Simons FE, et al. Risk of first-generation H(1)-antihista-mines: a GA(2)LEN position paper. Allergy 2010;65(4):459–66.

58. Weiner JM, Abramson MJ, Puy RM. Intranasal corticosteroids versus oral H1 re-ceptor antagonists in allergic rhinitis: systematic review of randomised controlled trials. BMJ 1998;317(7173):1624–9.

59. Pullerits T, Praks L, Skoogh BE, et al. Randomized placebo-controlled study comparing a leukotriene receptor antagonist and a nasal glucocorticoid in sea-sonal allergic rhinitis. Am J Respir Crit Care Med 1999;159(6):1814–8.

60. Ratner PH, Howland WC 3rd, Arastu R, et al. Fluticasone propionate aqueous nasal spray provided significantly greater improvement in daytime and nighttime nasal symptoms of seasonal allergic rhinitis compared with montelukast. Ann Al-lergy Asthma Immunol 2003;90(5):536–42.

61. Jen A, Baroody F, de Tineo M, et al. As-needed use of fluticasone propionate nasal spray reduces symptoms of seasonal allergic rhinitis. J Allergy Clin Immu-nol 2000;105(4):732–8.

62. Dykewicz MS, Kaiser HB, Nathan RA, et al. Fluticasone propionate aqueous nasal spray improves nasal symptoms of seasonal allergic rhinitis when used as needed (prn). Ann Allergy Asthma Immunol 2003;91(1):44–8.

63. Kaszuba SM, Baroody FM, deTineo M, et al. Superiority of an intranasal cortico-steroid compared with an oral antihistamine in the as-needed treatment of sea-sonal allergic rhinitis. Arch Intern Med 2001;161(21):2581–7.

64. Juniper EF, Guyatt GH, O'Byrne PM, et al. Aqueous beclomethasone dipropio-nate nasal spray: regular versus "as required" use in the treatment of seasonal allergic rhinitis. J Allergy Clin Immunol 1990;86(3 Pt 1):380–6.

65. Juniper EF, Guyatt GH, Archer B, et al. Aqueous beclomethasone dipropionate in the treatment of ragweed pollen-induced rhinitis: further exploration of "as needed" use. J Allergy Clin Immunol 1993;92(1 Pt 1):66–72.

66. Lieberman P. The role of antihistamines in the treatment of vasomotor rhinitis. World Allergy Organ J 2009;2(8):156–61.

67. Bernstein JA. Azelastine hydrochloride: a review of pharmacology, pharmacokinetics, clinical efficacy and tolerability. Curr Med Res Opin 2007;23(10):2441–52.

68. Taylor-Clark T, Sodha R, Warner B, et al. Histamine receptors that influence blockage of the normal human nasal airway. Br J Pharmacol 2005;144(6):867–74.

69. Cox JS. Disodium cromoglycate (FPL 670) ('Intal'): a specific inhibitor of reaginic antibody-antigen mechanisms. Nature 1967;216(5122):1328–9.

70. Nayak AS, Prenner B, Gates D, et al. Tolerability of concomitant administration of mometasone furoate and oxymetazoline nasal sprays administered once daily vs oxymetazoline twice daily, mometasone furoate once daily, and placebo in the treatment of subjects with seasonal allergic rhinitis. J Allergy Clin Immunol 2010;125(2):Ab175.

71. Greiner AN, Hellings PW, Rotiroti G, et al. Allergic rhinitis. Lancet 2011;378(9809): 2112–22.

72. van Adelsberg J, Philip G, Pedinoff AJ, et al. Montelukast improves symptoms of seasonal allergic rhinitis over a 4-week treatment period. Allergy 2003;58(12): 1268–76.

73. Wilson AM, O'Byrne PM, Parameswaran K. Leukotriene receptor antagonists for allergic rhinitis: a systematic review and meta-analysis. Am J Med 2004;116(5): 338–44.

74. Chen ST, Lu KH, Sun HL, et al. Randomized placebo-controlled trial comparing montelukast and cetirizine for treating perennial allergic rhinitis in children aged 2-6 yr. Pediatr Allergy Immunol 2006;17(1):49–54.

75. Keskin O, Alyamac E, Tuncer A, et al. Do the leukotriene receptor antagonists work in children with grass pollen-induced allergic rhinitis? Pediatr Allergy Immunol 2006;17(4):259–68.

76. Martin BG, Andrews CP, van Bavel JH, et al. Comparison of fluticasone propionate aqueous nasal spray and oral montelukast for the treatment of seasonal allergic rhinitis symptoms. Ann Allergy Asthma Immunol 2006;96(6):851–7.

77. National Asthma E, Prevention P. Expert Panel Report 3 (EPR-3): guidelines for the Diagnosis and Management of Asthma—Summary Report 2007. J Allergy Clin Immunol 2007;120(5 Suppl):S94–138.

78. Li JT, Pearlman DS, Nicklas RA, et al. Algorithm for the diagnosis and management of asthma: a practice parameter update: Joint Task Force on Practice Parameters, representing the American Academy of Allergy, Asthma and Immunology, the American College of Allergy, Asthma and Immunology, and the Joint Council of Allergy, Asthma and Immunology. Ann Allergy Asthma Immunol 1998;81(5 Pt 1):415–20.

79. Chauhan BF, Ben Salah R, Ducharme FM. Addition of anti-leukotriene agents to inhaled corticosteroids in children with persistent asthma. Cochrane Database Syst Rev 2013;(10):CD009585.

80. Wood CC, Fireman P, Grossman J, et al. Product characteristics and pharmacokinetics of intranasal ipratropium bromide. J Allergy Clin Immuno 1995;95(5 Pt 2): 1111–6.

81. Tran NP, Vickery J, Blaiss MS. Management of rhinitis: allergic and non-allergic. Allergy Asthma Immunol Res 2011;3(3):148–56.

82. Meltzer EO, Bernstein DI, Prenner BM, et al. Mometasone furoate nasal spray plus oxymetazoline nasal spray: short-term efficacy and safety in seasonal allergic rhinitis. Am J Rhinol Allergy 2013;27(2):102–8.

83. Baroody FM, Brown D, Gavanescu L, et al. Oxymetazoline adds to the effectiveness of fluticasone furoate in the treatment of perennial allergic rhinitis. J Allergy Clin Immunol 2011;127(4):927–34.

84. Vaidyanathan S, Williamson P, Clearie K, et al. Fluticasone reverses oxymetazoline-induced tachyphylaxis of response and rebound congestion. Am J Respir Crit Care Med 2010;182(1):19–24.

85. Graf P, Hallen H, Juto JE. The pathophysiology and treatment of rhinitis medicamentosa. Clin Otolaryngol Allied Sci 1995;20(3):224–9.

86. Petty DA, Blaiss MS. Intranasal corticosteroids topical characteristics: side effects, formulation, and volume. Am J Rhinol Allergy 2013;27(6):510–3.

87. Epstein TG, Liss GM, Murphy-Berendts K, et al. Immediate and delayed-onset systemic reactions after subcutaneous immunotherapy injections: ACAAI/AAAAI surveillance study of subcutaneous immunotherapy: year 2. Ann Allergy Asthma Immunol 2011;107(5):426–31.e1.

88. Zhang L, Cheng L, Hong J. The clinical use of cetirizine in the treatment of allergic rhinitis. Pharmacology 2013;92(1–2):14–25.

89. Yuen D, Buys YM, Jin YP, et al. Effect of beclomethasone nasal spray on intraocular pressure in ocular hypertension or controlled glaucoma. J Glaucoma 2013; 22(2):84–7.

90. Schenkel EJ, Skoner DP, Bronsky EA, et al. Absence of growth retardation in children with perennial allergic rhinitis after one year of treatment with mometasone furoate aqueous nasal spray. Pediatrics 2000;105(2):E22.

91. Bernstein JA, Prenner B, Ferguson BJ, et al. Double-blind, placebo-controlled trial of reformulated azelastine nasal spray in patients with seasonal allergic rhinitis. Am J Rhinol Allergy 2009;23(5):512–7.

92. Cross AJ, George J, Woodward MC, et al. Potentially inappropriate medications and anticholinergic burden in older people attending memory clinics in Australia. Drugs Aging 2016;33:37–44.

93. Collamati A, Martone AM, Poscia A, et al. Anticholinergic drugs and negative outcomes in the older population: from biological plausibility to clinical evidence. Aging Clin Exp Res 2015. [Epub ahead of print].

94. Hanlon JT, Semla TP, Schmader KE. Alternative medications for medications in the use of high-risk medications in the elderly and potentially harmful drug-disease interactions in the elderly quality measures. J Am Geriatr Soc 2015; 63(12):e8–18.

95. Gray SL, Anderson ML, Dublin S, et al. Cumulative use of strong anticholinergics and incident dementia: a prospective cohort study. JAMA Intern Med 2015; 175(3):401–7.

96. Braido F, Sclifo F, Ferrando M, et al. New therapies for allergic rhinitis. Curr Allergy Asthma Rep 2014;14(4):422.

97. Wambre E, DeLong JH, James EA, et al. Specific immunotherapy modifies allergen-specific CD4(+) T-cell responses in an epitope-dependent manner. J Allergy Clin Immunol 2014;133(3):872–9.e7.

Nonallergic Rhinitis
Mechanism of Action

Fuad M. Baroody, MD

KEYWORDS

- Nonallergic rhinitis • Neurogenic • Reactivity • Histamine • Cold-dry air

KEY POINTS

- Cellular inflammation is not a consistent finding in patients with nonallergic rhinitis.
- Neuropeptides play an important role in the pathophysiology of nonallergic rhinitis.
- Transient receptor potential ion channels have an important role in mediating the response of patients with nonallergic rhinitis to environmental stimuli.
- Patients with nonallergic rhinitis exhibit various degrees of nasal reactivity to certain nonspecific stimuli, such as histamine, cold-dry air, and capsaicin.

INTRODUCTION

Nonallergic rhinitis (NAR) is a chronic condition of the nasal mucosa that predominantly involves symptoms of nasal congestion and rhinorrhea with no evidence of allergic sensitization (ie, negative skin testing and/or serum-specific immunoglobulin E [IgE] testing). Although the primary and most common symptoms are congestion and anterior and posterior rhinorrhea, other associated symptoms include throat clearing, cough, eustachian tube dysfunction, sneezing, decreased sense of smell, and facial pain/pressure.[1] Itching of the eyes, throat, and ears is not a common symptom. The timing of symptoms may be perennial/persistent, intermittent, and/or precipitated by recognized triggers. Some of these include cold air, changes in environmental temperature and humidity, changes in barometric pressure, strong smells (perfumes, food, chemical odors), environmental tobacco smoke, pollutants and chemicals, ingestion of certain foods (gustatory rhinitis), and alcohol.

Unlike allergic rhinitis (AR), which is the most common chronic condition in children, NAR presents predominantly with adult onset; the female to male incidence varies

The author discloses that he does not have any financial or commercial conflicts of interest in relation to the submitted article. The author is currently funded by the Immune Tolerance Network (Grant ITN 057AD), for research unrelated to the content of this article.
Section of Otolaryngology, Head and Neck Surgery, Departments of Surgery and Pediatrics, The University of Chicago Medicine and Biological Sciences, 5841 South Maryland Avenue, MC1035, Chicago, IL 60637, USA
E-mail address: fbaroody@surgery.bsd.uchicago.edu

Immunol Allergy Clin N Am 36 (2016) 279–287
http://dx.doi.org/10.1016/j.iac.2015.12.005
0889-8561/16/$ – see front matter © 2016 Elsevier Inc. All rights reserved.

between 2:1 and 3:1. Data from rhinitis epidemiologic studies suggest that the prevalence of AR is around 3 times more than that of NAR (AR:NAR = 3:1).[2] Thus, based on our knowledge of the prevalence of AR in the United States and the aforementioned ratios, one can estimate the number of Americans with NAR as 20 million or 7% of the population.

The classification of NAR has been unsolidified over the years and its pathophysiology relatively unexplored. Although *vasomotor rhinitis* was a common term used to describe such an entity, this term is no longer favored and is mostly replaced by NAR. It is important to realize that there are other types of rhinitis that are nonallergic but have specific and identifiable precipitating factors and triggers. These types include chronic rhinosinusitis with and without nasal polyps; NAR with eosinophilia syndrome (NARES); aspirin-exacerbated rhinosinusitis; infectious rhinitis/rhinosinusitis such as triggered by viral, bacterial, or fungal infections; rhinitis of pregnancy; and drug-induced rhinitis. Furthermore, the presence of inflammation in the nasal mucosa of patients with NAR is not ubiquitous leading some investigators to consider the term *rhinopathy* instead of rhinitis to refer to this entity. In the following pages, the author attempts to discuss available information that pertains to the pathophysiology of this disease and mostly centers around a description of inflammation in the nasal mucosa in NAR as well as neurogenic mechanisms thought to be important for this disease process. The author also details various methods of nasal provocation the results of which might shed some light on pathophysiologic processes involved in NAR.

INFLAMMATION

Van Rijswijk and colleagues[3] performed nasal biopsies in patients with chronic rhinitis symptoms but negative evidence of allergic cause and compared those with the results of biopsies obtained from a normal control group with no nasal symptoms and negative skin test results. They evaluated various markers of lymphocytic cells, mast cells, Langerhans cells, macrophages, IgE+ cells, and eosinophils using immunohistochemistry. Most biopsies had a negligible number of eosinophils, which suggests that local AR and NARES were probably not a large contributor to this group. There were essentially no significant differences in the number of inflammatory cells between the rhinitis and control groups suggesting that cellular inflammation was not a prominent factor in this group of patients with NAR. The investigators also failed to show any relation between the number of immunocompetent cells in the nasal mucosa and nasal complaints in those patients when treated with either an intranasal corticosteroid or capsaicin.[4–6] In those studies, the intranasal corticosteroids resulted in a reduction of inflammatory cells but no improvement in symptoms and capsaicin reduced nasal symptoms without affecting the number of nasal inflammatory cells or mediators.

Powe and colleagues[7] performed similar investigations with different results. They evaluated nasal turbinate tissue obtained at the time of turbinectomies from patients with perennial allergic rhinitis, idiopathic rhinitis, and normal controls (undergoing surgery for mechanical, posttraumatic nasal obstruction) with no evidence of rhinitis. Using immunohistochemistry, they evaluated mast cells, IgE+ cells, eosinophils, and plasma cells and showed that both disease groups had essentially equivalent inflammatory cellular content, which was higher than that of the control, nonrhinitic subjects. The allergic group had a higher number of IgE+ cells and plasma cells compared with the group of patients with NAR. As mentioned earlier, the nonallergic group probably included subjects with local AR or NARES, as the number of eosinophils was equivalent in both rhinitis groups and was higher than the number of eosinophils found in the nonrhinitis control subjects. Another difference between this study and the previous one quoted, whereby there was no significant inflammation in the NAR group, is that the tissue was collected at the time of turbinectomies, which would indicate more severe disease that was mandating surgical intervention. A similar study by the same group evaluated the T-lymphocyte differences between similar subgroups and showed significant overlap in lymphocytic inflammation between the patients with allergic and NAR.[8] However, there were differences in some cells between the 2 groups with fewer antigen-presenting cells and more CD8+ cells in the NAR group compared with the subjects with perennial AR. Furthermore, in both groups with rhinitis, there was an association between lymphocytes and mast cells suggesting a common pathway in persistent nasal inflammation.

More recently, De Corso and colleagues[9] evaluated nasal inflammation in a large, well-characterized group of subjects presenting to their rhinology clinics over a 6-year time interval. NAR was diagnosed by history of symptoms of rhinitis for at least 12 weeks along with negative skin and/or serum allergy testing, negative response to allergen provocation, and negative nasal endoscopy and computed tomography scans to rule out paranasal sinus involvement. A nasal sample was obtained by scraping the inferior turbinates, and the cellular profile was used to subtype the subjects with NAR into NAR without inflammation (231 of 519 subjects, 44.5%) and NAR with inflammation (288 of 519 subjects, 55.49%). The group with inflammation was further subtyped into 4 different subgroups based on the predominant type of inflammatory cells: NAR with neutrophilia (32.95%), NAR with eosinophilia (15.61%), NAR with mast cells (3.66%), and NAR with mast cells and eosinophils (3.28%). The main finding from the study was that the groups of NAR without inflammation and NAR with neutrophils were fairly similar in that they had milder inflammation with fewer and milder symptoms compared with the groups of NAR with inflammation who reported more moderate or severe nasal symptoms. Also, the groups of NAR with eosinophils and mast cells were significantly more likely to have comorbidities than the NAR without inflammation and NAR with neutrophilia groups. This work suggests that a large portion of patients presenting with NAR have a significant inflammatory infiltrate and that the type of inflammatory infiltrate has a direct bearing on disease severity. The only issue that is not clarified in the study design was the number of allergens that were used in nasal challenges to confirm that these subjects had no local response to allergen.

As can be seen from the aforementioned information, studies on nasal cellular inflammation in patients with NAR do not yield uniform results probably related to the variations in clinical characterization of the subjects enrolled. Most investigators refer to the disease entity as idiopathic rhinitis and characterize the subjects by chronic nasal symptoms, such as nasal congestion and rhinorrhea, but carefully exclude infectious causes of such symptoms. Furthermore, all subjects enrolled in these studies had negative skin tests and/or specific IgE testing results.

Unfortunately, nasal challenge was not performed as part of the characterization of the subjects in all the studies, thus, potentially including a subset of subjects with what is now referred to as local or entopic AR.[10] In this entity, patients have an IgE-mediated, eosinophilic, nasal cellular infiltrate in the absence of evidence of positive skin or immunocap testing but do have a positive response to nasal provocation with relevant allergens and evidence of local IgE production. In contrast to NAR, these patients respond better to conventional therapies used to treat AR. This entity will be discussed in detail in a subsequent article (See Campo P, Salas M, Blanca-López N, et al: Local Allergic Rhinitis, in this issue).

NEUROGENIC MECHANISMS
Innervation of the Nasal Mucosa

The nasal neural supply is overwhelmingly sensory and autonomic (sympathetic, parasympathetic, and nonadrenergic noncholinergic). The sensory nasal innervation comes via both the ophthalmic and maxillary divisions of the trigeminal nerve and supplies the septum, the lateral walls, the anterior part of the nasal floor, and the inferior meatus.[11] The parasympathetic nasal fibers travel from their origin in the superior salivary nucleus of the midbrain via the nervus intermedius of the facial nerve to the geniculate ganglion where they join the greater superficial petrosal nerve that, in turn, joins the deep petrosal nerve to form the vidian nerve.[11] This nerve travels to the sphenopalatine ganglion where the preganglionic parasympathetic fibers synapse and postganglionic fibers supply the nasal mucosa. The sympathetic input originates as preganglionic fibers in the thoracolumbar region of the spinal cord, which pass into the vagosympathetic trunk and relay in the superior cervical ganglion. The postganglionic fibers end as the deep petrosal nerve, which joins the greater superficial nerve to form the vidian nerve. They traverse the sphenopalatine ganglion without synapsing and are distributed to the nasal mucosa.[11] Nasal glands receive direct parasympathetic nerve supply, and electrical stimulation of parasympathetic nerves in animals induces glandular secretions that are blocked by atropine. Furthermore, stimulation of the human nasal mucosa with methacholine, a cholinomimetic, produces an atropine-sensitive increase in nasal secretions.[12]

Parasympathetic nerves also provide innervation to the nasal vasculature, and stimulation of these fibers causes vasodilatation. Sympathetic fibers supply the nasal vasculature but do not establish a close relationship with nasal glands, and their exact role in the control of nasal secretions is not clear. Stimulation of these fibers in animals causes vasoconstriction and a decrease in nasal airway resistance. Adrenergic agonists are commonly used in man, both topically and orally, to decrease nasal congestion.

The presence of sympathetic and parasympathetic nerves and their transmitters in the nasal mucosa has been known for decades, but recent immunohistochemical studies have established the presence of additional neuropeptides. These neuropeptides are secreted by unmyelinated nociceptive C fibers (tachykinins, calcitonin gene-related peptide [CGRP], neurokinin A [NKA], gastrin-releasing peptide), parasympathetic nerve endings (vasoactive intestinal peptide [VIP], peptide histidine methionine), and sympathetic nerve endings (neuropeptide Y). Substance P (SP), a member of the tachykinin family, is often found as a cotransmitter with NKA and CGRP and has been found in high density in arterial vessels and to some extent in veins, gland acini, and epithelium of the nasal mucosa.[13] SP receptors (NK1 receptors) are located in epithelium, glands, and vessels.[13] CGRP receptors are found in high concentration on small muscular arteries and arterioles in the nasal mucosa.[14] The distribution of VIP fibers in human airways corresponds closely to that of cholinergic nerves.[15] In the human nasal mucosa, VIP is abundant and its receptors are located on arterial vessels, submucosal glands, and epithelial cells.[16] In addition to the identification of neuropeptides in the nasal mucosa, several studies support their potential contribution in the creation of nasal symptoms. VIP stimulates serous cell secretion,[16] dilates nasal vessels[17] and may regulate mucociliary clearance in dogs.[18] Nasal challenge with SP induces few changes in normal subjects but leads to a modest increase in vascular permeability, nasal airway resistance, and eosinophil and neutrophil chemotaxis in rhinitic subjects.[19]

Transient receptor potential (TRP) is one of a family of calcium ion channels involved in transducing external stimuli to sensory neurons.[20] Among those channels, TRP vanilloid-1 (TRPV1) is capsaicin sensitive and mediates the pungency of capsaicin and TRP ankyrin 1 (TRPA1) mediates the effects of noxious stimuli, such as cold temperatures, pungent natural compounds, and environmental irritants.[21] These channels are being recognized as increasingly important in mediating the nasal response to noxious chemical, mechanical, and osmotic stimuli and probably do so by mediating the release of neuropeptides from sensory nerve endings.[22] Therefore, their role in the pathophysiology of NAR is being investigated.

Contribution of Neurogenic Mechanisms to the Pathophysiology of Nonallergic Rhinitis

The sympathetic and parasympathetic components of the autonomic nervous system equally contribute input to the nasal efferent organs to maintain a delicate homeostasis between vasoconstriction and vasodilation of nasal vasculature and the secretion of nasal glands. An imbalance of these components is likely to contribute to glandular hypersecretion and increased nasal congestion, often seen in patients with NAR.[23–25]

Exposure to nonallergic triggers can precipitate rhinitis by activating TRPA1 and TRPV1 channels on nasal mucosal nerve fibers, which would lead to the release of neuropeptides, such as CGRP and SP, from sensory nerve endings.[26,27] These neuropeptides, in turn, will facilitate vasodilation and plasma extravasation causing edema and glandular hypersecretion. Evidence for the involvement of SP in the pathophysiology of NAR is indirect and relates to the beneficial effects on symptoms of the disease obtained by treatment with capsaicin, a substance known to deplete SP from sensory nerve endings and considered a TRPV1 agonist.[28,29] Another piece of supporting evidence was generated when symptoms and levels of SP in nasal lavage fluid were shown to increase significantly in subjects with NAR after hypertonic saline challenge.[30] In the same study, pretreatment with azelastine led to a reduction in SP levels as well as a significant improvement of nasal symptoms in the same subjects.

Van Gerven and colleagues[31] further investigated the role of TRP channels and SP in idiopathic rhinitis. They enrolled 14 subjects with idiopathic rhinitis and 12 controls and treated them with capsaicin for 12 weeks. There were significant reductions in symptoms of nasal obstruction, sneezing, and rhinorrhea after 4- and 12-week treatment with intranasal capsaicin coupled with a decrease in the nasal responsiveness to cold-dry air (CDA) provocation. More importantly, from a mechanistic standpoint, mRNA expression of TRPV1 and levels of SP were significantly higher in the nasal mucosa of subjects with idiopathic rhinitis at baseline compared with that from normal controls and were significantly reduced by capsaicin treatment. Levels of CGRP were not detectable and those of NKA showed no significant differences between subjects and controls. This study provides elegant support for the role of TRPV1 as well as SP in the pathophysiology of NAR and at least partially explains the mechanism by which capsaicin exerts its beneficial actions in patients with NAR.

RESPONSE TO NASAL PROVOCATION

Another way to try to elucidate some facets of the pathophysiology of rhinitic conditions is to evaluate the responsiveness of the nasal mucosa to different challenges. Nasal challenge with allergen has been very useful in elucidating cellular events that are associated with the generation of symptoms of patients with allergic rhinitis and has also been very useful in evaluating response to different therapeutic agents and the elucidation of their mechanisms of action. In the context of NAR, challenge with allergen has identified a group of subjects with local AR as mentioned earlier.[10] There are more limited data about other nasal provocation tests in NAR.

Histamine Challenge

Van De Heyning and colleagues[32] performed histamine nasal challenges in 53 subjects with chronic nasal symptoms and negative allergy testing and compared them to 11 subjects with no nasal complaints and negative allergy testing. The response to histamine provocation was measured by anterior rhinomanometry. Compared with normal controls, subjects with NAR had a higher nasal resistance at baseline and more reactivity to histamine as monitored by increase in the objective measure of nasal congestion. The dose of histamine that produced a 25% increase in nasal airway resistance was the best differentiator between subjects with NAR and controls and was significantly lower in the NAR group. A couple of other studies with smaller numbers and less rigorous characterization of study subjects suggested similar results.[33,34]

Cold-Dry Air Challenge

Many patients have significant history of nasal symptoms on exposure to CDA. This condition has been studied in the laboratory, and such patients will respond to a nasal challenge with CDA by generating nasal symptoms and releasing inflammatory mediators in nasal secretions, which include histamine, kinins, prostaglandins, and a marker of increased vascular permeability, suggesting a role for mast cell involvement.[35] Many responders to CDA do not have evidence of allergic disease and, thus, would qualify as having NAR in response to a specific trigger, CDA. In addition to investigating the pathophysiology of the CDA response in symptomatic individuals, CDA provocation has been used as a marker of nasal reactivity.

Braat and colleagues[36] compared CDA with histamine nasal challenge in differentiating patients with nonallergic, noninfectious perennial rhinitis from control subjects. The response was monitored by the weight of generated nasal secretions and nasal obstruction as measured by anterior rhinometry. The results suggested that CDA challenge was more suitable than histamine challenge in differentiating between NAR and controls as it had a much higher specificity than the histamine challenge. Van Gerven and colleagues[37] modified the protocol of CDA challenge by making it shorter and measuring symptoms and nasal peak flow after CDA, thus, simplifying the challenge and making it to be of potential use in clinical practice. They also demonstrate an increase in nasal obstruction (subjective and objective) after CDA in both patients with AR and NAR but not in healthy controls. Rhinorrhea and sneezing were not induced by this shortened challenge protocol. In another CDA provocation study, Shusterman and Tilles[38] demonstrated more symptoms and objective increase in nasal airway resistance in subjects with NAR compared with controls after CDA challenge. CDA challenge was successful in differentiating between the 2 groups if the subjects with NAR reported 2 or more triggers for their clinical symptoms. Similar results were obtained by Kim and Jang[39] who demonstrated a stronger response to CDA challenge in patients with both AR and NAR and the ability of nasal obstruction scores after CDA to differentiate between patients with NAR and controls.

Challenge with Capsaicin

Capsaicin has been used both to treat patients with NAR and as a challenge agent. It is a TRPV1 receptor agonist and has been shown to deplete neuropeptides in sensory nerves. If used for a prolonged period of time, it will lead to desensitization of the TRPV1 ion channels and improvement of the symptoms of NAR. Indeed, a recent

Cochrane review of available evidence shows that capsaicin seems to have beneficial effects on overall nasal symptoms up to 36 weeks after treatment, based on few small studies.[40] On the other hand, if used for short challenges, capsaicin generates significant symptoms and has been used to test nasal hyperreactivity.

Sanico and colleagues[41] performed nasal challenges with capsaicin in subjects with AR and NAR as well as normal controls and measured symptoms and levels of the glandular marker lactoferrin and the vascular permeability marker albumin in nasal secretions. They showed an increase in symptoms and lactoferrin in all 3 groups in response to capsaicin challenge and an increase in vascular permeability only in the allergic group, suggesting that NAR was not characterized by increased responsiveness to capsaicin. In contrast, Lambert and colleagues[42] challenged healthy controls and subjects with nonallergic irritant rhinitis with capsaicin and measured changes in nasal blood flow by optical rhinometry. Their results showed significantly higher optical density measurements in subjects with rhinitis compared with the healthy controls after capsaicin suggesting that this challenge could prove a viable option in the diagnosis of nonallergic irritant rhinitis. The difference between the two studies could be related to the different end points evaluated in response to capsaicin challenge. The first looked at glandular secretion and increased vascular permeability, whereas the second evaluated blood flow changes in the nasal mucosa. More work in this area would shed further light on the utility of capsaicin challenges in elucidating the mechanisms involved in the pathophysiology of NAR.

In summary, it is clear from the aforementioned information that the pathophysiologic events that underlie NAR have not been extensively investigated. In some subtypes, such as NARES and local AR, cellular inflammation is important akin to what investigators have shown in AR. In other subtypes, neurogenic factors and increased nasal reactivity to certain stimuli seem to be more important and dominant. Clearly, a more systematic effort is needed to elucidate the pathophysiology of NAR. This method would start by a careful phenotyping of these patients on multiple fronts, which would include type of symptoms and their temporal pattern; the type of environmental stimuli that trigger the symptoms; reactivity of the nasal mucosa to specific stimuli, such as histamine, CDA, and capsaicin; nasal cellular inflammation; prevalence of neuropeptides; and the role of the various TRP channels. Gaining this information would then allow better targeted therapies that would help relieve the symptoms in affected patients.

REFERENCES

1. Kaliner MA. Nonallergic rhinopathy (formerly known as vasomotor rhinitis). Immunol Allergy Clin N Am 2011;31:441–55.
2. Schatz M, Zeiger RS, Chen W, et al. The burden of rhinitis in a managed care organization. Ann Allergy Asthma Immunol 2008;101:240–7.
3. Van Rijswijk JB, Blom HM, KleinJan A, et al. Inflammatory cells seem not to be involved in idiopathic rhinitis. Rhinology 2003;41:25–30.
4. Blom HM, Godthelp T, Fokkens WJ, et al. The effect of nasal steroid aqueous spray on nasal complaint scores and cellular infiltrates in the nasal mucosa of patients with a non-allergic non-infectious perennial rhinitis. J Allergy Clin Immunol 1997;100:739–47.
5. Blom HM, Severijnen LA, Van Rijswijk JB, et al. The long-term effects of capsaicin aqueous spray on the nasal mucosa. Clin Exp Allergy 1998;28:1351–8.

6. Blom HM, Van Rijswijk JB, Garrelds IM, et al. Intranasal capsaicin is efficacious in non-allergic, non-infectious perennial rhinitis. A placebo-controlled study. Clin Exp Allergy 1997;27:796–801.

7. Powe DG, Huskisson RS, Carney AS, et al. Evidence for an inflammatory pathophysiology in idiopathic rhinitis. Clin Exp Allergy 2001;31:864–72.

8. Powe DG, Huskisson RS, Carney AS, et al. Mucosal T-cell phenotypes in persistent atopic and nonatopic rhinitis show an association with mast cells. Allergy 2004;59:204–12.

9. De Corso E, Battista M, Pandolfini M, et al. Role of inflammation in non-allergic rhinitis. Rhinology 2014;52:142–9.

10. Rondón C, Campo P, Togias A, et al. Local allergic rhinitis: concept, pathophysiology, and management. J Allergy Clin Immunol 2012;129(6):1460–7.

11. Proctor DF, Andersen IB. The nose-upper airway physiology and the atmospheric environment. Amsterdam (Netherlands): Elsevier Biomedical Press; 1982.

12. Baroody FM, Wagenmann M, Naclerio RM. A comparison of the secretory response of the nasal mucosa to histamine and methacholine. J Appl Physiol (1985) 1993;74(6):2661.

13. Baraniuk JN, Lundgren JD, Mullol J, et al. Substance P and neurokinin A in human nasal mucosa. Am J Respir Cell Mol Biol 1991;4:228.

14. Baraniuk JN, Castellino S, Merida M, et al. Calcitonin gene related peptide in human nasal mucosa. Am J Physiol 1990;258:L81.

15. Laitinen A, Partanen M, Hervonen A, et al. VIP-like immunoreactive nerves in human respiratory tract. Light and electron microscopic study. Histochemistry 1985;82:313.

16. Baraniuk JN, Okayama M, Lundgren JD, et al. Vasoactive intestinal peptide (VIP) in human nasal mucosa. J Clin Invest 1990;86:825.

17. Lung MA, Widdicombe JG. Lung reflexes and nasal vascular resistance in the anaesthesized dog. J Physiol 1987;386:465.

18. Nathanson I, Widdicombe JG, Barnes PJ. Effect of vasoactive intestinal peptide on ion transport across dog tracheal epithelium. J Appl Physiol Respir Environ Exerc Physiol 1983;55:1844.

19. Braunstein G, Fajac I, Lacronique J, et al. Clinical and inflammatory responses to exogenous tachykinins in allergic rhinitis. Am Rev Respir Dis 1991;144:630.

20. Eijkelkamp N, Quick K, Wood JN. Transient receptor potential channels and mechanosensation. Annu Rev Neurosci 2013;36:519–46.

21. Macpherson LJ, Dubin AE, Evans MJ, et al. Noxious compounds activate TRPA1 ion channels through covalent modification of cysteines. Nature 2007;445:541–5.

22. Van Gerven L, Boeckxstaeus G, Hellings P. Update on neuro-immune mechanisms involved in allergic and non-allergic rhinitis. Rhinology 2012;50:227–35.

23. Baraniuk JN. Neurogenic mechanisms in rhinosinusitis. Curr Allergy Asthma Rep 2001;1:252–61.

24. Lung MA. The role of the autonomic nerves in the control of nasal circulation. Biol Signals 1995;4:179–85.

25. Bernstein JA, Singh U. Neural abnormalities in nonallergic rhinitis. Curr Allergy Asthma Rep 2015;15:18.

26. Andre E, Campi B, Materazzi S, et al. Cigarette smoke-induced neurogenic inflammation is mediated by alpha, beta-unsaturated aldehydes and the TRPA1 receptor in rodents. J Clin Invest 2008;118(7):2574–82.

27. Stjarne P. Sensory and motor reflex control of nasal mucosal blood flow and secretion; clinical implications in non-allergic nasal hyperreactivity. Acta Physiol Scand Suppl 1991;600:1–64.

28. Bernstein JA, Davis BP, Picard JK, et al. A randomized, double-blind, parallel trial comparing capsaicin nasal spray with placebo in subjects with a significant component of nonallergic rhinitis. Ann Allergy Asthma Immunol 2011;107(2): 171–8.

29. Van Rijswijk JB, Boeke EL, Keizer JM, et al. Intranasal capsaicin reduces nasal hyperreactivity in idiopathic rhinitis: a double-blind randomized application regimen study. Allergy 2003;58(8):754–61.

30. Gawlik R, Jawor B, Rogala B, et al. Effect of intranasal azelastine on substance P release in perennial nonallergic rhinitis patients. Am J Rhinol Allergy 2013;27: 514–6.

31. Van Gerven L, Alpizar YA, Wouters MM, et al. Capsaicin treatment reduces nasal hyperreactivity and transient receptor potential cation channel subfamily V, receptor 1 (TRPV1) overexpression in patients with idiopathic rhinitis. J Allergy Clin Immunol 2014;133:1332–9.

32. Van De Heyning PH, Van Haesendonck J, Creten W, et al. Histamine nasal provocation test. An evaluation of active anterior rhinomanometry and of threshold criteria of provocative dose. Allergy 1989;44:482–6.

33. Ohm M, Juto JE. Nasal hyperreactivity. A histamine provocation model. Rhinology 1993;31(2):53–5.

34. Hallén H, Juto JE. A test for objective diagnosis of nasal hyperreactivity. Rhinology 1993;31(1):23–5.

35. Togias AG, Naclerio RM, Proud D, et al. Nasal challenge with cold, dry air results in release of inflammatory mediators. Possible mast cell involvement. J Clin Invest 1985;76(4):1375–81.

36. Braat JPM, Mulder PG, Fokkens WJ, et al. Intranasal cold dry air is superior to histamine challenge in determining the presence and degree of nasal hyperreactivity in nonallergic noninfectious perennial rhinitis. Am J Respir Crit Care Med 1998;157:1748–55.

37. Van Gerven L, Boeckxstaens G, Jorissen M, et al. Short-time cold dry air exposure: a useful diagnostic tool for nasal hyperresponsiveness. Laryngoscope 2012;122:2615–20.

38. Shusterman DJ, Tilles SA. Nasal physiological reactivity of subjects with nonallergic rhinitis to cold air provocation: a pilot comparison of subgroups. Am J Rhinol Allergy 2009;23:475–9.

39. Kim YH, Jang TY. Nasal provocation test using allergen extract versus cold dry air provocation test: which and when? Am J Rhinol Allergy 2013;27:113–7.

40. Gevorgyan A, Segboer C, Gorissen R, et al. Capsaicin for non-allergic rhinitis. Cochrane Database Syst Rev 2015;(7):CD010591.

41. Sanico AM, Philip G, Proud D, et al. Comparison of nasal mucosal responsiveness to neuronal stimulation in non-allergic and allergic rhinitis: effects of capsaicin nasal challenge. Clin Exp Allergy 1998;28:92–100.

42. Lambert EM, Patel CB, Fakhri S, et al. Optical rhinometry in nonallergic irritant rhinitis: a capsaicin challenge study. Int Forum Allergy Rhinol 2013;3(10): 795–800.

Nonallergic Rhinitis
Diagnosis

Justin Greiwe, MD[a,b], Jonathan A. Bernstein, MD[a,b],*

KEYWORDS

- Nonallergic rhinitis • Differential diagnosis • Triggers • Symptoms • Provocation
- Subtypes • Classification

KEY POINTS

- Nonallergic rhinitis (NAR) is a heterogeneous disorder that is difficult to characterize because there is very little consensus in the literature regarding its definition and mechanisms of action.
- The symptoms and physical findings of patients with allergic rhinitis (AR) are not pathognomonic, because patients with NAR often present with similar features and up to 50% suffer of AR patients have a non-allergic component termed mixed rhinitis (MR).
- NAR is currently diagnosed based exclusively on patients being nonatopic with symptoms in response to odorant and irritant triggers in the absence of a specific cause.
- Assessing treatment response remains a useful tool for differentiating among AR, MR, and NAR.
- More information regarding the mechanisms of NAR is needed, which will lead to more specific and effective therapeutic approaches.

INTRODUCTION

The practicing allergist manages several common clinical disorders, but none more prevalent than chronic rhinitis. Although asthma, atopic dermatitis, conjunctivitis, and sinusitis continue to afflict large proportions of the general population, they pale in scope to chronic rhinitis. This latter condition affects upward of 70 million individuals in the United States, making it one of the most prevalent medical disorders in the country.[1] Consequently, chronic rhinitis is associated with a considerable economic impact and can have major implications on quality of life, especially when one considers the various associated concomitant disorders. Although there is an

No funding was required for this research.

[a] Bernstein Allergy Group, 8444 Winton Rd, Cincinnati, OH 45231, USA; [b] Division of Allergy, Immunology and Rheumatology, University of Cincinnati, 231 Albert Sabin Way, Cincinnati, OH 45267, USA

* Corresponding author. Division of Allergy, Immunology and Rheumatology, University of Cincinnati, 231 Albert Sabin Way, ML 563, Cincinnati, OH 45267-0563.

E-mail address: Jonathan.Bernstein@uc.edu

Immunol Allergy Clin N Am 36 (2016) 289–303
http://dx.doi.org/10.1016/j.iac.2015.12.006
0889-8561/16/$ – see front matter © 2016 Elsevier Inc. All rights reserved.

extensive differential diagnosis for chronic rhinitis, the most ubiquitous and well known subtypes are seasonal and perennial allergic rhinitis (AR). In the United States, AR is estimated to affect approximately 10% to 30% of adults and 40% of children, with estimated direct costs of $11.2 billion, which overshadows other chronic illnesses, such as asthma, diabetes, and coronary heart disease.[2,3] Lost productivity at work estimated as a decrease of $600 per employee per year further magnifies the economic burden this condition has in the United States. A similar economic impact of AR has been reported for Europe and emerging economies.[4–6] Unfortunately, the economic and societal impact of chronic rhinitis is often underestimated and underappreciated.

Although millions of Americans believe they suffer from AR symptoms, the diagnosis of this condition is not always supported by serologic or skin testing identifying specific IgE responses to aeroallergens that correlate with their clinical history. In fact, a substantial proportion of patients that suffer from rhinitis symptoms turn out not to be sensitized, but instead suffer from a condition referred to as nonallergic rhinitis (NAR). NAR is a heterogeneous disorder that is difficult to characterize because there is very little consensus in the literature regarding its definition and mechanisms of action. However, emerging theories posit competing mechanisms including dysautonomia (autonomic dysfunction) resulting in diminished sympathetic activity and/or parasympathetic overactivity and altered expression or activity of transient receptor potential channels.[7]

A more detailed look at mechanism of action is addressed elsewhere (See Baroody FM: Non-Allergic Rhinitis: Mechanism of Action, in this issue). This article provides a framework for evaluation and accurate diagnosis of NAR. Development of a consensus opinion for diagnosis of this rhinitis subtype will improve clinical outcomes and provide a clearer pathway for investigation of underlying mechanisms and novel targeted therapies.

Classifying Chronic Rhinitis

Several attempts have been made to provide a classification system of chronic rhinitis subtypes to help guide the clinician in their diagnosis and treatment of these conditions. In 2009, a panel of key opinion leaders formed a consensus opinion on the classification of NAR subtypes based on the existing literature and consensus opinions.[8–10] They concluded that NAR should be classified into eight different subtypes because of their unique clinical presentation, summarized in **Box 1.**[4]

There are several other conditions excluded from this classification worth mentioning including mixed rhinitis (MR), localized AR or entopic rhinitis, rhinosinusitis with and without polyps, infectious rhinitis (bacterial and chronic rhinosinusitis), and occupational rhinitis, because they are not always purely nonallergic or are mediated through different mechanistic pathways that have been attributed to NAR. The lack of a consensus clinical phenotype for NAR may have hindered previous genetic studies that have investigated the role of cytokines (ie, interferon-γ and inducible T-cell tyrosine kinase) and olfactory receptor gene segments to establish more specific NAR endotypes.[11–14] The indeterminate results of these genetic studies may indicate that either these pathways in NAR or the clinical criteria used to enroll subjects may not be relevant or too heterogeneous, respectively. Therefore, one focus has been to determine better ways to characterize patients with NAR to make a more accurate diagnosis of this condition. This article reviews the different approaches that have been investigated to better differentiate NAR from other chronic rhinitis subtypes.

Box 1
World Allergy Organization classification of nonallergic rhinitis subtypes

1. Nonallergic rhinopathy: previously known as vasomotor rhinitis, irritant-induced rhinitis, and idiopathic rhinitis

2. Nonallergic rhinitis with eosinophila

3. Drug-induced rhinitis (ie, rhinitis medicamentosa)

4. Hormonal-induced rhinitis

5. Atrophic rhinitis

6. Senile rhinitis

7. Gustatory rhinitis (rhinorrhea associated with eating)

8. Cerebral spinal fluid leak manifesting as rhinorrhea

Adapted from Kaliner MA. Classification of nonallergic rhinitis syndromes with a focus on vasomotor rhinitis, proposed to be known henceforth as nonallergic rhinopathy. World Allergy Organ J 2009;2:99.

SYMPTOMS
Differences Between Allergic and Nonallergic Rhinitis

Several studies have attempted to identify the similarities and differences between AR and NAR to improve clinical diagnostic accuracy. Some argue that although NAR can present in a similar fashion to AR, these conditions have somewhat distinguishable characteristics that can help elucidate the correct diagnosis, summarized in **Table 1**.[15]

Table 1
Distinguishing features of nonallergic rhinitis and allergic rhinitis

Nonallergic Rhinitis	Allergic Rhinitis
• Onset of symptoms later in life, more common after age 20	• Usually presents in childhood
• No indication of a familial pattern	• Persuasive family history of atopy (asthma, rhinitis, and atopic dermatitis)
• More common in females	• Affects females and males equally
• Perennial symptoms in nature with very little seasonal variation[a]	• Most have seasonal exacerbation of symptoms
• Negative aeroallergen skin testing and/or serum IgE testing	• Positive aeroallergen skin testing and/or serum IgE testing
• Broad range of irritant triggers	• Aeroallergen triggers
• Symptoms include	• Symptoms include
○ Nasal congestion	○ Congestion, sneezing, rhinorrhea, and nasal itch
○ Postnasal drainage with or without cough	○ Ocular conjunctivitis, watering, and itch
○ Infrequent eye complaints	• Physical examination
○ Minimal itching	○ Nasal mucosa edematous, pale, and boggy
• Physical examination (more variable)	○ Allergic shiners (dark areas under the eyes)
○ Nasal mucosa can be normal with increased clear watery secretions, may be erythematous or atrophic	

[a] For NAR, patients often attribute seasonal worsening of symptoms to aeroallergen triggers (ie, tree and ragweed). These seasonal variations are not pollen related, but rather caused by changes in weather (ie, temperature, humidity, barometric pressure) causing acute worsening of perennial symptoms.

Adapted from Quillen DM, Feller DB. Diagnosing rhinitis: allergic vs. nonallergic. Am Fam Physician 2006;73(9):1587.

With such varied presentations it must be emphasized that the symptoms and physical findings of patients with AR are not pathognomonic, because patients with NAR often present with similar features.[16] Therefore, NAR and AR must not be considered mutually exclusive based on clinical symptoms alone, because these conditions can often overlap. In fact, studies have demonstrated that up to 50% of chronic rhinitis sufferers may have MR, defined as a combination of allergic and nonallergic triggers. One cross-sectional questionnaire designed to identify the prevalence of rhinitis subtypes reported that approximately 43% of the respondents had AR, 34% had MR, and 23% had NAR.[17]

To further investigate consistently dependable rhinitis features, Di Lorenzo and colleagues[18] examined several clinical and laboratory parameters to help reinforce or exclude the diagnosis of AR. They evaluated 1511 patients with rhinitis (aged 18–81 years) using skin prick testing (SPT), blood eosinophil counts, nasal eosinophil counts, peak nasal inspiratory flow measurement, and evaluation of nasal symptoms using a visual analog scale. They reported several distinguishing features that differentiated AR and NAR, summarized in **Box 2**. These findings are similar to other reports suggesting that clinical characteristics are important adjunctive criteria for accurately diagnosing NAR.

Questionnaire Diagnosis

Several questionnaire studies have been designed to help physicians recognize differences between AR and NAR subtypes. The National Rhinitis Classification Task Force attempted to categorize chronic rhinitis subtypes by distributing a questionnaire to assess the number of allergic and nonallergic triggers that induce rhinitis symptoms. The survey, which was performed in 15 allergy practices and enrolled 975 patients, revealed that NAR and MR occurred more commonly in adults, females, and on a perennial rather than seasonal basis.[17]

Box 2
Differences between allergic and nonallergic rhinitis in a large sample of adult patients with rhinitis symptoms

Allergic Rhinitis

- Higher nasal eosinophil count
- Lack of clinical response to antihistamines
- More sneezing and nasal pruritus
- More severe symptoms and recurrent conjunctivitis
- Peak nasal inspiratory flow, blood eosinophil counts, and visual analog scale of nasal symptoms were higher

Nonallergic Rhinitis

- Patients were older and predominately female subjects
- Characterized by nasal obstruction and rhinorrhea
- Slightly more frequent episodes of recurring headaches and olfactory dysfunction

10 variables were statistically different between AR and NAR: age, sneezing, nasal pruritus, mild symptoms, intermittent/severe nasal symptoms, visual analog scale, clinical response to antihistamines, conjunctivitis, peak nasal inspiratory flow, and nasal eosinophil counts.
Adapted from Di Lorenzo G, Pacor ML, Amodio E, et al. Differences and similarities between allergic and nonallergic rhinitis in a large sample of adult patients with rhinitis symptoms. Int Arch Allergy Immunol 2011;155(3):266.

Another survey distributed by Brandt and Bernstein to develop a model that could be used to predict a diagnosis of AR and NAR found that it was an especially useful tool for diagnosing NAR, whereas the questions asked of patients by physicians to diagnose AR do not correlate as well with physician diagnosis.[19] This study found that patients with symptom onset later in life (>35 years), no family history of allergies, no seasonality or cat-induced symptoms, and symptoms induced by perfumes and fragrances had greater than 95% likelihood of having a physician diagnosis of NAR before any type of testing to assess atopy.[19]

Despite noticeable and somewhat reproducible differences between AR and NAR in the aforementioned studies, subsequent research has demonstrated that clinical symptoms and triggers alone might not be as reliable for differentiating between rhinitis subtypes as once believed. In fact, an investigation of 634 patients with chronic rhinitis (AR = 496; NAR = 138) revealed that the AR population was more likely to experience anterior rhinorrhea but there was no difference between the two populations with respect to nasal congestion or postnasal drainage (**Table 2**).[20]

Subsequently, a more comprehensive analysis was undertaken to investigate the use of an Irritant Index Questionnaire that quantitated severity of symptoms in response to 21 nonallergic triggers.[21] This study, whose primary purpose was to investigate the relationship of headaches with rhinitis subtypes, enrolled 656 patients who were previously diagnosed using currently accepted physician consensus definitions of AR, MR, and NAR. The consensus physician definition used for AR was rhinitis symptoms that correlated with positive specific IgE testing (SPT or serum-specific IgE) and exposure to seasonal and/or perennial aeroallergens, whereas NAR was defined as rhinitis symptoms with negative specific IgE testing and symptoms in response to weather changes and/or odorants and irritants. MR was defined as rhinitis symptoms that correlated with specific IgE sensitization and exposure to seasonal and/or perennial allergens in addition to symptoms in response to weather and/or odorants and irritants. The diagnoses of these patients were then reclassified based on their IgE sensitization status to aeroallergens and their irritant index score. Based on these criteria there was significant reclassification of patients into different diagnostic categories.[21] Several patients with AR (N = 404) and MR (N = 129) were reclassified into low (N = 254) versus high (N = 279) irritant burden groups. Compared with the physician-diagnosed rhinitis subtype groups, reclassification found that the high irritant burden rhinitis group had more severe and frequent rhinitis symptoms and a significantly greater prevalence of physician-diagnosed asthma.[21] Similar outcomes in severity, frequency, and prevalence of physician-diagnosed asthma were found after the NAR population (N = 123) was reclassified based on having a high versus low irritant index score. Therefore, the Irritant Index Questionnaire resulted in

Table 2			
Prevalence of symptoms in patients characterized as allergic rhinitis and nonallergic rhinitis from the Cincinnati Headache/Rhinitis Database			
	Allergic Rhinitis[a] (n = 496)	Nonallergic Rhinitis (n = 138)	
Symptom	N (%)	N (%)	P Value
Stuffy nose	432 (87)	115 (83)	NS
Postnasal drainage	411 (83)	107 (78)	NS
Rhinorrhea	396 (80)	79 (57)	<0.01

[a] Allergic rhinitis includes seasonal and perennial allergic rhinitis.
Adapted from Bernstein JA. Characteristics of nonallergic vasomotor rhinitis. World Allergy Organ J 2009;2(6):103.

significant reclassification of physician-diagnosed patients with rhinitis into distinct subgroups with unique clinical differences that may represent more severe phenotypes than previously recognized by current diagnostic modalities.[21]

Some have postulated that patients with increased symptoms in response to odorants and irritants may exhibit increased differences in olfactory thresholds making them more susceptible to these triggers. However, using an automated olfactometer, which is modeled after the staircase approach for assessing olfaction, there was no difference identified in olfactory threshold responses among patients with AR, NAR, and MR.[22] Ultimately these studies demonstrate the clinical utility of standardized, validated questionnaires in clinical practice to objectively characterize chronic rhinitis subtypes, which can result in a more accurate diagnosis and focused treatment.[21]

Triggers

Currently there are no definitive tests available for the diagnosis of NAR. Unlike AR, which requires symptoms on exposure to sensitizing aeroallergen, NAR is currently diagnosed based exclusively on patients being nonatopic with symptoms in response to odorant and irritant triggers in the absence of a specific etiology (ie, infectious, immunologic, structural, hormonal). Therefore, focusing on pertinent irritant triggers has been considered an important diagnostic criterion for establishing a diagnosis of NAR (**Box 3**).[21] Common NAR triggers include changes in the environment (dry cold air, humidity, barometric pressure), airborne irritants including odors and fumes (cologne, perfume, cleaning products, cigarette smoke, diesel and car exhaust), certain medications (β-blockers, aspirin, and other nonsteroidal anti-inflammatory drugs), dietary factors (spicy food, alcohol), sexual arousal, exercise, strong emotions or stress, and hormone levels.

Box 3
Triggers of nonallergic rhinitis

- Changes in Environment
  - Cold, dry air
  - Hot air
  - Changes in temperature
  - Humidity
  - Barometric pressure changes

- Airborne irritants (odors, fumes)
  - Strong smells
    - Perfume, cologne, flowers, cooking smells, incense, newsprint, other fragrances
  - Cleaning products
    - Bleach
  - Tobacco smoke
  - Pollutants and chemicals
    - Volatile organics like diesel and car exhaust

- Medications
  - Alpha-blockers (clonidine, guanfacine)
  - Beta-blockers
  - Aspirin and other anti-inflammatory medicines
  - Angiotensin-converting enzyme inhibitors
  - Oral contraceptives (estrogens, progesterone)
  - Erectile dysfunction drugs (sildenafil)
  - Antidepressants, psychotropics, antiepileptics

- Dietary factors (gustatory)
  - Spicy food
  - Alcoholic beverages
  - Act of eating

- Sexual arousal

- Exercise

- Strong emotions or stress

- Changes in hormone levels
  - Pregnancy, puberty

- Occupational exposures

- Chronic health conditions

However, although irritant triggers are an important aspect for the evaluation of chronic rhinitis subtypes, this diagnostic criteria has its limitations. Recent studies found that a significant proportion of patients with NAR do not manifest symptoms in response to irritant or noxious odors, suggesting that the previously mentioned triggers are not a uniform clinical characteristic that can be used for establishing a diagnosis for all patients with NAR.[23] This observation in conjunction with the inability to differentiate rhinitis subtypes based on symptoms alone further confounds the ability to develop consensus definitions for rhinitis subtypes.[23]

Focused Physical Examination

A focused physical examination should always follow a comprehensive clinical history; however, examination alone is very unreliable for discriminating rhinitis subtypes. Certain signs/symptoms suggestive of seasonal allergic rhinitis include allergic shiners; mouth breathing; conjunctivitis; and edematous, pale, and boggy nasal mucosa. In addition, AR is often associated with other allergic conditions, such as asthma and atopic dermatitis. Physical examination of perennial allergic rhinitis and NAR is more variable. The nasal mucosa can be normal or erythematous, often with evidence of prominent postnasal drip with cobblestoning. Although fiberoptic nasal endoscopy provides the best visualization of intranasal structures, it is not always available or necessary and requires a certain amount of proficiency to operate and interpret. Therefore, physical examination is of limited utility in differentiating rhinitis subtypes.

Comorbidities

Poorly controlled chronic rhinitis can be accompanied by several different comorbidities, which can significantly impact its management and further impair quality of life.[24–30] Common associated conditions include acute and chronic sinusitis, tension and migraine headaches, asthma, chronic cough, conjunctivitis, Eustachian tube dysfunction, otitis media with or without effusion, nasal polyps, hearing impairment, nasal dyspnea and obstructive sleep apnea, and other sleep disturbances/related complications resulting in fatigue (**Box 4**).

Short- and long-term complications from chronic rhinitis are substantial, inflicting considerable physical and economic burdens on rhinitis sufferers. These impediments include poor cognitive functioning, sleep loss/daytime fatigue, reduced school/workplace productivity, and absenteeism all leading to overall decreased quality of life. One of the most frequent clinically relevant conditions resulting from poorly controlled rhinitis is postnasal drainage leading to chronic cough. These secretions likely stimulate cough receptors causing a persistent, refractory cough that needs to be differentiated from asthma and gastroesophageal reflux, which can also manifest as a chronic cough or occur concomitantly with postnasal drainage–induced cough.

DIAGNOSTIC TEST/IMAGING STUDY
Skin Prick and Allergen-specific IgE Antibody Testing

The most common diagnostic tests for chronic rhinitis include allergen skin testing or specific in vitro IgE testing to common seasonal and perennial aeroallergens. Skin testing involves introducing measured amounts of allergen in conjunction with a positive histamine and negative saline control onto the skin followed by a prick with the goal of eliciting an immediate wheal and flare response within 15 minutes indicating that the individual has specific IgE antibody directed to the allergen on high-affinity (FcER1) IgE receptors located on mast cells and basophils. Cross-linking of

---

Box 4
Comorbidities associated with chronic rhinitis

Medical Comorbidities

- Acute and chronic sinusitis
- Tension and migraine headaches
- Worsening of underlying asthma, increased propensity to develop asthma
- Chronic cough secondary to postnasal drip
- Conjunctivitis
- Acute and chronic otitis media
- Eustachian tube dysfunction
- Nasal polyps
- Sleep apnea and related complications
- Neuropsychiatric side effects from sedating antihistamines

Quality of Life Comorbidities

- Difficulty sleeping/sleep disturbances
- Nasal dyspnea
- Daytime fatigue, malaise
- Missed school days
- Missed work days, reduced productivity
- Decreased levels of cognitive function

---

the allergen to the specific IgE antibody binding regions results in cell activation and release of bioactive mediators resulting in the physiologic characteristics of AR. Percutaneous or skin SPT is considered the "gold standard" for detecting allergen-specific IgE and is usually preformed first for safety reasons followed in some cases if necessary by intracutaneous testing (ICT) if negative.[31,32] SPT requires experienced practitioners for accurate interpretation. Determination of serum-specific IgE antibodies directed toward a specific allergen is sometimes required if the patient is on medications that interfere with the histamine response (eg, antihistamines, tricyclic antidepressants), has a severe skin disease (eg, poorly controlled atopic dermatitis, chronic urticaria), or is dermatographic (**Table 3**). SPT is more sensitive than serum testing; however, in the absence of a reliable history, positive results with either test imply sensitization that needs to correlate with symptoms after exposure to be considered an allergy.

Intracutaneous Testing

SPT and serum-specific IgE testing are safe and convenient, with high levels of sensitivity, specificity, positive predictive values, and negative predictive values. ICT, however, has been met with more skepticism. Several studies have suggested that ICT is less diagnostically useful with higher sensitivity but less specificity than SPT, indicating that a positive ICT is not clinically relevant if previous percutaneous testing was unremarkable.[33–35] The concern is that extraneous IC testing could influence immunotherapy composition, increasing patient risk, discomfort, and cost.

Table 3
Advantages and disadvantages of skin prick versus allergen-specific IgE antibody testing

Skin Prick Testing	Serum Testing
• Advantages ○ More sensitive ○ Less expensive ○ Immediate results	• Advantages ○ Safer (especially in patients with severe allergy) ○ No experience required to perform test ○ No need to stop any medications ○ Suitable for patients with various skin conditions where clear skin is not available
• Disadvantages ○ Need trained staff to apply tests and interpret results ○ Potency of antigen extracts need to be maintained ○ Have to stop antihistamine medications 2–5 d before testing ○ Difficult in patients with chronic skin conditions that are poorly controlled ○ Young children sometimes cannot tolerate multiple pricks ○ May rarely cause severe allergic reactions in highly sensitive patients	• Disadvantages ○ Less sensitive ○ More expensive ○ Results are not immediate ○ Not all commercial tests for specific IgE provide reproducible, accurate data[12] ○ High levels of total IgE can cause false-positive results because of nonspecific binding

Data from Brasch-Andersen C, Haagerup A, Borglum AD, et al. Highly significant linkage to chromosome 3q13.31 for rhinitis and related allergic diseases. J Med Genet 2006;43:e10.

Imaging

Rarely is imaging part of the initial diagnostic work-up for chronic rhinitis. However, if the severity of the patient's condition necessitates diagnostic certainty, computerized tomography scan of the sinuses is an appropriate modality to further elucidate sinus anatomy and/or disease including the osteomeatal complexes and monitor progression of nasal polyps if applicable. Sinus plain films should not be performed because they are less sensitive than sinus computerized tomography scans, and are not dependable enough to assist with clinical decision making.

Additional Testing Modalities

Although it may not always be necessary to perform allergy testing before making a presumptive diagnosis of NAR, SPT or serum-specific IgE testing to indoor and outdoor allergens is helpful to establish MR subtypes or to confirm a diagnosis of NAR.[19] Even with a comprehensive clinical history and pertinent skin and/or serologic testing inconsistencies can occur, making the classification of rhinitis subtypes particularly challenging. To further complicate this issue, recent studies have identified a certain subset of patients with symptoms of AR but negative specific IgE-responses referred to as localized AR or "entopic" rhinitis.[36] This phenotype mimics AR with worsening symptoms on exposure to specific allergen triggers and response to avoidance measures, antihistamines, topical nasal corticosteroids, and/or possibly allergen immunotherapy. Localized AR symptoms can be reproduced by nasal provocation using specific allergens, but there is still debate in the literature on whether localized AR is in fact a unique disease process or rather the first step in the natural history of AR.[37] Rondón and colleagues[37] estimates that local AR affects 25.7% of the rhinitis population and more than 47% of patients previously diagnosed with NAR but these numbers have not been confirmed by other groups.

NAR therefore poses a unique challenge with a variety of possible disease mechanisms and a paucity of reliable and reproducible diagnostic tests. To address this problem additional methods for classifying and diagnosing rhinitis subtypes have been proposed, but have had varying degrees of reliability, success, and cost. In addition to ICT, less common diagnostic tools include nasal cytology for eosinophils or other cellular subtypes (using secretions, scraping, lavage, or biopsy), peak nasal inspiratory flow rates, anterior rhinomanometry, acoustic rhinometry, irritant index scales, specific biomarkers, nasal provocation testing with environmental exposure chambers, and nasolaryngoscopy (**Box 5**).

Proponents of the previously mentioned diagnostic tools suggest that the systematic use of these approaches in the work-up of chronic rhinitis will lead to more accurate subtyping, more focused treatment, and more favorable clinical outcomes. Although these techniques have been advocated by some, their use for the characterization of rhinitis subtypes in the outpatient setting is not always clinically practical. Difficulties with proper sampling and limitations in methodologies, such as nasal smears or scrapings for histology, nasal provocation to specific aeroallergens or measurement of local IgE in nasal lavage make these techniques more appropriate for clinical research and less feasible in clinical practice. In contrast, there are a few controversial tests without any diagnostic validity that should be avoided in clinical practice. These tests include cytotoxic tests, provocation-neutralization, electrodermal testing, applied kinesiology, iridology, and hair analysis.[10]

Box 5
Less common diagnostic tools for NAR

- Intracermal skin testing
- Nasal cytology
  - Several nonallergic subtypes have been proposed based on cytologic sampling including[38,39]
    - Nonallergic rhinitis with eosinophils
    - Nonallergic rhinitis with mast cells
    - Nonallergic rhinitis with neutrophils
    - Nonallergic rhinitis with eosinophils and mast cells
- Peak nasal inspiratory flow rates
- Anterior rhinomanometry
- Acoustic rhinometry
- Irritant index scale
- Specific biomarkers[36]
  - Peripheral blood cytokines and mediators
  - Nasal exhaled nitric oxide
  - Nasal exhaled breath condensate 8-isoprostane
  - Leukotriene B_4
  - Prostaglandin E_2
  - pH
  - Nasal-specific IgE (entopic rhinitis)
- Nasal provocation testing with environmental exposure chambers
- Nasolaryngoscopy

Data from Refs.[36,38,39]

TREATMENT RESPONSE

Affective rhinitis treatments are discussed at length in other articles in this issue however assessing treatment response remains a useful tool for differentiating among AR, MR, and NAR. Poor response to standard treatments in patients suspected of having AR often suggests incorrect usage of medications or poor technique, but in some cases may indicate a more complex diagnosis, such as MR or NAR. Unlike AR, pure NAR does not seem to be as responsive to second-generation H_1-antagonists, nasal corticosteroids, leukotriene-modifying agents, or allergen immunotherapy but instead responds better to topical nasal antihistamines, a combination of nasal corticosteroids and nasal antihistamines, nasal saline rinses, and oral first-generation H_1-antagonists because of their anticholinergic effect. These later medications should be dosed at bedtime to minimize their sedating side effects.[10] Gauging a patient's clinical response to these medications using an objective rhinitis control score between visits is helpful for determining if further characterization of patients incompletely controlled have a nonallergic component that requires an alternative treatment approach.[40]

DIFFERENTIAL DIAGNOSIS

The differential diagnosis for chronic rhinitis is summarized in **Box 6**.

FUTURE CONSIDERATIONS: ENVIRONMENTAL EXPOSURE CHAMBERS

It is clear that more information regarding the mechanisms of NAR is needed, which will lead to more specific and effective therapeutic approaches. The current consensus definition of NAR is based on recent clinical studies and is grounded on clinical symptoms, the absence of specific IgE responses to aeroallergens, and response to irritant nonallergic triggers; however, this classification may be too rudimentary. A major limitation of NAR diagnosis is that patients may under or over self-report irritant and other nonallergic triggers. Recent studies have demonstrated a relative disconnect between patient history and actual nasal end-organ objective responses by provocation to the suspected trigger. Thirty-seven patients were challenged to various triggers (cold dry air, temperature change, ozone, fragrance, and irritant) within a controlled environmental exposure chamber and clinical responses were measured subjectively using symptom diary cards and objectively using acoustic rhinometry to detect changes in nasal resistance. **Table 4** summarizes the discordance between perceived and actual symptoms elicited by each specific trigger emphasizing the importance of incorporating provocation into the phenotypic characterization of patients with NAR to further investigate disease mechanisms and novel therapies.[41] This study, which also demonstrated a heterogeneous response to single versus multiple triggers between subjects, and a previous study, which reported that more than half of patients with NAR studied report no known triggers, suggests that we should rethink how we define NAR in the future.[21]

Rather than focusing on cold dry air or other individual triggers, understanding the underlying mechanism for this condition will likely be more useful for ultimately making an accurate NAR diagnosis. As research tools for investigating suspected neurogenic pathways involved in NAR are developed, it may ultimately be realized that the various clinical presentations of NAR represent the same condition operating through a universal pathway distinguished only by subtle differences in ligand activation of specific receptors (ie, transient receptor potential-A, M V calcium ion channels).[41]

Box 6
Differential diagnosis of chronic rhinitis

- Allergic rhinitis (seasonal/perennial)
- Nonallergic rhinitis and various subtypes
- Mixed rhinitis
- Infectious rhinitis (viral, bacterial, and chronic rhinosinusitis)
- Episodic rhinitis
- Occupational rhinitis
- Localized AR or entopic rhinitis
- Rhinosinusitis with and without polyps
- Aspirin intolerance (aspirin triad)
- Drug-induced rhinitis
  - Rhinitis medicamentosa (decongestants)
  - β-Blockers
  - Birth control pills
  - Antihypertensives
- Rhinitis secondary to
  - Pregnancy
  - Hypothyroidism
  - Horner syndrome
  - Wegener granulomatosis
  - Sarcoidosis
  - Relapsing polychondritis
  - Sjögren syndrome
  - Midline granuloma
- Structural conditions causing rhinitis
  - Foreign body
  - Nasal polyps
  - Nasal septal deviation (intranasal cocaine, septal surgery)
  - Enlarged tonsils and adenoids
  - Nasal tumors
  - Cerebral spinal fluid rhinorrhea
  - Choanal atresia
  - Hypertrophic turbinates

Adapted from Kaliner MA. Classification of nonallergic rhinitis syndromes with a focus on vasomotor rhinitis, proposed to be known henceforth as nonallergic rhinopathy. World Allergy Organ J 2009;2:98–101.

Table 4
Concordance of NAR questionnaire & clinical response

	Cold Dry Air	Temp Change	Ozone	Fragrance	Irritant
Concordance between history and study[a,b]	(19/36) 53%	(25/36) 69%	(27/36) 75%	(19/36) 53%	(21/36) 58%
Percent of patients reporting symptoms to the triggers	(34/36) 94%	(34/36) 94%	(13/36) 36%	(22/36) 61%	(21/36) 58%

[a] n = 36 Patients who have completed all five challenges (19/36 = 53% female; 17/36 = 47% male).
[b] Some challenges had 37 patients participate in challenge.
Adapted from Bernstein JA, Salapatek AM, Lee JS, et al. Provocation of nonallergic rhinitis subjects in response to simulated weather conditions using an environmental exposure chamber model. Allergy Asthma Proc 2012;33:340; with permission.

SUMMARY

Even though chronic rhinitis continues to be one of the most ubiquitous conditions in medicine, affecting millions of patients throughout the United States, it remains a poorly managed and often difficult to treat condition. Unfortunately NAR is often suboptimally managed by clinicians because these patients are often treated in a similar manner to AR. Poor clinical outcomes occur when physicians take a "one size fits all" approach. Establishing the correct diagnosis requires a keen understanding of the unique underlying mechanisms involved in NAR, which is still evolving. Thus far, a detailed clinical history taking into account family history, age of onset, allergic and/or nonallergic triggers, seasonality, and response to treatment in addition to having a broad understanding of the differential diagnosis of chronic rhinitis subtypes is essential for establishing an accurate diagnosis. Ultimately epidemiologic studies that better define NAR prevalence and its economic burden on society are needed to convince funding agencies of the need for research to elucidate mechanisms and specific treatment approaches for this condition.

REFERENCES

1. Settipane RA, Charnock DR. Epidemiology of rhinitis: allergic and nonallergic. Clin Allergy Immunol 2007;19:23–34.
2. Schoenwetter WF, Dupclay L, Appajosyula S, et al. Economic impact and quality-of-life burden of allergic rhinitis. Curr Med Res Opin 2004;20(3):305–17.
3. Berger WE. Allergic rhinitis in children: diagnosis and management strategies. Paediatr Drugs 2004;6(4):233–50.
4. Kaliner MA. Classification of nonallergic rhinitis syndromes with a focus on vasomotor rhinitis, proposed to be known henceforth as nonallergic rhinopathy. World Allergy Organ J 2009;2:98–101.
5. Zuberbier T, Lötvall J, Simoens S, et al. Economic burden of inadequate management of allergic diseases in the European Union: a GA(2) LEN review. Allergy 2014;69(10):1275–9.
6. Hellgren J, Cervin A, Nordling S, et al. Allergic rhinitis and the common cold–high cost to society. Allergy 2010;65(6):776–83.
7. Bernstein JA, Singh U. Neural abnormalities in nonallergic rhinitis. Curr Allergy Asthma Rep 2015;15(4):511.
8. Scarupa MD, Kaliner MA. Nonallergic rhinitis, with a focus on vasomotor rhinitis: clinical importance, differential diagnosis, and effective treatment recommendations. J World Allergy Org 2009;2:20–5.
9. Greiner AN, Meltzer EO. Pharmacologic rationale for treating allergic and nonallergic rhinitis. J Allergy Clin Immunol 2006;118:985–96.
10. Wallace DV, Dykewicz MS, Bernstein DI, et al. The diagnosis and management of rhinitis, an updated practice parameter. J Allergy Clin Immunol 2008; 122(2 Suppl):S1–84.
11. Bernstein JA, Zhang G, Jin L, et al. Olfactory receptor gene polymorphisms and nonallergic vasomotor rhinitis. J Asthma 2008;45:287–92.
12. Brasch-Andersen C, Haagerup A, Borglum AD, et al. Highly significant linkage to chromosome 3q13.31 for rhinitis and related allergic diseases. J Med Genet 2006;43:e10.
13. Benson M, Mobini R, Barrenäs F, et al. A haplotype in the inducible T-cell tyrosine kinase is a risk factor for seasonal allergic rhinitis. Allergy 2009;64:1286–91.

14. Hussein YM, Ahmad AS, Ibrahem MM, et al. Interferon gamma gene polymorphism as a biochemical marker in Egyptian atopic patients. J Investig Allergol Clin Immunol 2009;19:292–8.

15. Quillen DM, Feller DB. Diagnosing rhinitis: allergic vs. nonallergic. Am Fam Physician 2006;73(9):1583–90.

16. Bernstein JA, Rezvani M. Mixed rhinitis: a new subclass of chronic rhinitis?. In: Kaliner M, editor. Current review of rhinitis. 2nd edition. Philadelphia: Current Medicine; 2006. p. 69–78.

17. Settipane RA, Lieberman P. Update on nonallergic rhinitis. Ann Allergy Asthma Immunol 2001;86:494–507.

18. Di Lorenzo G, Pacor ML, Amodio E, et al. Differences and similarities between allergic and nonallergic rhinitis in a large sample of adult patients with rhinitis symptoms. Int Arch Allergy Immunol 2011;155(3):263–70.

19. Brandt D, Bernstein JA. Questionnaire evaluation and risk factor identification for nonallergic vasomotor rhinitis. Ann Allergy Asthma Immunol 2006;96:526–32.

20. Bernstein JA. Characteristics of nonallergic vasomotor rhinitis. World Allergy Organ J 2009;2(6):102–5.

21. Bernstein JA, Levin LS, Al-Shuik E, et al. Clinical characteristics of chronic rhinitis patients with high vs low irritant trigger burdens. Ann Allergy Asthma Immunol 2012;109:173–8.

22. Rezvani M, Brandt D, Bernstein JA, et al. Investigation of olfactory threshold responses in chronic rhinitis subtypes. Ann Allergy Asthma Immunol 2007; 99(6):571–2.

23. Nathan RA, Meltzer EO, Derbery J, et al. The prevalence of nasal symptoms attributed to allergies in the United States: findings from the burden of rhinitis in America survey. Allergy Asthma Proc 2008;29:600–8.

24. Meltzer EO, Blaiss MS, Naclerio RM, et al. Burden of allergic rhinitis: allergies in America, Latin America, and Asia-Pacific adult surveys. Allergy Asthma Proc 2012;33(Suppl 1):S113–41.

25. Meltzer EO, Nathan RA, Derebery MJ, et al. Sleep, quality of life, and productivity impact of nasal symptoms in the United States: findings from the burden of rhinitis in America survey. Allergy Asthma Proc 2009;30:244–54.

26. Settipane RA. Complications of allergic rhinitis. Allergy Asthma Proc 1999;20: 209–13.

27. Accordini S, Corsico AG, Calciano L, et al. The impact of asthma, chronic bronchitis and allergic rhinitis on all-cause hospitalizations and limitations in daily activities: a population-based observational study. BMC Pulm Med 2015;15:10.

28. Fu QL, Ma JX, Ou CQ, et al. Influence of self-reported chronic rhinosinusitis on health-related quality of life: a population-based survey. PLoS One 2015;10(5): e0126881.

29. Position statement: allergen skin testing. J Allergy Clin Immunol 1993;92:636–7.

30. Bernstein IL, Storms WW. Practice parameters for allergy diagnostic testing. Ann Allergy Asthma Immunol 1995;75:553–624.

31. Szeinbach SL, Barnes JH, Sullivan TJ, et al. Precision and accuracy of commercial laboratories' ability to classify positive and/or negative allergen-specific IgE results. Ann Allergy Asthma Immunol 2001;86:373–81.

32. Nelson HS, Oppenheimer J, Buchmeier A, et al. An assessment of the role of intradermal skin testing in the diagnosis of clinically relevant allergy to timothy grass. J Allergy Clin Immunol 1996;97:1193–201.

33. Reddy PM, Nagaya H, Pascual HC, et al. Reappraisal of intracutaneous tests in the diagnosis of reaginic allergy. J Allergy Clin Immunol 1978;61:36–41.

34. Wood RA, Phipatanakul W, Hamilton RG, et al. A comparison of skin prick tests, intradermal skin tests, and RASTs in the diagnosis of cat allergy. J Allergy Clin Immunol 1999;103:773–9.
35. Derebery J, Meltzer EO, Nathan RA, et al. Rhinitis symptoms and comorbidities in the United States: burden of rhinitis in America survey. Otolaryngol Head Neck Surg 2008;139:198–205.
36. Bernstein JA. Characterizing rhinitis subtypes. Am J Rhinol Allergy 2013;27(6): 457–60.
37. Rondón C, Campo P, Zambonino MA, et al. Follow-up study in local allergic rhinitis shows a consistent entity not evolving to systemic allergic rhinitis. J Allergy Clin Immunol 2014;133(4):1026–31.
38. Gelardi M, Fiorella ML, Russo C, et al. Role of nasal cytology. Int J Immunopathol Pharmacol 2010;23(Suppl 1):45–9.
39. Gelardi M, Luigi Marseglia G, Licari A, et al. Nasal cytology in children: recent advances. Ital J Pediatr 2012;38:51.
40. Meltzer E, Schatz M, Nathan R, et al. Reliability, validity, and responsiveness of the Rhinitis Control Assessment Test in patients with rhinitis. J Allergy Clin Immunol 2013;131(2):379–86.
41. Bernstein JA, Salapatek AM, Lee JS, et al. Provocation of nonallergic rhinitis subjects in response to simulated weather conditions using an environmental exposure chamber model. Allergy Asthma Proc 2012;33:333–40.

Nonallergic Rhinitis

Treatment

Phillip L. Lieberman, MD[a,b,*], Peter Smith, MD[c]

KEYWORDS

- Nonallergic rhinitis • Vasomotor rhinitis • Nonallergic rhinopathy
- Noninfectious nonallergic rhinitis • Idiopathic rhinitis

KEY POINTS

- The therapy for nonallergic rhinitis is best based on the underlying pathology, which typically exists in a form whereby an abnormality of the autonomic nervous system is dominant or a form in which inflammation seems to be the cause of symptoms.
- In general nonallergic rhinitis is less responsive to treatment than its allergic counterpart.
- In most cases combination therapy with an intranasal corticosteroid and a topical nasal antihistamine is the most effective treatment.

DEFINITION

Chronic nonallergic rhinitis (NAR) is a syndrome rather than a specific disease. It is diagnosed by excluding other disorders. A lack of understanding of the pathogenesis of this condition has led to an imprecise terminology with several alternate names for this condition (**Table 1**).

NAR is best defined by the chronic presence of one or more symptoms of rhinitis, in the absence of a specific cause.

There is no consensus about how long symptoms should be present to establish chronicity, but many studies have required a minimum duration of more than 1 year.[1,2]

PATHOGENESIS

In order to understand the mechanisms of action of the medications used in the treatment of NAR, it is important to have some insight into the pathogenesis of this condition.

Disclosure Statement: Advisory board and speaker for Meda.
[a] Division of Allergy and Immunology, Department of Medicine, University of Tennessee, Memphis, TN, USA; [b] Department of Pediatrics, University of Tennessee, Memphis, TN, USA; [c] Qld Allergy Services, Clinical School of Medicine, Griffith University, 17/123 Nerang Street, Southport, Queensland 4215, Australia
* Corresponding author. 7205 Wolf River Boulevard, Suite 200, Germantown, TN 38138.
E-mail address: phillieberman@hotmail.com

Immunol Allergy Clin N Am 36 (2016) 305–319
http://dx.doi.org/10.1016/j.iac.2015.12.007
0889-8561/16/$ – see front matter © 2016 Elsevier Inc. All rights reserved.

Table 1
Treatment modalities for NAR

Treatment Modality	Comment
INS	It is the most useful in the inflammatory form of NAR. Not all studies have shown these agents to be effective. Efficacy may depend on triggers, with those patients who exhibit triggers only possibly responding to a lesser degree than those with triggers due to respiratory irritants (see text).
TA sprays	Azelastine is better studied than olopatadine, but one study of the latter indicated efficacy (see text). It is probably more effective in the inflammatory form. Effects are theoretically due to activities of these agents unrelated to their antagonism of H1 receptor stimulation.
Combination therapy with INS and TA	It is probably the most effective therapy to date. At least on a conceptual basis they should be more effective than either agent alone, and studies in allergic rhinitis have confirmed this.
Ipratropium bromide	It is effective only for rhinorrhea. It is of particular benefit in gustatory rhinitis and rhinitis due to exposure to cold.
Capsaicin	It is theoretically useful only in the noninflammatory form and thought to be effective because of desensitization or depletion of mediators. This effect seems to be mediated through TPV1.
Oral decongestants	There is a lack of good evidence of effect, but theoretically it may be helpful for nasal stuffiness only.
Nasal saline irrigation	It seems to have some modest effect in selected patients.
Oral antihistamines	Second-generation antihistamines theoretically should be of no benefit; but first-generation antihistamines, theoretically because of their anticholinergic activity, could be helpful in some patients.
Surgery	Numerous approaches have been studied, but reports are limited to case series. Of course, it is reserved for recalcitrant cases not responding to medical treatment.

Abbreviations: INS, intranasal corticosteroids; TA, topical antihistamine; TPV1, transient receptor potential cation channel subfamily V member 1.

Based on the fact that there seems to be many forms of this syndrome, there may be several different mechanisms underlying its clinical expression.[3–5] Several investigators have broadly divided NAR into noninflammatory and inflammatory forms.[6–33] The inflammatory form has been further divided into eosinophilic and noneosinophilic varieties.[1,2,6–33] With all forms of chronic NAR, there seems to be a component of autonomic dysregulation. In the noninflammatory form, these neurologic abnormalities are predominant.

For the purpose of this article, the authors have arbitrarily decided to use the inflammatory and noninflammatory classification in this brief discussion of NAR pathogenesis.

NONINFLAMMATORY FORMS

With the noninflammatory form, it is postulated that the disease results from abnormalities in the autonomic nervous system, which may include the adrenergic, cholinergic, and/or nonadrenergic, noncholinergic innervation of the nose.[8–11] Such abnormalities have also been demonstrated in the inflammatory form and, in that context, have been proposed to be secondary to the primary inflammatory process.[6,7,11,28] The nature and importance of these abnormalities has been clarified by Bernstein and colleagues[34] who evaluated the neurogenic responses to chemical/olfactory stimuli in patients with NAR using functional MRI. Subjects underwent MRI during exposure to different types of odors. They exhibited increased blood flow to several odor-sensitive regions of the brain in response to both pleasant (vanilla) and unpleasant (hickory smoke) odors. The neurologic responses were associated with the production of symptoms on exposure to hickory smoke.

Gustatory rhinitis is perhaps the prototype of noninflammatory NAR. In this condition eating, especially hot or spicy foods, produces profuse, watery rhinorrhea.[35] The underlying pathology seems to be a heightened cholinergic response.

Patients with noninflammatory NAR may display a variety of neurologic abnormalities, including heightened responses to cold, methacholine, and other stimuli designed to activate cholinergic responses[6,9,28] as well as diminished responses to vasoconstrictive stimuli[36] and increased concentrations of intranasal neuropeptides.[15]

Of growing importance in the pathogenesis of NAR is the recognition that a superfamily of 28 chemical, thermal, and nociceptors transmit the neural stimuli that trigger symptoms. The transient receptor potential (TRP) receptors, TRP vanilliod 1 (TRPV1) and TRP ankyrin 1 (TRPA1), are perhaps of particular note. TRPV1 is the receptor for capsaicin. Several triggers activate TRPA1, including cold dry air as well as dietary isothiocyanates (mustard, wasabi, horseradish), allicin (garlic and onion), environmental isothiocyanates, formalin, toluene, ozone, chlorite, and noxious components of smoke (acrolein, methacrolein, croton aldehyde).[37–54] TRPV1 and TRPA1 sensitization and activation patterns are summarized in **Fig. 1**.

INFLAMMATORY FORMS

Nasal eosinophilia occurs in a significant number of individuals with NAR. Nasal biopsies from these patients commonly show increased eosinophils as well as increased numbers of mast cells and prominent mast cell degranulation.[2,18] The cellular inflammatory infiltrate may have dominant cells other than eosinophils. Nasal cytology in some cases shows a predominance of mast cells and neutrophils.[55,56] These histologic findings may be associated with different clinical manifestations.[55] For example, eosinophilia can indicate responsiveness to glucocorticoids, whereas when mast cells are the predominant cell type, nasal itching is often a characteristic feature.[55]

The inflammatory cytokine pattern in chronic NAR may differ from that in normal nonrhinitis patients. In a study comparing patients with allergic rhinitis, NAR, and controls (45 included in each group), both the patient groups had increased levels of interleukins 16 and 17 compared with controls.[57]

By definition patients with chronic NAR have negative skin and in vitro tests for allergen-specific immunoglobulin E (IgE) and, thus, lack evidence of systemic production of allergen-specific IgE. However, IgE production has been shown to occur locally in the nasal tissue in some patients with NAR.[2,58–61] One group has shown that as many as one-half of patients with chronic NAR react to nasal challenge with allergen, especially dust mite allergen, with symptoms and signs similar to those experienced by patients with allergic rhinitis.[59,62,63] Because of these findings some investigators suggest performing an allergen-specific nasal challenge and measuring nasal-specific IgE levels in addition to standard allergy tests in this subgroup of patients. In addition, they recommend repeating allergy testing "after a time interval" because patients formerly diagnosed with NAR may develop allergic disease.[64–66]

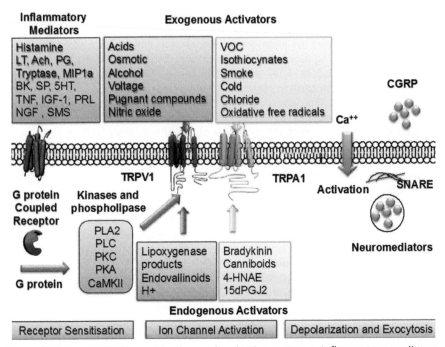

Fig. 1. TRPV1 and TRPA1 sensitization and activation patterns. Inflammatory mediators, neurokinins, hormones including histamine, LT, acetylcholine, prostaglandins, proteases including tryptase, bradykinin, MIP1 alpha, tumor necrosis factor (TNF) alpha, insulin growth factor 1 (IGF-1), prolactin, nerve growth factor (NGF), somatostatin, and calcitonin gene-related peptide (CGRP) act via their receptors to activate kinase and phospholipase systems, which prime TRPV1. Priming of TRPA1 is less defined. Once primed, the receptors become more susceptible to activation by endogenous and exogenous compounds. Activation results in a preferential influx of calcium and, in the case of sensory nerves, depolarization. This process promotes active exocytosis of neuromediators at the peripheral nerve terminals. The later process is reported to comprise the major component of neurogenic inflammation. BK, bradykinin; LT, Leukotriene; MIP1, Macrophage Inflammatory Protein; PC, phospholipase C; PG, prostaglandin; SP, substance P; VOC, volatile organic compound.

These observations have prompted the question as to whether the production of local allergen-specific IgE in patients with symptoms of rhinitis is simply premonitory to the development of the systemic production of these IgE antibodies. In this case one would expect the appearance of positive skin tests and serum-specific IgE in the future. A prospective 10-year follow-up study with initial cohorts of 194 patients with local allergic rhinitis and 130 healthy controls was designed to answer this question. After 5 years of follow-up, skin prick tests and/or serum-specific IgE became positive in 6.81% of patients with local allergic rhinitis and in 4.5% of controls. The investigators interpreted these findings as indicating local allergic rhinitis is a separate condition from classic allergic rhinitis and not simply a premonitory phase of this disorder.[67]

Contrary to these observations, other researchers were unable to demonstrate consistent responses to nasal allergen challenge in patients with NAR,[68] challenging the concept that NAR results from a localized, IgE-mediated mechanism. Furthermore, localized allergic rhinitis (LAR) patients respond to medications conventionally used to treat allergic rhinitis, which are characteristically not as effective in NAR.

TREATMENT
Overview

The basic medications that we use to treat NAR are similar but not identical to those used for allergic rhinitis. These medications include intranasal glucocorticoids (INS), topical antihistamine (TA) sprays, combination therapy with INS and TA, ipratropium bromide, capsaicin, oral and intranasal decongestants, nasal saline irrigation, first-generation oral antihistamines, and surgery.

As can be seen in **Table 1**, and as mentioned earlier, knowledge of the pathogenesis of NAR is helpful in the choice of treatment. In the inflammatory form of this disease, INS and TA are probably the most helpful compounds; in the noninflammatory variety, ipratropium bromide and capsaicin play an important role.

Unfortunately patients with chronic NAR are in general less responsive to pharmacologic therapy than those with allergic rhinitis.[7,69] For example, second-generation oral antihistamines are usually not helpful.[70,71] In contrast, first-generation antihistamines may be more effective in the noninflammatory form because of their anticholinergic activity, which helps reduce postnasal drainage. The 2 classes of medications most useful in treating the total symptom complex of chronic NAR[72–83] are intranasal corticosteroids (INS) and topical nasal antihistamines (TA). Additionally ipratropium bromide is specifically effective in the therapy for rhinorrhea.[84,85] Nasal decongestants, both topically and orally, can be used to treat patients who have continued nasal congestion in spite of the use of intranasal corticosteroids. They can be applied as adjunctive agents in this regard (see later discussion).

Patients with mild disease may be adequately treated with either an INS or TA. There are no comparative studies specifically designed to compare these two agents. Those with moderate to severe disease tend to respond better to the combination of an INS and TA.[86]

Specific Agents

Intranasal corticosteroids

Several INS preparations have been shown to be effective for most patients in multiple randomized controlled studies.[75,76,78,87] Multiple preparations are available. The largest report demonstrating a treatment effect with INS was a combined analysis of 3 double-blind, randomized, prospective, placebo-controlled studies of 983 patients with NAR. Included in this evaluation were subjects with and without nasal eosinophilia (674 were classified as without nasal eosinophils).[87] Intranasal fluticasone propionate at doses of 200 or 400 µg was more effective than placebo in both groups, as assessed by total nasal symptom scores for nasal obstruction, postnasal drip, and rhinorrhea.

However, not all patients with NAR have been shown to respond to INS. A large study showed no significant impact on symptoms.[7] A subsequent multicenter trial was performed to assess the effects of INS therapy on a subset of patients with symptoms triggered predominantly by weather and temperature changes.[88] In this randomized study, which excluded patients triggered by respiratory irritants, 699 patients with NAR triggered by weather factors were treated with either fluticasone furoate or placebo for 4 weeks. There were no significant differences between the two groups. Thus, although patients with NAR as a group respond to INS, there may be subgroups of nonresponders that require further study. Specifically, based on this study, those with symptoms triggered by respiratory irritants may respond to a greater extent than those with problems related only to weather conditions.

Topical antihistamine sprays

Two topical antihistamine sprays have been studied in NAR. These sprays are azelastine and olopatadine.

Azelastine is the best studied of the two and the only one to be evaluated in a double-blind, multicenter, placebo-controlled trial.[77] It is available as Astelin in a 0.1% preparation containing 137 mcg per actuation that is dosed 2 actuations each nostril twice daily in adults and one actuation twice daily in children. It is also available in a 0.15% concentration (Astepro, containing 205 mcg per actuation), one to 2 actuations per nostril twice daily and decreasing the dose as symptoms improve. The 0.15% version contains sucralose as a taste-masking agent. It decreases the incidence of taste perversion (bad taste), which is one of the most common side effects of this drug. Both concentrations are available as generic preparations.

Olopatadine hydrochloride nasal spray (0.06%) is available as Patanase (containing 665 mcg per actuation) that is dosed 2 actuations twice daily in adults and one actuation twice daily for children down to 6 years of age. Patanase has not been approved for use in NAR.

As monotherapy, azelastine has been shown to be effective in randomized controlled studies.[77,89] In 2 multicenter randomized open-label trials, approximately 80% to 85% of more than 200 subjects with NAR responded favorably to azelastine.[77] Significant improvement was seen in all symptoms evaluated.

The improvement in symptoms with azelastine is likely in part due to its antiinflammatory properties. These effects are multiple. They include the ability to diminish eosinophil activation and adhesion molecule expression and suppression of inflammatory cytokine generation.[81,82,90] Azelastine may also reduce neurogenic excitation from olfactory stimuli. In the previously mentioned study in which subjects with NAR were exposed to pleasant and unpleasant odors, the administration of azelastine significantly attenuated exaggerated blood flow to odor-sensitive regions of the brain as assessed by MRI.[34] More recently, an in vitro cell study found that azelastine, like capsaicin, can activate TRPV1 receptors and with continuous cell exposure can desensitize these receptors. A similar effect was seen with the antihistamine bepotastine but not with olopatadine or fluticasone.[91]

Olopatadine and azelastine (0.1%) were compared for the treatment of NAR in a multicenter, randomized parallel group study lasting 14 days.[92] Both reduced congestion, rhinorrhea, postnasal drip, and sneezing; there were no statistically significant differences between their effects. In addition, there was no difference in the side-effect profile of the two agents. But this study did not contain a placebo arm and was powered only to assess noninferiority. In another placebo-controlled study, olopatadine reduced the exaggerated response to hyperosmolar challenge in patients with prominent vasomotor symptoms.[93] This drug, like azelastine, also seems to have clinically significant antiinflammatory activity unrelated to its antagonism of histamine receptor 1 stimulation.[93]

Combination therapy with intranasal corticosteroids and azelastine

The most effective treatment of NAR uses the combination of INS and azelastine. Based on several studies in allergic rhinitis the combined treatment is more effective than either agent alone. Combination therapy can be achieved either by using 2 separate nasal sprays or a combination product. A combination spray containing azelastine hydrochloride 137 mcg and fluticasone propionate 50 mcg (Dymista) became available in the United States in 2012 and is approved for children down to age 5 years and adults for seasonal allergic rhinitis. The dose is one actuation per nostril, twice daily. This combination product has been studied in patients with seasonal allergic rhinitis and has been shown to be superior to single treatment with either agent alone.[94] Also in a post hoc analysis of a 1-year, randomized, open-label, active-controlled, parallel-group study in 612 subjects aged 12 years and older with perennial allergic rhinitis (424 subjects) or NAR (188 subjects), Dymista was found to be effective in both groups. Efficacy was assessed by change from baseline in PM reflective total nasal symptom score (rTNSS), time to first achieve 100% PM rTNSS reduction from baseline, and percentage of symptom-free days.[95]

The conclusion one draws from these investigations is that combination treatment with azelastine and fluticasone seems to be at this time the treatment of choice in most individuals with NAR.

Ipratropium bromide

When rhinorrhea is the only symptom or the dominant symptom, as in gustatory or skiers/joggers rhinitis, ipratropium bromide (0.03% or 0.06%) nasal spray is recommended and is the treatment of choice.[35,96] Ipratropium bromide is usually used at a dose of one or 2 sprays each nostril up to 3 times a day. Alternatively, it can also be used as needed or an hour before exposures that cause rhinorrhea, such as cold air or before eating. The concentration of 0.06% is usually intended only for short-term use (eg, treatment of rhinorrhea associated with the common cold). Two multicenter placebo-controlled trials have demonstrated the effectiveness of ipratropium bromide to control rhinorrhea.[84,85]

The administration of ipratropium bromide nasal spray (0.03%) for 1 year among 285 patients with perennial NAR resulted in significant improvement in rhinorrhea as well as a decreased need for additional medications to control symptoms.[84] In addition, in a study of 253 patients with perennial NAR, ipratropium nasal spray significantly reduced rhinorrhea versus that observed with placebo.[85] However, this drug has little if any effect on any manifestation of rhinitis other than anterior rhinorrhea.

Adjunctive therapies

Adjunctive therapies include topical capsaicin, oral or topical decongestants, nasal saline sprays and irrigations, and oral antihistamines. Studies of antileukotriene drugs and intranasal chromones in the treatment of NAR are lacking, but clinical consensus is these medications are relatively ineffective for this condition.

Topical capsaicin

Topical capsaicin has been shown to diminish the symptoms of NAR, but irritation of the nasal mucosa can be a limiting factor.[97,98] A randomized trial of 42 patients with NAR evaluated the effects of a diluted capsaicin nasal spray to which eucalyptol was added to reduce the burning sensation caused by this agent (Sinus Buster Nasal Spray [Akorn, Incorporated, Lake Forest, IL, USA]).[99] After 2 weeks of therapy with this preparation (dosed up to 12 actuations daily), patients reported significant improvements in total nasal symptom scores compared with placebo and good tolerability. This preparation is available without a prescription. A recent Cochrane Review of the use of capsaicin concluded "Capsaicin may be an option in the treatment of idiopathic non-allergic rhinitis." It is given in the form of brief treatments, usually during the same day. It seems to have beneficial effects on overall nasal symptoms up to 36 weeks after treatment, based on a few small studies (low-quality evidence). Well-conducted randomized controlled trials are required to further advance our understanding of the effectiveness of capsaicin in NAR, especially in patients with NAR of different types and severity, and using different methods of capsaicin application.[100]

Oral and intranasal decongestants

Although there are no specific studies examining the clinical efficacy of decongestants for NAR, they can used as needed only for congestion not responsive to the use of a nasal glucocorticoid, topical nasal antihistamine, or a combination of both. An oral decongestant, such as pseudoephedrine or phenylephrine, can be added to the treatment regimen. The usual dosing of pseudoephedrine is 30 or 60 mg, up to 3 times daily on symptomatic days. A sustained-release preparation of 120 mg used twice daily is also available. Phenylephrine hydrochloride is less effective and in some studies has not been superior to placebo at the 10-mg dose that is commonly available without prescription.[101,102] Intranasal decongestants when used as monotherapy for extended periods of time can cause rebound nasal congestion or tolerance (tachyphylaxis). However, several recent studies of perennial and seasonal allergic rhinitis have indicated this agent can be used for longer periods of time without inducing tolerance if used in conjunction with an intranasal corticosteroid. This combination therapy has yet to be investigated in NAR; however, clinical experience indicates it is effective and well tolerated for this condition as well.[103–105]

Nasal saline irrigation

A large body of observational reports and one prospective controlled clinical study has found that nasal lavage can be helpful in NAR.[106,107] In the only prospective study the use of nasal irrigation significantly improved nasal symptoms.[107] Intranasal saline sprays have been found effective in relieving postnasal drip, sneezing, and congestion.[72,108] Saline sprays may be somewhat less effective than larger-volume nasal lavage, although they may be more convenient for some patients.[109] A variety of over-the-counter devices, including bulb syringes and bottle sprayers, are effective, provided the system delivers an adequate volume of solution (>200 mL per side) into the nose.

Oral antihistamines

Clinical experience and limited data suggest that the newer nonsedating H1 antihistamines are not as effective in NAR, compared with allergic rhinitis.[70,71] Older, first-generation H1 antihistamines (eg, chlorpheniramine) have anticholinergic properties that may be helpful to some patients with persistent and bothersome postnasal drip and/or anterior rhinorrhea despite the use of the aforementioned therapies.[110] However, these medications are sedating; but if dosed at night the carryover effect during the day is minimal making these agents well tolerated in most patients.

Role of surgery

Several surgical approaches have been used in patients with severe chronic NAR.[96,111–114] These approaches have been reported as uncontrolled case series. Such interventions can be considered in patients with recalcitrant symptoms not responding to standard therapies, such as topical nasal steroids in combination with TA and/or decongestants and/or ipratropium bromide. Six to 12 months of medical management should be allowed before surgical options are considered.

A turbinectomy can be performed when congestion is predominant. With this technique there has been concern about the destruction and/or elimination of the mucosal surface. However, laser turbinectomy has been reported to preserve normal nasal cytology as well as normal ciliary activity.[113]

Several other surgical procedures have been tried in the past, including vidian nerve resection, electrocoagulation of anterior ethmoidal nerve, sphenopalatine ganglion block, and others.[114–116] None of these techniques has been shown to have long-term benefits, and the potential risks (eg, persistent pain) have to be considered carefully because they may outweigh any possible benefits.

Other alternative and complementary therapies have been evaluated, such as acupuncture and topical silver nitrate, although these cannot be recommended at this time.

Prognosis

NAR is a persistent condition, usually present lifelong. In one study, 180 patients with NAR were reevaluated 3 to 7 years after the initial diagnosis was made.[117] Patients with NAR generally experienced worsening disease (52%), with an increase in the persistence (12%) and severity (9%) of nasal symptoms. In addition, 24% developed new comorbidities over time. Asthma was the most frequently developed comorbidity at the reevaluation, increasing from 32% to 55% of the subjects. There was also an increase in the development of sinusitis. This longitudinal study emphasizes the need for research to further elucidate relevant mechanistic pathways for NAR, which could potentially lead to novel, more effective therapeutic strategies.

REFERENCES

1. Blom HM, Godthelp T, Fokkens WJ, et al. Mast cells, eosinophils and IgE-positive cells in the nasal mucosa of patients with vasomotor rhinitis. An immunohistochemical study. Eur Arch Otorhinolaryngol 1995;252(Suppl 1):S33.
2. Powe DG, Huskisson RS, Carney AS, et al. Evidence for an inflammatory pathophysiology in idiopathic rhinitis. Clin Exp Allergy 2001;31:864.
3. Bousquet J, Fokkens W, Burney P, et al. Important research questions in allergy and related diseases: nonallergic rhinitis: a GA2LEN paper. Allergy 2008;63: 842.
4. Wallace DV, Dykewicz MS, Bernstein DI, et al. The diagnosis and management of rhinitis: an updated practice parameter. J Allergy Clin Immunol 2008;122:S1.
5. van Rijswijk JB, Blom HM, Fokkens WJ. Idiopathic rhinitis, the ongoing quest. Allergy 2005;60:1471.
6. Numata T, Konno A, Hasegawa S, et al. Pathophysiological features of the nasal mucosa in patients with idiopathic rhinitis compared to allergic rhinitis. Int Arch Allergy Immunol 1999;119:304.
7. Blom HM, Godthelp T, Fokkens WJ, et al. The effect of nasal steroid aqueous spray on nasal complaint scores and cellular infiltrates in the nasal mucosa of patients with nonallergic, noninfectious perennial rhinitis. J Allergy Clin Immunol 1997;100:739.
8. Malcomson KG. The vasomotor activities of the nasal mucous membrane. J Laryngol Otol 1959;73:73.
9. Jones AS, Lancer JM. Vasomotor rhinitis. Br Med J (Clin Res Ed) 1987;294:1505.
10. Wilde AD, Cook JA, Jones AS. The nasal response to isometric exercise. Clin Otolaryngol Allied Sci 1995;20:345.
11. Wolf G. New aspects in the pathogenesis and therapy of hyperreflexive rhinopathy. Laryngol Rhinol Otol (Stuttg) 1988;67:438.
12. Moneret-Vautrin DA, Hsieh V, Wayoff M, et al. Nonallergic rhinitis with eosinophilia syndrome a precursor of the triad: nasal polyposis, intrinsic asthma, and intolerance to aspirin. Ann Allergy 1990;64:513.
13. Baraniuk JN. Neural control of human nasal secretion. Pulm Pharmacol 1991;4: 20.
14. Lundblad L, Hua XY, Lundberg JM. Mechanisms for reflexive hypertension induced by local application of capsaicin and nicotine to the nasal mucosa. Acta Physiol Scand 1984;121:277.

15. Lacrois JS, Pochon N, Lundberg JM. Increased concentration of sensory neuro-peptide in the nasal mucosa from patients with nonallergic chronic rhinitis. In: Passall D, editor. The new frontier of otorhinolaryngology in Europe. Sorrento (Italy): Monduzzi Editore; 1992. p. 59.
16. Borson DB. Roles of neutral endopeptidase in airways. Am J Physiol 1991;260: L212.
17. Trotter CM, Hall GH, Salter DM, et al. Histology of mucous membrane of human inferior nasal concha. Clin Anat 1990;3:307.
18. Berger G, Goldberg A, Ophir D. The inferior turbinate mast cell population of patients with perennial allergic and nonallergic rhinitis. Am J Rhinol 1997;11:63.
19. Bachert C, Prohaska P, Pipkorn U. IgE-positive mast cells on the human nasal mucosal surface in response to allergen exposure. Rhinology 1990;28:149.
20. Otsuka H, Inaba M, Fujikura T, et al. Histochemical and functional characteris-tics of metachromatic cells in the nasal epithelium in allergic rhinitis: studies of nasal scrapings and their dispersed cells. J Allergy Clin Immunol 1995;96:528.
21. Fokkens WJ, Godthelp T, Holm AF, et al. Dynamics of mast cells in the nasal mucosa of patients with allergic rhinitis and non-allergic controls: a biopsy study. Clin Exp Allergy 1992;22:701.
22. Ying S, Durham SR, Jacobson MR, et al. T lymphocytes and mast cells express messenger RNA for interleukin-4 in the nasal mucosa in allergen-induced rhinitis. Immunology 1994;82:200.
23. Varney VA, Jacobson MR, Sudderick RM, et al. Immunohistology of the nasal mucosa following allergen-induced rhinitis. Identification of activated T lympho-cytes, eosinophils, and neutrophils. Am Rev Respir Dis 1992;146:170.
24. Godthelp T, Holm AF, Fokkens WJ, et al. Dynamics of nasal eosinophils in response to a nonnatural allergen challenge in patients with allergic rhinitis and control subjects: a biopsy and brush study. J Allergy Clin Immunol 1996; 97:800.
25. Connell JT. Nasal mastocytosis. J Allergy 1969;43:182.
26. Drake-Lee AB, Moriarty B, Smallman LA. Mast cell numbers in the mucosa of the inferior turbinate in patients with perennial allergic rhinitis: a light microscopic study. J Laryngol Otol 1991;105:736.
27. Ruhno J, Howie K, Anderson M, et al. The increased number of epithelial mast cells in nasal polyps and adjacent turbinates is not allergy-dependent. Allergy 1990;45:370.
28. Malm L, Wihl JA, Lamm CJ, et al. Reduction of methacholine-induced nasal secretion by treatment with a new topical steroid in perennial non-allergic rhinitis. Allergy 1981;36:209.
29. Humbert M, Menz G, Ying S, et al. The immunopathology of extrinsic (atopic) and intrinsic (non-atopic) asthma: more similarities than differences. Immunol Today 1999;20:528.
30. Humbert M, Grant JA, Taborda-Barata L, et al. High-affinity IgE receptor (FcepsilonRI)-bearing cells in bronchial biopsies from atopic and nonatopic asthma. Am J Respir Crit Care Med 1996;153:1931.
31. Kroegel C, Jäger L, Walker C. Is there a place for intrinsic asthma as a distinct immunopathological entity? Eur Respir J 1997;10:513.
32. Togias AG, Proud D, Lichtenstein LM, et al. The osmolality of nasal secretions increases when inflammatory mediators are released in response to inhalation of cold, dry air. Am Rev Respir Dis 1988;137:625.
33. Howarth PH, Salagean M, Dokic D. Allergic rhinitis: not purely a histamine-related disease. Allergy 2000;55(Suppl 64):7.

34. Bernstein JA, Hastings L, Boespflug EL, et al. Alteration of brain activation patterns in nonallergic rhinitis patients using functional magnetic resonance imaging before and after treatment with intranasal azelastine. Ann Allergy Asthma Immunol 2011;106:527.

35. Raphael G, Raphael MH, Kaliner M. Gustatory rhinitis: a syndrome of food-induced rhinorrhea. J Allergy Clin Immunol 1989;83:110.

36. Papon JF, Brugel-Ribere L, Fodil R, et al. Nasal wall compliance in vasomotor rhinitis. J Appl Physiol (1985) 2006;100:107.

37. Story GM, Peier AM, Reeve AJ, et al. ANKTM1, a TRP-like channel expressed in nociceptive neurons, is activated by cold temperatures. Cell 2003;112:819–29.

38. Trevisani M, Siemens J, Materazzi S, et al. 4-Hydroxynonenal, an endogenous aldehyde, causes pain and neurogenic inflammation through activation of the irritant receptor TRPA1. Proc Natl Acad Sci U S A 2007;104(33):13519–24.

39. Bautista DM, Jordt SE, Nikai T, et al. TRPA1 mediates the inflammatory actions of environmental irritants and proalgesic agents. Cell 2006;124(6):1269–82.

40. Taylor-Clark TE, Undem BJ, Macglashan DW Jr, et al. Prostaglandin-induced activation of nociceptive neurons via direct interaction with transient receptor potential A1 (TRPA1). Mol Pharmacol 2008;73(2):274–81.

41. Bandell M, Story GM, Hwang SW, et al. Sensitization of TRPA1: a molecular mechanism of inflammatory pain. Brain 2008;131(Pt 5):1241–51.

42. Corey DP, Garcia-Anoveros J, Holt JR, et al. TRPA1 mediates formalin-induced pain. Proc Natl Acad Sci U S A 2007;104(33):13525–30.

43. Patapoutian A. Noxious cold ion channel TRPA1 is activated by pungent compounds and bradykinin. Neuron 2004;41(6):849–57.

44. Bautista DM, Movahed P, Hinman A, et al. Pungent products from garlic activate the sensory ion channel TRPA1. Proc Natl Acad Sci U S A 2005;102(34):12248–52.

45. Jordt SE, Bautista DM, Chuang HH, et al. Mustard oils and cannabinoids excite sensory nerve fibres through the TRP channel ANKTM1. Nature 2004;427:260–5.

46. Macpherson LJ, Geierstanger BH, Viswanath V, et al. The pungency of garlic: activation of TRPA1 and TRPV1 in response to allicin. Curr Biol 2005;15(10):929–34.

47. Macpherson LJ, Xiao B, Kwan KY, et al. An ion channel essential for sensing chemical damage. J Neurosci 2007;27(42):11412–5.

48. Namer B, Seifert F, Handwerker HO, et al. TRPA1 and TRPM8 activation in humans: effects of cinnamaldehyde and menthol. Neuroreport 2005;16(9):955–9.

49. Merrill AW, Cuellar JM, Judd JH, et al. Effects of TRPA1 agonists mustard oil and cinnamaldehyde on lumbar spinal wide-dynamic range neuronal responses to innocuous and noxious cutaneous stimuli in rats. J Neurophysiol 2008;99(2):415–25.

50. Puig S, Sorkin LS. Formalin-evoked activity in identified primary afferent fibers: systemic lidocaine suppresses phase-2 activity. Pain 1996;64(2):345–55.

51. Koizumi K, Iwasaki Y, Narukawa M, et al. Diallyl sulfides in garlic activate both TRPA1 and TRPV1. Biochem Biophys Res Commun 2009;382(3):545–8.

52. Escalera J, von Hehn CA, Bessac BF, et al. TRPA1 mediates the noxious effects of natural sesquiterpene deterrents. J Biol Chem 2008;283:24136–44.

53. Bessac BF, Sivula M, von Hehn CA, et al. TRPA1 is a major oxidant sensor in murine airway sensory neurons. J Clin Invest 2008;118:1899–910.

54. Andre E, Campi B, Materazzi S, et al. Cigarette smoke-induced neurogenic inflammation is mediated by alpha, beta-unsaturated aldehydes and the TRPA1 receptor in rodents. J Clin Invest 2008;118:2574–82.

55. Maselli Del Giudice A, Barbara M, Russo GM, et al. Cell-mediated non-allergic rhinitis in children. Int J Pediatr Otorhinolaryngol 2012;76:1741.

56. Gelardi M, Luigi Marseglia G, Licari A, et al. Nasal cytology in children: recent advances. Ital J Pediatr 2012;38:51.

57. Cai J, Guan S, Mai Z, et al. Analysis of the level and significance of IL-16 and IL-17 in nasal secretion and in serum of patients with allergic rhinitis and non-allergic rhinitis. Lin Chung Er Bi Yan Hou Tou Jing Wai Ke Za Zhi 2014;28(11): 821–3 [in Chinese].

58. Klein Jan A, Vinke JG, Severijnen LW, et al. Local production and detection of (specific) IgE in nasal B-cells and plasma cells of allergic rhinitis patients. Eur Respir J 2000;15:491.

59. Rondón C, Romero JJ, López S, et al. Local IgE production and positive nasal provocation test in patients with persistent nonallergic rhinitis. J Allergy Clin Immunol 2007;119:899.

60. Rondón C, Fernández J, López S, et al. Nasal inflammatory mediators and specific IgE production after nasal challenge with grass pollen in local allergic rhinitis. J Allergy Clin Immunol 2009;124:1005.

61. Rondón C, Campo P, Togias A, et al. Local allergic rhinitis: concept, pathophysiology, and management. J Allergy Clin Immunol 2012;129:1460.

62. Rondón C, Campo P, Herrera R, et al. Nasal allergen provocation test with multiple aeroallergens detects polysensitization in local allergic rhinitis. J Allergy Clin Immunol 2011;128:1192.

63. Rondón C, Campo P, Galindo L, et al. Prevalence and clinical relevance of local allergic rhinitis. Allergy 2012;67:1282.

64. Klimek L, Bardenhewer C, Spielhaupter M, et al. Local allergic rhinitis to Alternaria alternata: evidence for local IgE production exclusively in the nasal mucosa. HNO 2015;63(5):364–72 [in German].

65. Klimek L, von Bernus L, Pfaar O. Local (exclusive) IgE production in the nasal mucosa. Evidence for local allergic rhinitis. HNO 2013;61(3):217–23 [in German].

66. Campo P, Rondón C, Gould HJ, et al. Local IgE in non-allergic rhinitis. Clin Exp Allergy 2015;45(5):872–81.

67. Rondón C, Campo P, Zambonino MA, et al. Follow-up study in local allergic rhinitis shows a consistent entity not evolving to systemic allergic rhinitis. J Allergy Clin Immunol 2014;133(4):1026–31.

68. Wierzbicki DA, Majmundar AR, Schull DE, et al. Multiallergen nasal challenges in nonallergic rhinitis. Ann Allergy Asthma Immunol 2008;100:533.

69. Philip G, Togias AG. Nonallergic rhinitis. Pathophysiology and models for study. Eur Arch Otorhinolaryngol 1995;252(Suppl 1):S27.

70. Mullarkey MF. Eosinophilic nonallergic rhinitis. J Allergy Clin Immunol 1988;82:941.

71. Rinne J, Simola M, Malmberg H, et al. Early treatment of perennial rhinitis with budesonide or cetirizine and its effect on long-term outcome. J Allergy Clin Immunol 2002;109:426.

72. Settipane RA, Lieberman P. Update on nonallergic rhinitis. Ann Allergy Asthma Immunol 2001;86:494.

73. Kondo H, Nachtigal D, Frenkiel S, et al. Effect of steroids on nasal inflammatory cells and cytokine profile. Laryngoscope 1999;109:91.

74. Malm L, Wihl JA. Intra-nasal beclomethasone dipropionate in vasomotor rhinitis. Acta Allergol 1976;31:245.
75. Wight RG, Jones AS, Beckingham E, et al. A double blind comparison of intra-nasal budesonide 400 micrograms and 800 micrograms in perennial rhinitis. Clin Otolaryngol Allied Sci 1992;17:354.
76. Small P, Black M, Frenkiel S. Effects of treatment with beclomethasone dipropionate in subpopulations of perennial rhinitis patients. J Allergy Clin Immunol 1982;70:178.
77. Banov CH, Lieberman P, Vasomotor Rhinitis Study Groups. Efficacy of azelastine nasal spray in the treatment of vasomotor (perennial nonallergic) rhinitis. Ann Allergy Asthma Immunol 2001;86:28.
78. Scadding GK, Lund VJ, Jacques LA, et al. A placebo-controlled study of fluticasone propionate aqueous nasal spray and beclomethasone dipropionate in perennial rhinitis: efficacy in allergic and non-allergic perennial rhinitis. Clin Exp Allergy 1995;25:737.
79. Pipkorn U, Berge T. Long-term treatment with budesonide in vasomotor rhinitis. Acta Otolaryngol 1983;95:167.
80. Takao A, Shimoda T, Matsuse H, et al. Inhibitory effects of azelastine hydrochloride in alcohol-induced asthma. Ann Allergy Asthma Immunol 1999;82:390.
81. Ciprandi G, Pronzato C, Passalacqua G, et al. Topical azelastine reduces eosinophil activation and intercellular adhesion molecule-1 expression on nasal epithelial cells: an antiallergic activity. J Allergy Clin Immunol 1996;98:1088.
82. Yoneda K, Yamamoto T, Ueta E, et al. Suppression by azelastine hydrochloride of NF-kappa B activation involved in generation of cytokines and nitric oxide. Jpn J Pharmacol 1997;73:145.
83. Tamaoki J, Yamawaki I, Tagaya E, et al. Effect of azelastine on platelet-activating factor-induced microvascular leakage in rat airways. Am J Physiol 1999;276: L351.
84. Grossman J, Banov C, Boggs P, et al. Use of ipratropium bromide nasal spray in chronic treatment of nonallergic perennial rhinitis, alone and in combination with other perennial rhinitis medications. J Allergy Clin Immunol 1995;95:1123.
85. Bronsky EA, Druce H, Findlay SR, et al. A clinical trial of ipratropium bromide nasal spray in patients with perennial nonallergic rhinitis. J Allergy Clin Immunol 1995;95:1117.
86. Hampel FC, Ratner PH, Van Bavel J, et al. Double-blind, placebo-controlled study of azelastine and fluticasone in a single nasal spray delivery device. Ann Allergy Asthma Immunol 2010;105:168.
87. Webb DR, Meltzer EO, Finn AF Jr, et al. Intranasal fluticasone propionate is effective for perennial nonallergic rhinitis with or without eosinophilia. Ann Allergy Asthma Immunol 2002;88:385.
88. Jacobs R, Lieberman P, Kent E, et al. Weather/temperature-sensitive vasomotor rhinitis may be refractory to intranasal corticosteroid treatment. Allergy Asthma Proc 2009;30:120.
89. Lieberman P, Kaliner MA, Wheeler WJ. Open-label evaluation of azelastine nasal spray in patients with seasonal allergic rhinitis and nonallergic vasomotor rhinitis. Curr Med Res Opin 2005;21:611.
90. Lieberman P. Intranasal antihistamines for allergic rhinitis: mechanism of action. Allergy Asthma Proc 2009;30:345.
91. Singh U, Bernstein JA, Haar L, et al. Azelastine desensitization of transient receptor potential vanilloid 1: a potential mechanism explaining its therapeutic effect in nonallergic rhinitis. Am J Rhinol Allergy 2014;28:215–24.

92. Lieberman P, Meltzer EO, LaForce CF, et al. Two-week comparison study of olopatadine hydrochloride nasal spray 0.6% versus azelastine hydrochloride nasal spray 0.1% in patients with vasomotor rhinitis. Allergy Asthma Proc 2011;32:151.
93. Smith PK, Collins J. Olopatadine 0.6% nasal spray protects from vasomotor challenge in patients with severe vasomotor rhinitis. Am J Rhinol Allergy 2011; 25:e149.
94. Carr W, Bernstein J, Lieberman P, et al. A novel intranasal therapy of azelastine with fluticasone for the treatment of allergic rhinitis. J Allergy Clin Immunol 2012; 129:1282.
95. Price D, Shah S, Bhatia S, et al. A new therapy (MP29-02) is effective for the long-term treatment of chronic rhinitis. J Investig Allergol Clin Immunol 2013; 23(7):495–503.
96. Georgalas C, Jovancevic L. Gustatory rhinitis. Curr Opin Otolaryngol Head Neck Surg 2012;20:9.
97. Blom HM, Van Rijswijk JB, Garrelds IM, et al. Intranasal capsaicin is efficacious in non-allergic, non-infectious perennial rhinitis. A placebo-controlled study. Clin Exp Allergy 1997;27:796.
98. Marabini S, Ciabatti PG, Polli G, et al. Beneficial effects of intranasal applications of capsaicin in patients with vasomotor rhinitis. Eur Arch Otorhinolaryngol 1991;248:191.
99. Bernstein JA, Davis BP, Picard JK, et al. A randomized, double-blind, parallel trial comparing capsaicin nasal spray with placebo in subjects with a significant component of nonallergic rhinitis. Ann Allergy Asthma Immunol 2011;107:171.
100. Gevorgyan A, Segboer C, Gorissen R, et al. Capsaicin for non-allergic rhinitis. Cochrane Database Syst Rev 2015;(7):CD010591.
101. Hatton RC, Winterstein AG, McKelvey RP, et al. Efficacy and safety of oral phenylephrine: systematic review and meta-analysis. Ann Pharmacother 2007; 41:381.
102. Horak F, Zieglmayer P, Zieglmayer R, et al. A placebo-controlled study of the nasal decongestant effect of phenylephrine and pseudoephedrine in the Vienna Challenge Chamber. Ann Allergy Asthma Immunol 2009;102:116.
103. Baroody FM, Brown D, Gavanescu L, et al. Oxymetazoline adds to the effectiveness of fluticasone furoate in the treatment of perennial allergic rhinitis. J Allergy Clin Immunol 2011;127(4):927–34.
104. Meltzer EO, Bernstein DI, Prenner BM, et al. Mometasone furoate nasal spray plus oxymetazoline nasal spray: short-term efficacy and safety in seasonal allergic rhinitis. Am J Rhinol Allergy 2013;27(2):102–8.
105. Vaidyanathan S, Williamson P, Clearie K, et al. Fluticasone reverses oxymetazoline-induced tachyphylaxis of response and rebound congestion. Am J Respir Crit Care Med 2010;182(1):19–24.
106. Harvey R, Hannan SA, Badia L, et al. Nasal saline irrigations for the symptoms of chronic rhinosinusitis. Cochrane Database Syst Rev 2007;(3):CD006394.
107. Tomooka LT, Murphy C, Davidson TM. Clinical study and literature review of nasal irrigation. Laryngoscope 2000;110:1189.
108. Spector SL. The placebo effect is nothing to sneeze at. J Allergy Clin Immunol 1992;90:1042.
109. Pynnonen MA, Mukerji SS, Kim HM, et al. Nasal saline for chronic sinonasal symptoms: a randomized controlled trial. Arch Otolaryngol Head Neck Surg 2007;133:1115.

110. Meltzer EO. An overview of current pharmacotherapy in perennial rhinitis. J Allergy Clin Immunol 1995;95:1097.
111. el-Guindy A. Endoscopic transseptal vidian neurectomy. Arch Otolaryngol Head Neck Surg 1994;120:1347.
112. Dong Z. Anterior ethmoidal electrocoagulation in the treatment of vasomotor rhinitis. Zhonghua Er Bi Yan Hou Ke Za Zhi 1991;26:358.
113. Mladina R, Risavi R, Subaric M. CO2 laser anterior turbinectomy in the treatment of non-allergic vasomotor rhinopathia. A prospective study upon 78 patients. Rhinology 1991;29:267.
114. Fernandes CM. Bilateral transnasal vidian neurectomy in the management of chronic rhinitis. J Laryngol Otol 1994;108:569.
115. Prasanna A, Murthy PS. Vasomotor rhinitis and sphenopalatine ganglion block. J Pain Symptom Manage 1997;13:332.
116. Prianikov PD, Svistushkin VM, Egorov VI, et al. The modern approach to the treatment of the patients presenting with vasomotor rhinitis with the use of the electrosurgical technique. Vestn Otorinolaringol 2015;2:63–6.
117. Rondón C, Doña I, Torres MJ, et al. Evolution of patients with nonallergic rhinitis supports conversion to allergic rhinitis. J Allergy Clin Immunol 2009;123:1098.

Local Allergic Rhinitis

Paloma Campo, MD, PhD[a], María Salas, MD, PhD[a],
Natalia Blanca-López, MD, PhD[b], Carmen Rondón, MD, PhD[a],*

KEYWORDS

- Local allergic rhinitis • Asthma • Nasal allergen provocation test • Local IgE
- Natural evolution • Allergen immunotherapy

KEY POINTS

- Local allergic rhinitis (LAR) is a rhinitis phenotype defined by a nasal allergic response in patients with negative skin prick test and nondetectable serum specific immunoglobulin E (sIgE) antibodies.
- Patients from different countries, ethnic groups, and ages may be affected. Impairment of quality of life and association with conjunctivitis and asthma are frequent.
- Diagnosis is based on clinical history, the demonstration of a positive response to nasal allergen provocation test and/or the detection of nasal sIgE. A positive basophil activation test may support the diagnosis.
- Allergen immunotherapy is a clinically effective immune-modifying treatment for LAR.

DEFINITION OF LOCAL ALLERGIC RHINITIS

Local allergic rhinitis (LAR) is a clinical entity characterized by symptoms suggestive of allergic rhinitis (AR) owing to a localized allergic response in the nasal mucosa in the absence of systemic atopy assessed by conventional diagnostic tests such as skin prick test or determination of specific immunoglobulin E (sIgE) in serum.[1–17]

UNDERLYING IMMUNE MECHANISMS

A better understanding of the underlying immune mechanisms is essential for developing diagnostic methods and targeted therapies. The immune characteristics of LAR (**Fig. 1**) include:

- Nasal T-helper 2 cell allergic inflammation[4–6,18,19]
- Positive response to nasal allergen provocation test (NAPT)[3,5,11,20]
- Nasal production of sIgE[5,6,8,9,18,19] and inflammatory mediators[8,21,22]
- Allergen-specific basophil activation[23,24]
- No detectable sIgE antibodies in serum[16,17]

Disclosure Statement: The authors declare that they have no conflicts of interest.
[a] Regional University Hospital of Malaga, Plaza Hospital Civil s/n pabellon 6, Málaga 29009, Spain; [b] Allergy Service, Hospital Infanta Leonor, Gran Vía del Este, 80, Madrid 28031, Spain
* Corresponding author. Allergy Unit, Hospital Civil, pabellon 6, Plaza del Hospital Civil, Málaga 29009, Spain.
E-mail address: carmenrs61@gmail.com

Immunol Allergy Clin N Am 36 (2016) 321–332
http://dx.doi.org/10.1016/j.iac.2015.12.008
0889-8561/16/$ – see front matter © 2016 Elsevier Inc. All rights reserved.

immunology.theclinics.com

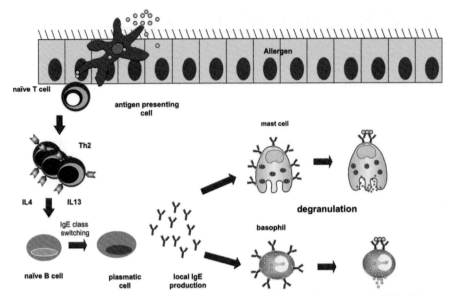

Fig. 1. Local allergic immune response. IgE, immunoglobulin E; IL, interleukin; Th2, T-helper 2 cell. (*Adapted from* Rondón C, Fernandez F, Canto G, et al. Local allergic rhinitis: concept, clinical manifestations, and diagnostic approach. J Investig Allergol Clin Immunol 2010;20:366.)

T-helper 2 Cell Nasal Immunologic Response

Natural exposure to aeroallergens induces a nasal T-helper 2 cell inflammatory response in LAR with increased eosinophils, basophils, mast cells, CD3[+], and CD4[+] T cells.[5,6] T cells may play a role in eosinophil recruitment and IgE production.

Positive Response to the Nasal Allergen Provocation Test

NAPT studies have helped to increase our understanding of the pathophysiology of LAR,[13] confirming the characteristic immediate/early and late phases of the allergic response in LAR patients.[21,22] The response to NAPT has been confirmed objectively by acoustic rhinometry,[5,6,8,20–22] anterior rhinomanometry,[3] and by nasal secretion of sIgE[5,6,8,9,21,22] and inflammatory mediators[5,6,8,21,22] as well as subjectively by nasal and ocular symptoms.[3,5,6,20–22]

In LAR, aeroallergen exposure induces local sIgE production, mast cells, and eosinophil activation with nasal secretion of tryptase and eosinophil cationic protein (ECP).[21,22] The maximum secretion of tryptase occurs 15 minutes after NAPT, returning to baseline at 6 hours (immediate responders), or 24 hours (dual responders). Nasal secretion of ECP is long lasting, increasing progressively from 15 minutes to 24 hours.[21,22] A recent study showed that 83% of LAR subjects sensitized to *Olea europaea* pollen responded to NAPT with nOle e 1, demonstrating that purified allergens can also induce an allergic response with secretion of ECP potentially acting as a confirmatory biomarker of this inflammatory response.[24]

Local Specific Immunoglobulin E Production

Mechanistic studies have shown nasal production of sIgE in AR[25–28] and LAR.[2,5,6,8,9,19,21,22] The local production of sIgE in target organs may explain why some atopic subjects develop rhinitis, and others asthma, conjunctivitis, and/or eczema alone or in combination.[29] Conversely the absence of local sIgE could explain why up to 50% of the population, who demonstrate positive skin prick test/serum sIgE, have no clinical manifestations of allergy.[29]

Since the first detection of nasal sIgE in nonatopic rhinitis patients by Huggins and Brostoff in 1975,[2] several studies have confirmed the presence of nasal sIgE in LAR patients after natural exposure,[5,6] after controlled exposure to aeroallergens by NAPT,[8,9,21,22] as well as during periods of nonexposure to aeroallergens.[21,22]

Cellular studies have confirmed the expression of epsilon germline gene transcripts and messenger RNA for the epsilon heavy chain of IgE in nasal mucosal B cells.[26] In addition, the localization of free light chains of IgE in tissue and nasal secretions of patients with AR and with NAR suggests that they could mediate immune responses involving mast cells.[30,31]

Basophil Activation

Recent studies have shown that local sIgE production with binding to the high-affinity receptor for IgE of basophils could take place without detectable circulating sIgE in LAR patients sensitized to dust mites and pollens.[23,24] Furthermore, wortmanin experiments demonstrated that the activation of basophils is IgE mediated.[23] These findings suggest that, after local IgE production, basophils might be the first cells for sIgE leaked from the target organ to the circulation.

CLINICAL FEATURES AND EPIDEMIOLOGIC DATA
Clinical Features of Local Allergic Rhinitis

Studies performed in well-phenotyped rhinitis patients have shown that some clinical features are similar between AR and LAR. However, several clinical–demographic features may be useful for identifying LAR patients among those subjects with rhinitis symptoms and absence of atopy[11–13] (**Box 1**).

Epidemiologic Studies

There are several epidemiologic studies for LAR (**Table 1**). Early reports studying small populations showed frequencies of 47% of LAR sensitized to betula[20] and 62% to *Dermatophagoides pteronyssinus*[3] among adult patients previously labeled as NAR. A recent study performed in children with rhinitis detected positive nasal sIgE to *Alternaria*.[32] Another study of 219 elderly subjects with rhinitis (65–89 years of age) revealed that 21% of patients had LAR, 40.2% had AR, and 38.8% had NAR diagnosed by NAPT.[8]

In a recent prospective study of 428 rhinitis subjects in Spain, we found a LAR prevalence of 25.7%[11] diagnosed by NAPT. Two independent studies in different geographic areas with high allergenic load (grass pollen and house dust mites) revealed a frequency of 61% and 72%, respectively,[33,34] using NAPT. Taken together, these studies show that LAR is common in several populations, and in children and adults.[7–10,20,35] However, larger population studies using established LAR diagnosis protocols are required to fully determine its prevalence and incidence.

COMORBIDITIES AND LOCAL ALLERGIC RESPIRATORY DISEASE

As with AR, LAR frequently presents with other diseases such as asthma and conjunctivitis.[11–13]

Box 1
Clinical-demographic features for identifying LAR

Clinical Similarities Between LAR and AR

- Nasal pruritus, watery rhinorrhea, and sneezing are the most common clinical features
- Association with conjunctivitis
- Accompanied by lower airway symptoms
- Mostly moderate to severe symptoms
- Not limited to adults: 36% of subjects develop it in childhood
- Tendency to worsen over time

Differential Characteristics of LAR Compared with NAR

- Significantly younger
- Nonsmokers
- More likely female
- Family history of atopy
- More severe symptoms

Abbreviations: AR, allergic rhinitis; LAR, local allergic rhinitis; NAR, nonallergic rhinitis.
   Data from Refs.[11–13]

Local Immunoglobulin E in Lower Airways

More than 30% of subjects with LAR also report asthmatic symptoms.[11,12,36] IgE may play an important role in nonatopic asthma, and may be produced locally as in the nasal mucosa of LAR subjects.[37] Several studies have demonstrated the local synthesis of IgE in the bronchial mucosa of atopic and nonatopic asthmatics, with increased expression of the IgE epsilon heavy chain germ line and mature gene transcripts (epsilon chain messenger RNA) and local IgE class switching.[38,39] There is also a similar cellular infiltrate in bronchial mucosa in both atopic and nonatopic asthmatics, with a similar increase in cytokines and their receptors such as interleukin-4, -5, and -13.[40,41] However, the possible role of allergens in the bronchial symptoms of LAR patients requires further clarification. Researchers have demonstrated the presence of *D pteronyssinus* sIgE in the sputum of nonatopic asthmatics after bronchial allergen challenge, even though subjects did not respond clinically to the allergen,[42] and have also demonstrated a correlation with periostin.[43] Pillai and colleagues[44] have also found elevated levels of total IgE in tissues of both atopic and nonatopic patients, but only demonstrated allergen sIgE in atopic subjects. Preliminary results obtained by our group revealed positive bronchial responses to *D pteronyssinus* demonstrated by bronchial allergen provocation test in 8 of 16 subjects with LAR, with increased eosinophils and ECP in induced sputum, providing more evidence for a possible equivalent to LAR in the lower airways.[45]

Conjunctivitis and Local Immunoglobulin E

Ocular symptoms are often found in LAR patients.[11–13] The existence of an ocular local allergic response has been demonstrated through specific conjunctival provocation tests and determination of sIgE in ocular secretions.[46,47] In some cases, the ocular allergic response was demonstrated in patients clinically suggestive of LAR.[47] Investigators have reported a lack of correlation between serum sIgE and ocular allergy, suggesting that the sIgE detected in the eye is most likely produced locally.[48]

Table 1
Epidemiologic studies for LAR

Author, Year	Country	Study Groups	Group Age	Allergens	Positive NAPT Response, n (%)
Carney et al,[3] 2002	UK/ Australia	21 IR (perennial)	Adults	DP/DF Cats/Dogs Grass	13/21 (61.9)
Wedback et al,[20] 2005	Sweden	15 IR (seasonal)	Adults	Birch Timothy	7/15 (46.7)
Rondon et al,[5] 2007	Spain	50 IR (perennial)	Adults	DP	27/50 (54)
Rondon et al,[6] 2008	Spain	32 IR (seasonal)	Adults	Grass Olive	21/32 (65.6)
Fuiano et al,[32] 2012	Italy	36 IR (perennial)	Children (4–18 y)	Alternaria	25/36 (69.4)
Cruz Niesvaara et al,[33] 2012	Spain	30 IR (perennial)	Adults	DP	19/30 (63.3)
Rondon et al,[11] 2012	Spain	158 IR (seasonal/ perennial)	Adults	DP Alternaria Grass Olive Cat Dog	110/158 (69.6)
Cheng et al,[10] 2013	China	147 IR (perennial)	Adults	DF	12/147 (8.1)
Chang et al,[7] 2014	Korea	62 IR	Adults	DP	22/62 (35.5)
Bozek et al,[8] 2015	Poland	131 IR (perennial)	Adults >65 y	DP Phleum Molds Trees Cat	46/131 (351)
Klimek et al,[9] 2015	Germany	2 IR (perennial)	Adults	Alternaria	2 (case report)
Adinoff et al,[63] 2015	USA	30 IR (seasonal/ perennial)	Adults/ children	Trees Weeds Timothy grass Cat	11/30 (36.7)
Jang et al,[64] 2015	Korea	110 IR (perennial)	Adults	DP	12/110 (10.9)
Buntarickpornpan et al,[65] 2015	Thailand	25 IR (perennial)	Children (8–18 y)	DP	0/25 (0)
Refaat et al,[66] 2015	Egypt	40 IR	Adults	DP	25/40 (62.5)
Blanca-López,[34] 2016	Spain	61 IR (seasonal)	Adults/ Children	Phleum	37/61 (61)

Abbreviations: DP, Dermatophagoides pteronyssinus; IR, idiopathic rhinitis; LAR, local allergic rhinitis; NAPT, nasal allergen provocation test.
Data from Refs.[3,5–11,20,32–34,63–66]

NATURAL HISTORY AND RISK FACTORS

The characterization of LAR has generated important clinical questions as to whether it develops into AR with systemic atopy, or is a risk factor for asthma.[36] The results of the first longitudinal study revealed that LAR is a well-differentiated disease with a similar low rate of conversion to AR as for healthy controls (6.25% vs 5.2%) after 5 years of evolution.[12] This study periodically evaluated a cohort of 149 LAR patients and 130 controls using questionnaires, skin tests, serum sIgE, lung function, and NAPTs.[12] LAR patients worsened over time, with impairment in quality of life, an increase in rhinitis persistence and severity, the use of emergency assistance, and new associations with conjunctivitis and asthma.

Previously, a retrospective study had detected a 24% conversion rate from NAR to AR, indirectly suggesting that a long-term conversion from LAR to AR might be possible[49]; however, this study did not differentiate between NAR and LAR patients.

In 2015, a retrospective study performed in 19 LAR patients reevaluated by skin prick test or intracutaneous testing reported a 21% long-term conversion rate from LAR to AR after more than 7 years of evolution.[50] This figure was very close to the 17% conversion rate detected in 7930 healthy subjects evaluated in the region where the study was conducted.[51] However, the retrospective design, lack of healthy controls, surveillance bias, small number of patients included, and great variability in patient age and time interval between evaluations must be considered when interpreting the results.[52] It will be interesting to compare these results with our 10-year longitudinal follow-up study in LAR subjects, which will be completed in the next 2 years.

Diagnostic Test and Differential Diagnosis

The diagnosis of LAR must always be considered for patients with symptoms of AR but no evidence of systemic atopy as measured by conventional methods (skin testing/serum sIgE).[1,16,17,36] By conducting a detailed clinical history, a thorough nasal exploration (anterior rhinoscopy/endoscopy) and/or imaging (CT scan), a differential diagnosis can be established (**Box 2**). The prototype LAR patient is a young female nonsmoker with family history of atopy and clear symptoms of AR.[11,12] However, to confirm a diagnosis of LAR it is necessary to perform a specific allergological evaluation[1,16,17,36] (**Fig. 2**).

The diagnosis of LAR starts with the demonstration of an allergen-specific nasal response by means of NAPT and/or sIgE in nasal secretions or tissue.[5,6,11–13,16,36] NAPT is considered the gold standard for AR and LAR diagnosis,[11,16,36,53,54] with a higher sensitivity than allergen-sIgE measurement in nasal secretions.[13,21,36] NAPT with multiple allergens may be useful as an initial screening method for LAR and NAR.[54] The presence of nasal sIgE has been demonstrated in nasal biopsies,[25] but in clinical practice noninvasive methods for diagnosis are recommended.[13,36] However, the measurement of sIgE in nasal secretions can vary depending on the technique used. Although highly specific, sensitivity is rather low when measured by nasal lavage, ranging from 22% to 40%,[5,6,21,22] most likely owing to dilutional effects. Other techniques such as the direct application to the ostium of a cellulose device coupled to the allergen,[32] nasal brushing[55] and sinus packs or filter disks[56] used in AR need to be tested in LAR subjects.

The basophil activation test has proved to be useful for LAR diagnosis. In patients with LAR to D pteronyssinus, it has a sensitivity of 50% with greater than 90% specificity.[23] For patients with LAR to O europaea, the sensitivity is 66% with greater than 90% specificity.[24] Therefore, basophil activation test can be a useful adjunctive tool to diagnose LAR to inhalant allergens.

Box 2
Differential diagnosis of local allergic rhinitis

- Nasal polyposis

- Chronic rhinosinusitis

- Known causes of nonallergic rhinitis
  - Drug-related
  - Hormonal
  - Systemic diseases
    - Cystic fibrosis
    - Primary ciliary dyskinesia
    - Granulomatosis
    - Sarcoidosis
    - Amyloidosis
  - Atrophic rhinitis
  - Occupational (irritant)

- Anatomic alterations
  - Septal deviation
  - Turbinate hypertrophy
  - Adenoidal hypertrophy
  - Cerebrospinal fluid leaking

Data from Refs.[1,11,12,17,36]

Establishing the correct diagnosis of LAR will allow for the identification of the allergen(s) that trigger the allergic response and the administration of a specific treatment.[13,16,36] This diagnostic approach should also be applied to workers with nasal respiratory symptoms clearly related to occupational exposure but who have negative immunologic tests, especially for high molecular weight agents.[37]

THERAPEUTICS OPTIONS

Given the clinical–immunologic similarities between AR and LAR, it is reasonable to think that these patients will benefit from the same therapeutic approaches.[13,16,36] This includes education, allergen avoidance measures, pharmacologic treatment with intranasal corticosteroids, oral and intranasal antihistamines, and allergen immunotherapy (AIT).[57] Information based on the clinical evolution of LAR patients shows a similar response in terms of symptomatic relief and disease control with oral antihistamines and intranasal corticosteroids.[5,6,12]

AIT has the ability to modify the natural course of AR, increasing immunologic tolerance, and reducing the clinical symptoms and the use of medication.[58,59] The most relevant question is how beneficial AIT may be in LAR patients, and which immunologic effects it may produce. According to ARIA guidelines, AIT is indicated in children and adults with moderate to severe, persistent or intermittent AR and/or allergic asthma,[57,58,60] so the question is this: Should LAR be considered a new indication for AIT?

An observational study with grass pollen[14] and a double-blind, placebo-controlled clinical trial with *D pteronyssinus* subcutaneous immunotherapy[15] have demonstrated the clinical and immunologic effect of AIT in LAR. The former study was conducted in a group of LAR patients sensitized to grass pollen.[14] It showed that grass pollen subcutaneous immunotherapy induces a significant improvement in nasal tolerance to NAPTs, and clinical symptoms in response to the natural exposure to the allergen, with reduced use of rescue medication.[14] These findings have been recently confirmed in a 2 years

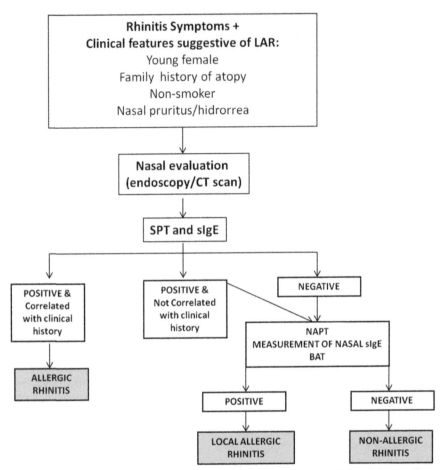

Fig. 2. Diagnostic approach in local allergic rhinitis (LAR). BAT, basophil activation test; CT, computed tomography; NAPT, nasal allergen provocation test; sIgE, specific immunoglobulin E; SPT, skin prick test. (*Adapted from* Rondón C, Fernandez F, Canto G, et al. Local allergic rhinitis: concept, clinical manifestations, and diagnostic approach. J Investig Allergol Clin Immunol 2010;20:368.)

phase II randomized double-blind, placebo-controlled clinical trial with *D pteronyssinus* subcutaneous immunotherapy.[15] In this study, AIT had a short-term and sustained clinical effect reducing symptom and medication scores, and increasing the number of medication-free days[15] as occurs with AR.[61,62] The immunologic effects were demonstrated by the production of allergen sIgG4 and a decrease in serum sIgE with a significant improvement in nasal allergen tolerance. At the end of the study, two-thirds of patients treated with AIT tolerated a concentration of Der p1 10 times higher by NAPT than basal concentration, and NAPT was negative in 50% of patients.[15] These results support the indication for AIT in LAR.

FUTURE CONSIDERATIONS AND SUMMARY

LAR constitutes an interesting model of allergic inflammation localized in the target organ. Despite recent achievements in the investigation of this disease, there remain many unanswered questions. Future research will focus on the study of the pathophysiologic mechanisms of LAR, elucidation of lower airway and ocular responses, AIT studies with different allergens, the improvement of sIgE detection in nasal secretion and the further development of reproducible in vitro tests that can be performed readily in the clinical setting.

REFERENCES

1. Papadopoulos NG, Bernstein JA, Demoly P, et al. Phenotypes and endotypes of rhinitis and their impact on management: a PRACTALL report. Allergy 2015;70: 474–94.
2. Huggins KG, Brostoff J. Local production of specific IgE antibodies in allergic-rhinitis patients with negative skin tests. Lancet 1975;2:148–50.
3. Carney AS, Powe DG, Huskisson RS, et al. Atypical nasal challenges in patients with idiopathic rhinitis: more evidence for the existence of allergy in the absence of atopy? Clin Exp Allergy 2002;32:1436–40.
4. Powe DG, Jagger C, Kleinjan A, et al. 'Entopy': localized mucosal allergic disease in the absence of systemic responses for atopy. Clin Exp Allergy 2003;33:1374–9.
5. Rondon C, Romero JJ, Lopez S, et al. Local IgE production and positive nasal provocation test in patients with persistent nonallergic rhinitis. J Allergy Clin Immunol 2007;119:899–905.
6. Rondon C, Dona I, Lopez S, et al. Seasonal idiopathic rhinitis with local inflammatory response and specific IgE in absence of systemic response. Allergy 2008; 63:1352–8.
7. Chang GU, Jang TY, Kim KS, et al. Nonspecific hyper-reactivity and localized allergy: cause of discrepancy between skin prick and nasal provocation test. Otolaryngol Head Neck Surg 2014;150:194–200.
8. Bozek A, Ignasiak B, Kasperska-Zajac A, et al. Local allergic rhinitis in elderly patients. Ann Allergy Asthma Immunol 2015;114:199–202.
9. Klimek L, Bardenhewer C, Spielhaupter M, et al. Local allergic rhinitis to alternaria alternata: evidence for local IgE production exclusively in the nasal mucosa. HNO 2015;63:364–72.
10. Cheng KJ, Xu YY, Liu HY, et al. Serum eosinophil cationic protein level in Chinese subjects with nonallergic and local allergic rhinitis and its relation to the severity of disease. Am J Rhinol Allergy 2013;27:8–12.
11. Rondon C, Campo P, Galindo L, et al. Prevalence and clinical relevance of local allergic rhinitis. Allergy 2012;67:1282–8.
12. Rondon C, Campo P, Zambonino MA, et al. Follow-up study in local allergic rhinitis shows a consistent entity not evolving to systemic allergic rhinitis. J Allergy Clin Immunol 2014;133:1026–31.
13. Campo P, Rondon C, Gould HJ, et al. Local IgE in non-allergic rhinitis. Clin Exp Allergy 2015;45:872–81.
14. Rondon C, Blanca-Lopez N, Aranda A, et al. Local allergic rhinitis: allergen tolerance and immunologic changes after preseasonal immunotherapy with grass pollen. J Allergy Clin Immunol 2011;127:1069–71.
15. Rondon C, Campo P, Blanca-Lopez N, et al. Subcutaneous allergen immunotherapy in patient with "Local Allergic Rhinitis" sensitized to Dermatophagoides Pteronyssinus. J Allergy Clin Immunol 2015;135(2):AB171.
16. Rondon C, Canto G, Blanca M. Local allergic rhinitis: a new entity, characterization and further studies. Curr Opin Allergy Clin Immunol 2010;10:1–7.

17. Rondón C, Fernandez F, Canto G, et al. Local allergic rhinitis: concept, clinical manifestations, and diagnostic approach. J Investig Allergol Clin Immunol 2010;20:364–71.
18. Powe DG, Huskisson RS, Carney AS, et al. Evidence for an inflammatory pathophysiology in idiopathic rhinitis. Clin Exp Allergy 2001;31:864–72.
19. Powe DG, Huskisson RS, Carney AS, et al. Mucosal T-cell phenotypes in persistent atopic and nonatopic rhinitis show an association with mast cells. Allergy 2004;59:204–12.
20. Wedback A, Enbom H, Eriksson NE, et al. Seasonal non-allergic rhinitis (SNAR)–a new disease entity? A clinical and immunological comparison between SNAR, seasonal allergic rhinitis and persistent non-allergic rhinitis. Rhinology 2005;43: 86–92.
21. Lopez S, Rondon C, Torres MJ, et al. Immediate and dual response to nasal challenge with Dermatophagoides pteronys sinus in local allergic rhinitis. Clin Exp Allergy 2010;40:1007–14.
22. Rondon C, Fernandez J, Lopez S, et al. Nasal inflammatory mediators and specific IgE production after nasal challenge with grass pollen in local allergic rhinitis. J Allergy Clin Immunol 2009;124:1005–11.e1.
23. Gomez E, Campo P, Rondon C, et al. Role of the basophil activation test in the diagnosis of local allergic rhinitis. J Allergy Clin Immunol 2013;132:975–6.e1–5.
24. Campo P, Villalba M, Barrionuevo E, et al. Immunologic responses to the major allergen of Olea europaea in local and systemic allergic rhinitis subjects. Clin Exp Allergy 2015;45(11):1703–12.
25. Coker HA, Durham SR, Gould HJ. Local somatic hypermutation and class switch recombination in the nasal mucosa of allergic rhinitis patients. J Immunol 2003; 171:5602–10.
26. Durham SR, Gould HJ, Thienes CP, et al. Expression of epsilon germ-line gene transcripts and mRNA for the epsilon heavy chain of IgE in nasal B cells and the effects of topical corticosteroid. Eur J Immunol 1997;27:2899–906.
27. Platts-Mills TA. Local production of IgG, IgA and IgE antibodies in grass pollen hay fever. J Immunol 1979;122:2218–25.
28. Takhar P, Smurthwaite L, Coker HA, et al. Allergen drives class switching to IgE in the nasal mucosa in allergic rhinitis. J Immunol 2005;174:5024–32.
29. James LK, Durham SR. Rhinitis with negative skin tests and absent serum allergen-specific IgE: more evidence for local IgE? J Allergy Clin Immunol 2009;124:1012–3.
30. Powe DG, Groot Kormelink T, Sisson M, et al. Evidence for the involvement of free light chain immunoglobulins in allergic and nonallergic rhinitis. J Allergy Clin Immunol 2010;125:139–45.e1–3.
31. Rondon C, Canto G, Fernandez J, et al. Are free light chain immunoglobulins related to nasal local allergic rhinitis? J Allergy Clin Immunol 2010;126:677 [author reply: 8].
32. Fuiano N, Fusilli S, Incorvaia C. A role for measurement of nasal IgE antibodies in diagnosis of Alternaria-induced rhinitis in children. Allergol Immunopathol (Madr) 2012;40:71–4.
33. Cruz Niesvaara D, Rondon C, Almeida Quintana L, et al. Evidence of local allergic rhinitis in areas with high and permanent aeroallergens exposure. J Allergy Clin Immunol 2012;129:AB111.
34. Blanca-Lopez N, Campo P, Salas M, et al. Seasonal local allergic rhinitis in areas with high concentration of grass pollen. J Investig Allergol Clin Immunol 2016; 26(2).

35. Kim YH, Jang TY. Clinical characteristics and therapeutic outcomes of patients with localized mucosal allergy. Am J Rhinol Allergy 2010;24:e89–92.

36. Rondon C, Campo P, Togias A, et al. Local allergic rhinitis: concept, pathophysiology, and management. J Allergy Clin Immunol 2012;129:1460–7.

37. Gómez F, Rondón C, Salas M, et al. Local allergic rhinitis: mechanisms, diagnosis and relevance for occupational rhinitis. Curr Opin Allergy Clin Immunol 2015; 15(2):111–6.

38. Ying S, Humbert M, Meng Q, et al. Local expression of epsilon germ line gene transcripts and RNA for the epsilon heavy chain of IgE in the bronchial mucosa in atopic and non-atopic asthma. J Allergy Clin Immunol 2000;107:686–92.

39. Takhar P, Corrigan CJ, Smurthwaite L, et al. Class switch recombination to IgE in the bronchial mucosa of atopic and nonatopic patients with asthma. J Allergy Clin Immunol 2007;119:213–8.

40. Bentley AM, Durham SR, Kay AB. Comparison of the immunopathology of extrinsic, intrinsic and occupational asthma. J Investig Allergol Clin Immunol 1994;4:222–32.

41. Humbert M, Durham SR, Ying S, et al. IL-4 and IL-5 mRNA and protein in bronchial biopsies from patients with atopic and nonatopic asthma: evidence against "intrinsic" asthma being a distinct immunopathologic entity. Am J Respir Crit Care Med 1996;154:1497–504.

42. Mouthuy J, Detry B, Sohy C, et al. Presence in sputum of functional dust mite-specific IgE antibodies in intrinsic asthma. Am J Respir Crit Care Med 2011; 184(2):206–14.

43. Mouthuy J, Viart S, Ladjemi MZ, et al. Mite allergen-specific IgE is detectable in bronchial secretions of patients with nonatopic asthma and correlates with mucosal expression of periostin. J Allergy Clin Immunol 2015;136(6):1685–8.e2.

44. Pillai P, Fang C, Chan YC, et al. Allergen-specific IgE is not detectable in the bronchial mucosa of nonatopic asthmatic patients. J Allergy Clin Immunol 2014;133(6):1770–2.e1.

45. Campo P, Antunez C, Rondon C, et al. Positive bronchial challenges to D. pteronyssinus in asthmatic subjects in absence of systemic atopy. J Allergy Clin Immunol 2011;127(Suppl 2):AB6.

46. Leonardi A, Battista MC, Gismondi M, et al. Antigen sensitivity evaluated by tear-specific and serum-specific IgE, skin tests, and conjunctival and nasal provocation tests in patients with ocular allergic diseases. Eye 1993;7:461–4.

47. Ballow M, Mendelson L, Donshik P, et al. Pollen specific IgE antibodies in tears of patients with allergic-like conjunctivitis. J Allergy Clin Immunol 1984;73:376–80.

48. Hoffmann-Sommergruber K, Ferreira FD, Ebner C, et al. Detection of allergen-specific IgE in tears of grass pollen-allergic patients with allergic rhinoconjunctivitis. Clin Exp Allergy 1996;26:79–87.

49. Rondon C, Dona I, Torres MJ, et al. Evolution of patients with nonallergic rhinitis supports conversion to allergic rhinitis. J Allergy Clin Immunol 2009;123: 1098–102.

50. Sennekamp J, Joest I, Filipiak-Pittroff B, et al. Local allergic nasal reactions convert to classic systemic allergic reactions: a long-term follow-up. Int Arch Allergy Immunol 2015;166:154–60.

51. Nicolai T, Bellach B, Mutius EV, et al. Increased prevalence of sensitization against aeroallergens in adults in West compared with East Germany. Clin Exp Allergy 1997;27:886–92.

52. Rondon C, Campo P, Blanca-Lopez N, et al. More research is needed for local allergic rhinitis. Int Arch Allergy Immunol 2015;167:99–100.

53. Scadding G, Hellings P, Alobid I, et al. Diagnostic tools in rhinology EAACI position paper. Clin Transl Allergy 2011;1:2.

54. Rondon C, Campo P, Herrera R, et al. Nasal allergen provocation test with multiple aeroallergens detects polysensitization in local allergic rhinitis. J Allergy Clin Immunol 2011;128:1192–7.

55. Reisacher WR, Bremberg MG. Prevalence of antigen-specific immunoglobulin E on mucosal brush biopsy of the inferior turbinates in patients with nonallergic rhinitis. Int Forum Allergy Rhinol 2014;4(4):292–7.

56. De Schryver E, Devuyst L, Derycke L, et al. Local immunoglobulin e in the nasal mucosa: clinical implications. Allergy Asthma Immunol Res 2015;7(4):321–31.

57. Bousquet J, Khaltaev N, Cruz AA, et al. Allergic Rhinitis and its Impact on Asthma (ARIA) 2008 update (in collaboration with the World Health Organization, GA(2) LEN and AllerGen). Allergy 2008;63(Suppl 86):8–160.

58. Bousquet J, Lockey R, Malling HJ. Allergen immunotherapy: therapeutic vaccines for allergic diseases. A WHO position paper. J Allergy Clin Immunol 1998;102:558–62.

59. Frew AJ, Powell RJ, Corrigan CJ, et al. Efficacy and safety of specific immunotherapy with SQ allergen extract in treatment-resistant seasonal allergic rhinoconjunctivitis. J Allergy Clin Immunol 2006;117:319–25.

60. Brozek JL, Bousquet J, Baena-Cagnani CE, et al. Allergic Rhinitis and its Impact on Asthma (ARIA) guidelines: 2010 revision. J Allergy Clin Immunol 2010;126: 466–76.

61. Tabar AI, Echechipia S, Garcia BE, et al. Double-blind comparative study of cluster and conventional immunotherapy schedules with Dermatophagoides pteronyssinus. J Allergy Clin Immunol 2005;116:109–18.

62. Varney VA, Tabbah K, Mavroleon G, et al. Usefulness of specific immunotherapy in patients with severe perennial allergic rhinitis induced by house dust mite: a double-blind, randomized, placebo-controlled trial. Clin Exp Allergy 2003;33: 1076–82.

63. Adinoff AD, Tsai KS, Steffen M. Entopy: where art thou entopy? J Allergy Clin Immunol 2015;135(2):AB190.

64. Jang TY, Kim YH. Nasal provocation test is useful for discriminating allergic, nonallergic, and local allergic rhinitis. Am J Rhinol Allergy 2015;29(4):e100–4.

65. Buntarickpornpan P, Veskitkul J, Pacharn P, et al. The prevalence and clinical characteristics of local allergic rhinitis in Thai children. J Allergy Clin Immunol 2015;135(2):AB282.

66. Refaat M, Melek N, Shahin R, et al. Study for assessing prevalence of local allergic rhinitis among rhinitis patients. J Allergy Clin Immunol 2015;135(2): AB140.

Occupational Rhinitis

Leslie C. Grammer III, MD

KEYWORDS

- Occupational rhinitis • Allergic occupational rhinitis
- Nonallergic occupational rhinitis • High molecular weight • Low molecular weight
- Laboratory animals • Flour • Acid anhydrides

KEY POINTS

- Occupational exposures associated with a high prevalence of occupational rhinitis (OR) are laboratory animals, flour, other foods, acid anhydrides, cleaning products, and strong irritants.
- OR is rhinitis developing as a result of workplace exposure in a previously asymptomatic individual.
- OR can be divided into allergic OR, which has an immunologic basis, and nonallergic OR, which does not.
- The primary therapy for OR is avoidance of the implicated exposure.
- In those with OR, the possibility of coexisting occupational asthma should be considered.

INTRODUCTION

Occupational rhinitis (OR) is 1 of 2 forms of work-related rhinitis (**Fig. 1**). The other form is work-exacerbated rhinitis, in which the individual has preexisting rhinitis made worse by exposures in the workplace.[1] The European Academy of Allergy and Clinical Immunology published a consensus definition of OR in 2009, "an inflammatory disease of the nose, which is characterized by intermittent or persistent symptoms (ie, nasal congestion, sneezing, rhinorrhea and itching) and/or variable nasal airflow limitation and/or hypersecretion owing to causes and conditions attributable to a particular work environment and not to stimuli encountered outside the workplace."[2] OR can be further subdivided into allergic and nonallergic rhinitis. Allergic OR has an immunologic basis and is associated with a latency period. Allergic OR can be caused by high-molecular-weight (HMW) or low-molecular-weight (LMW) agents. Nonallergic OR has no latency and can occur with one high level exposure to irritants such as chlorine gas, giving rise to reactive upper airway dysfunction syndrome.[2] In contrast,

This work was supported by The Ernest S. Bazely grant to Northwestern University and Northwestern Memorial Hospital.
The author has no financial conflicts of interest.
Division of Allergy-Immunology, Department of Medicine, Northwestern University Feinberg School of Medicine, 211 East Ontario Street Suite 1000, Chicago, IL 60611, USA
E-mail address: l-grammer@northwestern.edu

Immunol Allergy Clin N Am 36 (2016) 333–341
http://dx.doi.org/10.1016/j.iac.2015.12.009
0889-8561/16/$ – see front matter © 2016 Elsevier Inc. All rights reserved.

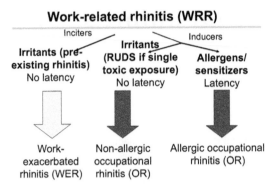

Fig. 1. There are 2 major forms of work-related rhinitis (WRR): (1) work-exacerbated rhinitis (WER) in those with preexisting rhinitis and (2) occupational rhinitis (OR). OR can be divided into 2 types. One type, called nonallergic OR, has no latency period and is caused by irritants. The other type, called allergic OR, has a latency period and is caused by sensitizers that can be either high or low molecular weight. RUDS, reactive upper airway dysfunction syndrome.

multiple exposures to irritants at a more moderate level is probably the most common cause of irritant-induced OR.

Irritant-induced OR has a range of severity, from annoying, reversible irritation to chronic erosive rhinitis. A number of different chemicals have been associated with irritant-induced OR, among those reported include ammonia, bleach, chlorine, volatile organic solvent vapors, aldehydes, sulfur dioxide, nitrogen dioxide, and hydrogen sulfide. When encountering a new chemical to which a worker is exposed, obtaining a material safety data sheet for the chemical can be helpful. Whether or not the agent is a known respiratory sensitizer or respiratory irritant will be stated under the section entitled Health Hazard and Toxicologic Data.

EPIDEMIOLOGY

The epidemiology of occupational diseases, in general, and OR, specifically, is unclear. In the United States, OR is not a reportable condition. There is also the issue of the "healthy worker effect," in which those who are not affected by a given workplace exposure stay in the job and those who are made ill are likely to simply leave and find alternative employment.

It is clear that certain exposures, such as flour and laboratory animals, seem to be 2 agents commonly reported to cause OR.[3] The range of the prevalence of OR among bakers in Norway has been estimated to be between 23% and 50%.[4] Among laboratory animal handlers, one review reported a range of 10% to 42% of exposed individuals had OR.[5] In a skin test study of sensitization, it was found that 16% of laboratory animal handlers were sensitized as compared with 3% of nonhandlers.[6] In a 1997 Finnish study, it was reported that the risk of developing OR was highest in the following occupations: bakers, food processing workers, farmers, veterinarians, furriers, livestock breeders, electronic product assemblers, and boat builders.[7]

RISK FACTORS

Risk factors for OR include the particular agent, level of exposure, and atopy. The relationship between smoking and OR is not clear.[2] As reviewed, some agents such as flour and other foods as well as animal dander, are more likely than other exposures to result in OR. The level of exposure and the relationship to immunoglobulin (Ig)

E-mediated sensitization has been reported for several HMW agents, such as detergent enzymes,[8] flour,[9] laboratory animals,[10] and latex.[11] In most reports, the correlation between exposure and IgE-mediated sensitization is clear, but the relationship to OR is less clear. In any event, IgE sensitization seems to be a strong predictor of developing rhinitis as well as asthma symptoms. In some cases of LMW agents, in particular acid anhydrides, this relationship between exposure level and IgE sensitization has been reported.[12,13]

The prevalence of OR reported in selected exposures in various industries is shown in **Table 1**. In a number of studies of HMW agents including laboratory animals and flour, atopy has been associated with an increased risk of sensitization. Atopy is also associated with an increased risk of OR from those HMW agents.[31] The results of studies assessing atopy as a risk factor for OR caused by LMW agents has been inconsistent.[2]

PATHOPHYSIOLOGY

The pathophysiology of IgE-mediated OR is thought to be the same as IgE-mediated rhinitis from nonoccupational causes such as pollens. This has been studied extensively using nasal allergen challenges and evaluating nasal airway resistance, nasal lavage cells, and mediators.[32] In 1 nasal lavage study comparing 22 patients with asthma and rhinitis owing to house dust mites, 25 patients with OR and asthma owing to laboratory animal allergens, and 15 healthy subjects, those with OR actually had higher levels of eosinophils, basophils, and albumin in lavage fluid compared with normal subjects as well as compared with those with nonoccupational house dust mite allergy.[33] Other immune mechanisms may also cause OR; in particular, IgG or other agents of the adaptive immune system have been speculated as causal.[34,35]

Nonimmunologic OR has been studied very little. A number of agents including biocides and cleaning agents have been reported to cause non–IgE-mediated rhinitis, but their mechanisms remain unclear.[36] In a study of nasal smears from 27 indoor pool workers with OR and 49 control subjects, it was reported that the OR subjects had more epithelial cells and more eosinophils than the control subjects.[37] Others have

Table 1
Prevalence, selected industries and exposures associated with occupational rhinitis

Industry/Exposure	Prevalence (%)	References
Laboratory animal workers	10–42	5
Bakers	23–50	4
Latex exposed workers	0.12–20	11,14
Foodstuffs (spices, vegetables, lupin) workers	5–54	15–17
Seafood (shrimp, crab, turbot) workers	5–50	18,19
Wood dusts (processing, carpentry)	10–78	20–22
Detergent enzymes (production, hospital use)	2–19	8,23
Organic acid anhydrides (epoxy resin production)	10–28	12,13
Diisocyanates (2 component paints, polyurethane workers)	1–54	24,25
Platinum workers	28–43	26
Nondomestic cleaners (janitors, hotel housekeepers)	35	27
Hairdressers	18–27	28,29
Swine confinement workers	8–23	30

Data from Refs.[4,5,8,11–30]

proposed mechanisms involving neurokinin release, nociceptors and epithelial damage and may reflect the mechanisms discussed for non-allergic rhinitis (See Baroody FM: Non-allergic rhinitis: mechanism of action, in this issue).[38–40]

CLINICAL FEATURES

The clinical manifestations of OR are similar to non-OR. The individuals generally have symptoms of nasal congestion, sneezing, rhinorrhea, and/or postnasal drip. Those with IgE-mediated disease often also have pruritus. Those with IgE-mediated disease have a latency, with usual onset of symptoms being 1 to 5 years after initial exposure. Those individuals with nonimmunolgic disease may have symptoms with the first exposure. Once the disease of OR is established, the individual generally develops symptoms within a short period of time (ie, a few minutes to an hour or so) after exposure to the causal agent.

On physical examination, an individual with OR will have findings of rhinitis such as boggy turbinates and increased nasal secretions may be visualized. Individuals with OR may also have associated ocular or chest symptoms owing to occupational conjunctivitis or occupational asthma.[2]

ACUTE MANAGEMENT

Avoidance is the principal strategy used to reduce signs and symptoms of OR over time. Acutely, the same pharmacologic therapies that are used in non-OR may be of benefit, as outlined in the current guidelines.[1] The most effective class of medications for control of rhinitis is intranasal glucocorticoids and intranasal antihistamines.[41] Nasal cromolyn could benefit some patients; nasal saline irrigation may be helpful. H1 antihistamines and leukotriene inhibitors may also be useful. Sedating antihistamines should, of course, be used cautiously, especially for workers who are involved in dangerous work processes.[42] Although immunotherapy is used in nonoccupational IgE-mediated rhinitis, it has not been adequately studied for OR and, therefore, is generally not advised.

CHRONIC MANAGEMENT

The chronic management of OR involves avoidance strategies, once the implicated agent has been identified.[43] In some cases, the employee can be moved to another location and complete avoidance can be achieved. In other cases, personal protective equipment such as a mask or respirator may suffice. Sometimes, improved ventilation or containment of a process may be useful. Whether reduction of exposure is sufficient is an area of controversy. If reduction rather than avoidance of exposure is implemented, careful surveillance for persistent symptoms or the progression to OA is in order.

DIFFERENTIAL DIAGNOSIS

The differential diagnosis of OR is rhinitis owing to any other causes. The clinical history alone has a relatively low specificity for verifying the diagnosis of OR, and therefore additional evaluation is generally necessary.[44] **Fig. 2** presents an algorithm for the evaluation of a patient with rhinitis symptoms related to work. Of course, the evaluation starts with a careful history, focusing on the onset of symptoms and their temporal relationship to possible workplace exposures. Material safety data sheets can be obtained for LMW agents to determine whether the exposures are known respiratory sensitizers or irritants. Most HMW exposures do not have material safety data

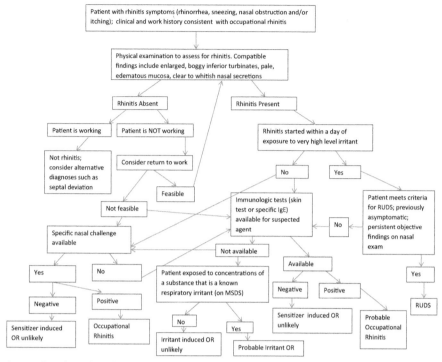

Fig. 2. This algorithm shows a general approach to the patient who has symptoms and exposure history compatible with occupational rhinitis (OR). IgE, immunoglobulin E; MSDS, material safety data sheet; RUDS, reactive upper airway dysfunction syndrome.

sheets. It should be recognized that any process that results in aerosolization of foreign proteins can result in sensitization to those foreign proteins.

IgE-mediated disease has a latency; in contrast, neither irritant-induced OR nor reactive upper airway dysfunction syndrome have a latency period.[45] On physical examination, the patient should have evidence of rhinitis: erythema, edema, and rhinorrhea. Given the known association of OR and OA, all OR patients should have a chest examination and objective screening for asthma, which may be subclinical. If the OR is thought to be IgE mediated, an in vitro or in vivo test of specific IgE could be performed, with the caveat that sensitization does not necessarily mean disease. Nasal provocation tests are the gold standard for the diagnosis of OR.[2,44] However, nasal challenge studies are limited by the availability of appropriately characterized reagents, the lack of agreed upon criteria for a positive result, and the number of centers with expertise to perform well-controlled provocation testing.

PROGNOSIS

If avoidance of the causative agent can be achieved, the prognosis of individuals with OR is generally good. In a report of greenhouse employees with OR, those who avoided exposure reported a significantly improved quality of life as compared with those individuals who continued exposure.[46] In a prospective study of 20 individuals with allergic or nonallergic OR, when causative exposures were eliminated, the individuals noted both decreased nasal symptoms and improved quality of life.[47]

AREAS REQUIRING FURTHER INVESTIGATION

OR remains an underrecognized and poorly investigated condition. The clinical features and pathophysiologic mechanism of nonallergic OR are unclear. The epidemiology and contribution of OR to the general burden of rhinitis is also unknown. Furthermore, a validated questionnaire to identify OR in epidemiologic surveys has not yet been developed. This lack has directly impeded the ability to identify the relevance of risk factors, such as smoking and other clinical characteristics for OR.

Standardization of occupational allergen extracts for in vitro or in vivo testing to confirm occupational allergen-specific IgE in workers suspected of HMW-induced OR are generally unavailable, as are standardized methodologies for performing nasal provocation tests to occupational agents and meaningful clinical endpoints are lacking. It has been speculated, but not proven, that OR can result from local allergic rhinitis.[48] Finally, understanding the magnitude of exposure reduction to the inciting agent(s) is needed that results in a good prognosis; at present, absolute avoidance is the recommended therapy.

FUTURE CONSIDERATIONS AND SUMMARY

Rhinitis affects up to 30% of individuals in Westernized societies.[49,50] The prevalence and incidence of OR and the clinical and economic burden it has on industrialized countries is unknown. OR can be allergic or nonallergic. Some agents are frequently causal and exposure level seems to be a risk factor. Agents known to cause OR, such as lactase, can appear in previously undescribed environmental settings.[51]

OR can be associated with occupational asthma. New causes of immunologic occupational asthma are often associated with symptoms of OR.[52] A diagnosis of OR cannot be made with clinical history alone. The prognosis seems to be good with avoidance of the offending exposure. However, OR is understudied and many questions and challenges remain, including criteria for nasal provocation tests and availability of standardized agents for testing.

REFERENCES

1. Wallace DV, Dykewicz MS, Bernstein DI, et al. The diagnosis and management of rhinitis: an updated practice parameter. J Allergy Clin Immunol 2008;122: S1–84.
2. Moscato G, Vandenplas O, Van Wijk RG, et al. EAACI position paper on occupational rhinitis. Respir Res 2009;10:16.
3. Ameille J, Hamelin K, Andujar P, et al. Occupational Asthma and Occupational Rhinitis: The United Airways Disease Model Revisited. Occup Environ Med 2013;70:471–5.
4. Storaas T, Steinsvag SK, Florvaag E, et al. Occupational rhinitis: diagnostic criteria, relation to lower airway symptoms and IgE sensitization in bakery workers. Acta Otolaryngol 2005;125:1211–7.
5. Folletti I, Forcina A, Marabini A, et al. Have the prevalence and incidence of occupational asthma and rhinitis because of laboratory animals declined in the last 25 years? Allergy 2008;63:834–41.
6. Ferraz E, Arruda LK, Bagatin E, et al. Laboratory animals and respiratory allergies: the prevalence of allergies among laboratory animal workers and the need for prophylaxis. Clinics (Sao Paulo) 2013;68:750–9.
7. Hytonen M, Kanerva L, Malmberg H, et al. The risk of occupational rhinitis. Int Arch Occup Environ Health 1997;69:487–90.

8. Cullinan P, Harris JM, Newman Taylor AJ, et al. An outbreak of asthma in a modern detergent factory. Lancet 2000;356:1899–900.

9. Houba R, Heederik D, Doekes G. Wheat sensitization and work related symptoms in the baking industry are preventable. Am J Respir Crit Care Med 1998;158:1499–503.

10. Heederik D, Venables KM, Malmberg P, et al. Exposure-response relationships for work related sensitization in workers exposed to rat urinary antigens. J Allergy Clin Immunol 1999;103:678–84.

11. Vandenplas O, Larbanois A, Vanassche F, et al. Latex-induced occupational asthma: time trend in incidence and relationship with hospital glove policies. Allergy 2009;64:415–20.

12. Nielsen J, Welinder H, Bensryd I, et al. Ocular and airway symptoms related to organic acid anhydride exposure-a prospective study. Allergy 2006;61:743–9.

13. Grammer LC, Ditto AM, Tripathi A, et al. Prevalence and onset of rhinitis and conjunctivitis in subjects with occupational asthma caused by trimellitic anhydride (TMA). J Occup Environ Med 2002;44:1179–81.

14. Larese Filon F, Bochdanovits L, Capuzzo C, et al. Ten years incidence of natural rubber latex sensitization and symptoms in a prospective cohort of health care workers using non-powdered latex gloves 2000-2009. Int Arch Occup Environ Health 2014;87:463–9.

15. Campbell CP, Jackson AS, Johnson AR, et al. Occupational sensitization to lupin in the workplace: occupational asthma, rhinitis and work-aggravated asthma. J Allergy Clin Immunol 2007;119:1133–9.

16. vander Walt A, Lopata AL, Nieuwenhuizen NE, et al. Work-related allergy and asthma in spice mill workers: the impact of processing dried spices on IgE reactivity patterns. Int Arch Allergy Immunol 2010;152:271–8.

17. Patiwael JA, Jong NW, Burdorf A, et al. Occupational allergy to bell pepper pollen in greenhouses in the Netherlands, an 8-year follow-up study. Allergy 2010;65:1423–9.

18. Perex Carral C, Martin-Lazaro J, Ledesma A, et al. Occupational asthma caused by turbot allergy in 3 fish-farm workers. J Investig Allergol Clin Immunol 2010;20: 349–51.

19. Bonlokke JH, Gautrin D, Sigsgaard T, et al. Snow crab allergy and asthma among Greenlandic workers—a pilot study. Int J Circumpolar Health 2012;71:19126.

20. Aranda A, Campo P, Palacin A, et al. Antigenic proteins involved in occupational rhinitis and asthma caused by obeche wood (Triplochiton scleroxylon). PLoS One 2013;8:e53926.

21. Schlunssen V, Kespohl S, Jacobsen G, et al. Immunoglobulin E-mediated sensitization to pine and beech dust in relation to wood dust exposure levels and respiratory symptoms in the furniture industry. Scand J Work Environ Health 2011;37:159–67.

22. Aguwa EN, Okeke TA, Asuzu MC. The revalence of occupational asthma and rhinitis among woodworkers in southeastern Nigeria. Tanzan Health Res Bull 2007;9:52–5.

23. van Rooy FG, Houba R, Palmen N, et al. A cross-sectional study among detergent workers exposed to liquid detergent enzymes. Occup Environ Med 2009; 66:759–65.

24. Bernstein DI, Korbee L, Stauder T, et al. The low prevalence of occupational asthma and antibody-dependent sensitization to diphenylmethan diisocyanate in a plant engineered for minimal exposure to diisocyanates. J Allergy Clin Immunol 1993; 92:387–96.

25. Sastre J, Poltronieri A, Mahillo-Fernandez I, et al. Nasal response in patients with diisocyante asthma. Rhinology 2014;52:431–6.

26. Baker DB, Gann PH, Brooks SM, et al. Cross-sectional study of platinum salts sensitization among precious metals refinery workers. Am J Ind Med 1990;18: 653–64.
27. de Fatima Macaira E, Algranti E, Medine Coeli Mendonca E, et al. Rhinitis and asthma symptoms in non-domestic cleaners from the Sao Paulo metropolitan area, Brazil. Occup Environ Med 2007;64:446–53.
28. Diab KK, Truedsson L, Albin M, et al. Persulphate challenge in female hairdressers with nasal hypersensitivity suggests immune cell, but no IgE reaction. Int Arch Occup Environ Health 2009;82:771–7.
29. Lysdal SH, Mosbech H, Johansen JD, et al. Asthma and respiratory symptoms among hairdressers in Denmark: results from a register based questionnaire study. Am J Ind Med 2014;57:1368–76.
30. May S, Romberger DJ, Poole JA. Respiratory health effects of large animal farming environments. J Toxicol Environ Health B Crit Rev 2012;15:524–41.
31. Gautrin D, Malo JL. Risk factors, predictors and markers for work-related asthma and rhinitis. Curr Allergy Asthma Rep 2010;10:365–72.
32. Castano R, Maghni K, Castellanos L, et al. Proinflammatory mediators in nasal lavage of subjects with occupational rhinitis. Otolaryngol Head Neck Surg 2010;143:301–3.e1.
33. Krakowiak A, Ruta U, Gorski P, et al. Nasal lavage fluid examination and rhinomanometry in the diagnostics of occupational airway allergy to laboratory animals. Int J Occup Med Environ Health 2003;16:125–32.
34. Grammer LC, Shaughnessy MA, Lowenthal M. Hemorrhagic rhinitis. An immunologic disease due to hexahydrophthalic anhydride. Chest 1993;104:1792–4.
35. Hox V, Steelant B, Fokkens W, et al. Occupational upper airway disease: how work affects the nose. Allergy 2014;69:282–91.
36. Siracusa A, Folletti I, Moscato G. Non-IgE-mediated and irritant-induced work-related rhinitis. Curr Opin Allergy Clin Immunol 2013;13:159–66.
37. Erkul E, Yaz A, Cingi C, et al. Effects of indoor swimming pools on the nasal cytology of pool workers. J Laryngol Otol 2014;128:442–6.
38. Meggs WJ. Hypothesis for induction and propagation of chemical sensitivity based on biopsy studies. Environ Health Perspect 1997;105(Suppl 2):473–8.
39. Castano R, Malo JL. Occupational rhinitis and asthma: where do we stand, where do we go? Curr Allergy Asthma Rep 2010;10:135–42.
40. Zhao YA, Shusterman D. Occupational rhinitis and other work-related upper respiratory tract conditions. Clin Chest Med 2012;33:637–47.
41. Rodrigo GJ, Yanez A. The role of antileukotriene therapy in seasonal allergic rhinitis: a systematic review of randomized trials. Ann Allergy Asthma Immunol 2006;96:779–86.
42. Banerji A, Long AA, Camargo CA Jr. Diphenhydramine versus nonsedating antihistamines for acute allergic reactions: a literature review. Allergy Asthma Proc 2007;28:418–26.
43. Moscato G, Rolla G, Siracusa A. Occupational rhinitis: consensus on diagnosis and medicolegal implications. Curr Opin Otolaryngol Head Neck Surg 2011;19: 36–42.
44. Nguyen SB, Castano R, Labrecque M. Integrated approach to diagnosis of associated occupational asthma and rhinitis. Can Respir J 2012;19:385–7.
45. Meggs WJ, Elsheik T, Metzger WJ, et al. Nasal pathology and ultrastructure in patients with chronic airway inflammation (RADS and RUDS) following an irritant exposure. J Toxicol Clin Toxicol 1996;34:383–96.

46. Gerth van Wijk R, Patiwael JA, de Jong NW, et al. Occupational rhinitis in bell pepper greenhouse workers: determinants of leaving work and the effects of subsequent allergen avoidance on health-related quality of life. Allergy 2011;66:903–8.

47. Castano R, Trudeau C, Castellanos L, et al. Prospective outcome assessment of occupational rhinitis after removal from exposure. J Occup Environ Med 2013;55: 579–85.

48. Gomez F, Rondon C, Salas M, et al. Local allergic rhinitis: mechanisms, diagnosis and relevance for occupational rhinitis. Curr Opin Allergy Clin Immunol 2015;15: 111–6.

49. Moscato G, Siracusa A. Rhinitis guidelines and implications for occupational rhinitis. Curr Opin Allergy Clin Immunol 2009;9:110–5.

50. Shusterman D. Occupational irritant and allergic rhinitis. Curr Allergy Asthma Rep 2014;14:425.

51. Stocker B, Grundmann S, Mosters P, et al. Occupational sensitization to lactase in the dietary supplement industry. Arch Environ Occup Health 2015;70:191–9.

52. Cartier A. New causes of immunologic occupational asthma, 2012-2014. Curr Opin Allergy Clin Immunol 2015;15:117–23.

Rhinitis in the Elderly

Alan P. Baptist, MD, MPH[a],*, Sharmilee Nyenhuis, MD[b]

KEYWORDS

- Rhinitis • Allergic rhinitis • Nonallergic rhinitis • Atrophic rhinitis • Elderly
- Older adults

KEY POINTS

- Symptoms of rhinitis are common, and affect approximately 32% of older adults.
- Nonallergic and atrophic rhinitis are more common among older adults than younger populations. Determining the rhinitis subtype can help to provide the most appropriate therapy.
- Special considerations regarding treatment need to be made because comorbidities, limited income, memory loss, and side effects of medications frequently occur and may impact outcomes.

EPIDEMIOLOGY OF RHINITIS IN THE ELDERLY

Unfortunately, older adults are routinely excluded from large epidemiologic studies on rhinitis. For example, both National Health and Nutrition Examination Survey III and the European Swiss Study on Air Pollution and Lung Disease in Adults study (which each had more than 8000 participants) excluded anyone over the age of 60 when analyzing rhinitis outcomes and prevalence.[1] Allergic rhinitis (AR) seems to decrease with age, and older literature has suggested a prevalence of approximately 12%.[2] However, more recent literature suggests that this figure may underestimate significantly the current rhinitis prevalence rate.[3] Results from the National Health and Nutrition Examination Survey from 2005 and 2006 found that the self-reported prevalence of rhinitis was approximately 32% among those between the age of 54 and 89, which was no different than younger adult populations (**Fig. 1**).[4] However, in that study adults aged 54 to 89 had significantly lower rates of allergic sensitization compared with younger age groups (although approximately 33% of older adults were positive for inhalant allergen sensitivity on skin testing). Overall, it seems that non-AR (NAR) increases with age, and the highest prevalence is seen in the elderly.[5]

Funding Support: National Institute on Aging 1 R01 AG043401-01A1.
[a] Division of Allergy and Clinical Immunology, University of Michigan, 24 Frank Lloyd Wright Drive, Suite H-2100, Ann Arbor, MI 48106, USA; [b] Division of Pulmonary, Critical Care, Sleep and Allergy, University of Illinois at Chicago, 840 S. Wood Street MC 719, Chicago, IL 60612, USA
* Corresponding author.
E-mail address: abaptist@med.umich.edu

Immunol Allergy Clin N Am 36 (2016) 343–357
http://dx.doi.org/10.1016/j.iac.2015.12.010
0889-8561/16/$ – see front matter © 2016 Elsevier Inc. All rights reserved.

immunology.theclinics.com

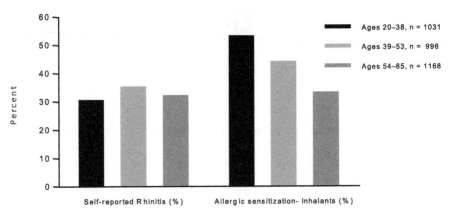

Fig. 1. Self-reported rhinitis and allergic sensitization among participants in the National Health and Nutrition Examination Survey 2005-2006 study. (*Data from* Shargorodsky J, Garcia-Esquinas E, Galán I, et al. Allergic sensitization, rhinitis and tobacco smoke exposure in US adults. PLoS One 2015;10(7):e0131957.)

TYPES OF RHINITIS IN THE ELDERLY
Allergic Rhinitis

AR is characterized by intermittent or persistent symptoms of nasal congestion, rhinorrhea, nasal/ocular pruritus, sneezing, and postnasal drainage. These symptoms are a result of immunoglobulin (Ig)E-mediated allergic inflammation in the nasal mucosa triggered by various allergens. Triggering allergens may be seasonal or perennial. The seasonal allergens include pollen and mold, and perennial allergens include dust mites, pet dander, and pests (eg, cockroaches, mice). A key component to diagnosing AR is objective evidence of allergen sensitivity. Allergy skin testing (prick and intracutaneous) or serum testing for specific IgE is used to assess allergen sensitization to environmental allergens. Allergen sensitization as well as total IgE have been shown to diminish with age.[6–8]

Recent reports have revealed a subset of rhinitis patients with a positive nasal provocation to allergens despite negative skin prick tests.[9,10] It has been hypothesized that these patients have localized AR. Further studies are needed to gain a better understanding of the immunopathology, prevalence, practical diagnostic tests, and management of localized AR, especially in older adults.

Nonallergic Rhinitis

NAR is characterized by symptoms of nasal congestion, rhinorrhea, and postnasal drainage in the absence of specific IgE-dependent events.[11] The diagnosis of NAR is based on clinical history and exclusion of other causes of rhinitis. The symptoms of NAR may be persistent, intermittent, seasonal (climatic), and/or elicited by recognized triggers. These triggers include cold air, changes in climate, strong odors, pollutants, chemicals, and exercise, to name a few. Gustatory rhinitis is a form of NAR triggered by eating, which can be a frequent complaint of older rhinitis patients.[12]

Mixed Rhinitis

NAR frequently co-occurs in 44% to 87%of patients with AR. This condition (NAR and AR) is called mixed rhinitis and has multiple triggers (eg, pollens, change in weather, strong odors).[13] The clinical presentation of mixed rhinitis can be variable and is characterized by intermittent or persistent rhinitis symptoms that are not fully explained by specific IgE sensitization (**Fig. 2**). Despite the often similar clinical presentation, it is important to assess for the presence of both by identifying symptom triggers. Recognition of co-occurrence of these 2 common conditions, will help clinicians to provide the most effective and appropriate treatment and help to reduce significant morbidity associated with both diseases.

Atrophic Rhinitis

Atrophic rhinitis is a type of rhinitis that is more prevalent in older adult populations.[14] This type of rhinitis is manifested by symptoms of congestion, nasal crusting, and fetor. Decreased blood flow to the nasal mucosa contributes to the local atrophy and leads to the enlargement of nasal space with paradoxical nasal congestion.[14] Atrophic rhinitis can overlap with both AR and NAR (see **Fig. 1**).

DIFFERENTIAL DIAGNOSIS OF RHINITIS

It is important, especially in the older adult, to examine for comorbidities that may cause or contribute to rhinitis. The differential is varied from granulomatous diseases such as Wegener's granulomatosis and sarcoidosis to nasal polyposis, hypothyroidism, cerebrospinal fluid leak, and malignancy (**Box 1**). Many medications that are widely used in older adults, such as antihypertensives, psychotropics, alpha-adrenergic antagonists, and phosphodiesterase 5 inhibitors can cause a drug-induced rhinitis (**Box 2**).

SPECIAL CONSIDERATIONS IN OLDER ADULTS
Age-related Nasal Changes

With normal aging, there are several changes that occur in the nasal anatomy and physiology that may impact the presence and severity of rhinitis symptoms. Structural changes include loss of nasal tip support owing to weakening of fibrous connective tissue at the upper and lower lateral cartilages and collagen fiber atrophy that leads to a dropped nasal tip.[15,16] Furthermore, fragmentation and weakening of septal cartilage and nasal columella retraction causes changes in the nasal cavity.[16] The

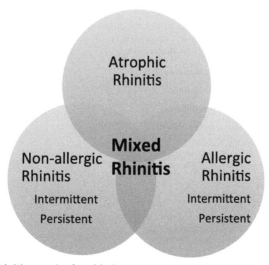

Fig. 2. Types of rhinitis seen in the elderly.

Box 1
Differential diagnosis for rhinitis in older adults

- Allergic rhinitis
  - Intermittent
  - Persistent

- Nonallergic rhinitis
  - Vasomotor rhinitis
  - Gustatory rhinitis
  - Infectious
  - Nonallergic rhinitis with eosinophilia syndrome (NARES)

- Occupational rhinitis
  - Caused by protein and chemical allergens, immunoglobulin E–mediated
  - Caused by chemical respiratory sensitizers, immune mechanism uncertain
  - Work-aggravated rhinitis

- Other rhinitis syndromes
  - Hormonally induced
  - Drug induced
  - Atrophic rhinitis

- Rhinitis associated with inflammatory–immunologic disorders
  - Granulomatous infections
  - Wegener granulomatosis
  - Sarcoidosis
  - Midline granuloma
  - Churg–Strauss syndrome
  - Relapsing polychondritis
  - Amyloidosis

- Cerebrospinal fluid leak

- Nasopharyngeal malignancy

Adapted from Wallace DV, Dykewicz MS, Bernstein DI, et al. The diagnosis and management of rhinitis, an updated practice parameter. J Allergy Clin Immunol 2008;122(Suppl):S10; with permission.

Box 2
Medications that can cause or contribute to rhinitis

- Aspirin/nonsteroidal anti-inflammatory drugs
- Alpha blockers (doxazosin, terazosin)
- Angiotensin-converting enzymes inhibitors
- β-Blockers (carvedilol, labetalol, nadolol)
- Calcium channel blockers
- Diuretics
- Oxymetolazone
- Oral contraceptives
- Phosphodiesterase 5 inhibitors (sildenafil, tadalafil, vardanafil)
- Psychotropics (risperidone, chlorpromazine, amitriptyline)
- Phentolamine

changes associated with the natural aging process may decrease nasal airflow and account for the symptoms of nasal congestion often found in older adults.

In addition to structural changes in the nose, mucosal changes are found with normal aging. The mucosal epithelium becomes atrophic and dry. A decrease in mucosal blood flow has been found with increasing age.[17] The decreased blood flow can contribute to decreased humidification of the nasal passages, because the submucosal vessels are not able to warm and moisten the inspired air sufficiently.[17] The decreased humidification of the nose leads to dryness, crusting, and irritation.

There are also change in the viscoelastic properties of nasal mucus that account for the excessively thick mucus in older adults.[18] Thick mucus mixed with impaired mucociliary function leads to the rhinitis symptoms of chronic postnasal drainage, nasal drainage, and cough.[18] Additionally, there is an increase in cholinergic activity in the nose with age that causes an increase in postnasal drainage.[19]

Aging is associated with decreases in olfaction, with the greatest decline occurring usually after the seventh decade. Seiberling and Conley[20] demonstrated that both the sense of smell and ability to distinguish between 2 smells diminishes with age. Diminished olfaction is also commonly found in rhinitis patients. One study found that 71% of patients with dysosmia had evidence of allergic sensitization.[21] The dysosmia that occurs in AR is attributed to obstruction of the nasal passages, although Sivam and colleagues[22] demonstrated that inflammation of the olfactory cleft might be the cause. Older adults with rhinitis thus have 2 contributing factors to olfactory dysfunction.

Immunosenescence and Rhinitis

There is a growing body of evidence describing changes in the function of immune cells with aging, a phenomenon referred to as "immunosenescence." Because rhinitis is a disease of inflammation, alterations in immune cell function with age may impact rhinitis in older adults. With normal aging, the thymus rapidly involutes, resulting in a decline in total T cells ($CD3^+$) involving both $CD4^+$ and $CD8^+$ subsets. In addition, a decrease in naïve T cells and an increase in the production of memory T cells. Despite the increase in memory T cells, their responses and T-cell proliferative responses to antigens and mitogens are diminished.[23–25] Finally, with aging, an increase in $FOXP3^+$ $CD4^+$ regulatory T cells exerting suppressive effects on T-cell function along with a shift in cytokine pattern from T-helper type 1 to T-helper type 2 cells also have been described.[26,27] These changes in cytokine patterns may explain late onset rhinitis and the decreases in T-cell response may be associated with the increase in infections found in older adults.

B-cell function also changes with aging. The peripheral B-cell population remains constant, although there is less IgG isotype class switching and then the total number of antigen-specific antibodies decreases.[28,29] This may be one explanation for why older adults are more prone to infection and have decreased immune response to vaccines. These aberrations in B cells may contribute to the symptoms of rhinitis, including infectious rhinitis.

Impact of Comorbidities

As people age, it is not surprising that the number of medical conditions and medications to manage these conditions increases. In the United States, 40% of those older than 65 use 5 or more prescription medications on a daily basis.[30] Patients with multiple chronic medical problems have several challenges to ensure optimal management of each of their conditions. There can be interactions between conditions, difficulties in determining which medical problem is primarily active when the symptoms are similar, decreased compliance with multiple medications, and conflicting recommendations in self-care management.[31]

Medication and self-management costs can increase exponentially in elderly patients with multiple comorbidities, and therefore certain conditions may receive suboptimal care owing to a lower prioritization by the individual.[32] Previous research has demonstrated that physicians often ignore and underdiagnose rhinitis.[33] This may owing to competing medical conditions and limited time spent during an examination, which is especially relevant among older adults with multiple comorbidities. Although rhinitis is typically not a life-threatening condition, it can significantly affect quality of life[34] and is deserving of care among older adults.

A few specific comorbidities deserve special mention when considering rhinitis in the elderly. Depression has been associated with anosmia, rhinitis, and chronic sinonasal disease in a number of studies.[35–38] Although the exact cause is unknown, theories for the association include sleep disturbance, inflammatory cytokine upregulation, and common etiologic pathogenic factors. Depression and depressive syndromes have an extremely high prevalence among the elderly population, with rates ranging from 15% to 35%.[39,40] One study found that, compared with placebo, treatment of depression and/or anxiety with escitalopram improved nasal symptoms, although participants in this study were younger than 50 years.[41] It is also important to note that multiple psychiatric medications can cause nasal drying or rhinitis, and therefore knowledge of the side effects of drugs that each patient is taking (even when prescribed by another physician) is critically important.

A second common comorbidity among the elderly is gastroesophageal reflux disease (GERD). The prevalence of this condition is thought to increase with age,[42] and among the elderly up to 22% of individuals have GERD.[43] A recent 10-year prospective cohort study found that those with nocturnal GERD were 60% more likely to develop rhinitis symptoms, although this study was not conducted among older adults.[44] Another recent study that included subjects up to the age of 75 also found a link between GERD and rhinitis symptoms.[45] The exact underlying mechanisms of the GERD–rhinitis association, and whether treatment of GERD will improve rhinitis symptoms in the elderly merits further investigation.

Sleep disturbance, and in particular obstructive sleep apnea (OSA), are also common in older adults. Similar to GERD, OSA symptoms increase with age. Among adults over the age of 70, approximately 25% are thought to have OSA, by far greater than any other age group.[46] Two recent studies evaluated the effects of AR treatment for OSA, and both found significant improvements in OSA symptomatology.[47,48] Underlying mechanisms of the improvement were thought to be related to improvements in nasal inflammation with a resultant decreased nasal obstruction. Although the mean age of the participants in these studies was approximately 49 years, the results may also be applicable to older adults, although again, further studies are needed.

Limited Income and Poverty

Among older adults, poverty is common. Data from the US Census Bureau found that approximately 10% of older adults lived below the poverty line.[49] Unfortunately, this number has been increasing over the past 10 years owing to a variety of factors, such as increased medical costs, loss of pension or retirement benefits, spending down assets to qualify for Medicaid and state-sponsored supplemental insurance coverage, and economic recessions requiring spending of retirement savings.[50] Currently, multiple antihistamines and intranasal corticosteroids (INS) have moved from prescription to over-the-counter (OTC) status. One study examining this switch for antihistamines found a 65% decrease in medication use,[51] and similar decreases in use have been seen in other prescription-to-OTC medication changes. Studies have not been conducted to examine the impact of prescription-to-OTC changes on rhinitis quality of life and symptom control associated with decreased use. It is important for the physician caring for older adults with rhinitis to inquire about the ability to afford both prescription and OTC medications, and to offer prescription assistance programs or social work referral as appropriate.

Complementary and Alternative Medicine for Rhinitis Among the Elderly

Complementary and alternative medicine (CAM) is defined as a group of diverse medical and health care systems, practices, and products that are not generally considered part of the conventional allopathic medical practices. Patients often use CAM therapy because of low cost, concerns of medication side effects, belief that adverse effects are not encountered with CAM therapy, and effectiveness (although such claims are often not based on clinical trials).[52] Examples of CAM used for allergic disease include herbal therapies, traditional Chinese medicine, acupuncture, nasal powders, and others.

Overall, CAM use has been increasing steadily, and 40% of population in the United States has used some form of CAM therapy.[53] Similarly high levels of CAM use for rhinitis have also been seen in both children and adults.[54,55] Older adults are often more likely than younger adults to use CAM therapy,[56] although this has not been examined specifically in rhinitis therapy. Additionally, older adults with atopic conditions such as asthma rarely tell their physician about CAM use, and physicians typically do not ask.[57] Although CAM use is typically thought to be safe by patients, adverse event monitoring is typically poor, and interactions with allopathic medications can occur. It is therefore important for the physician caring for the older adult with rhinitis to assess CAM use, and to work with the patient on a strategy that is both patient centered and effective.

Dementia, Memory Loss, and Medication Compliance in Older Adults

A cornerstone in the management of a chronic disease such as AR is compliance with a daily medical regimen. Unfortunately, memory loss owing to conditions such as dementia and neurovascular complications can make such a task difficult. Dementia and/or memory loss are common among older adults. For adults over the age of 60, approximately 13% note some degree of memory loss[58]; among those over age 85, the rate of dementia is 37%.[59] Additionally, the number of people in the United States with Alzheimer's dementia is expected to increase dramatically over the next 30 years as the population ages.[60]

Although the different methods of screening an older adult for memory loss and dementia are beyond the scope of this article, once such a patient is identified there are steps the physician can implement to help maximize medication compliance. These steps include prescribing as few medicines as possible, tailoring dose regimens to personal habits, and coordinating all drug dosing schedules as feasible.[61] The health care provider must assess the patient's level of self-efficacy and particular living situation when searching for the optimal medication adherence strategy, and at times may need to enlist a family member or other individual to accommodate medication delivery. Along with memory loss, other factors can affect compliance. Poor coordination, hand weakness, and arthritis may influence the ability to use nasal sprays. Health care providers should review the use of nasal sprays at each visit to ensure proper use.

TREATMENT OF RHINITIS IN THE ELDERLY
Allergic Rhinitis

One of the mainstays of AR treatment is avoidance of the offending allergens. In some cases, avoidance may reduce or eliminate the patient's symptoms. Implementing avoidance measures may be difficult in older adults owing to physical limitations to regular cleaning, financial constraints, or communal living situations. Older adults living in communal living situations such as nursing homes or assisted living may have little control to make changes in their environmental surroundings.

Second-generation antihistamines are standard treatment for mild AR. This class of medications is effective for the symptoms of ocular and nasal pruritus, rhinorrhea, and sneezing, but is less effective in reducing nasal congestion.[62] Medications in this class are generally safe in older adults with rhinitis. First-generation antihistamines should be avoided in older adults when possible because they have adverse effects on the central nervous system and interact with other medications. Additionally, studies have shown that the first generation antihistamines can affect driving performance, disturb the normal sleep cycle, and impact cognition, which can further worsen conditions prevalent in the geriatric population.[63,64] Topical antihistamines are an alternative to oral antihistamines. They are as effective as oral antihistamines and may decrease nasal congestion more so than oral antihistamines. Azelastine, a topical antihistamine, is well tolerated in older adults with rhinitis.[65,66]

INS are the first-line therapy for moderate to severe persistent AR.[62] They are effective in reducing all the symptoms of AR including nasal congestion, rhinorrhea, and nasal pruritus, but may not be as effective in NAR. They are generally effective and well-tolerated in older adults.[67] Side effects include epistaxis, nasal dryness, and mucosal crusting. Patients should be monitored periodically to assess for these adverse effects.

Immunotherapy is deemed the only treatment that can at least partly modify the natural course of the disease during its initial stages. Its use in older adults is still debated. Subcutaneous immunotherapy can be considered an effective therapeutic option in otherwise healthy older adults with short disease duration whose symptoms cannot be adequately controlled by medications alone.[68,69] One study also describes that sublingual immunotherapy reduces symptoms, drug consumption, and the progression of the disease in both young and older adults allergic to house dust mites and with persistent rhinitis and mild bronchial asthma.[70]

Nonallergic Rhinitis

Evidence-based guidance for the treatment of NAR in older adults is lacking. The treatment of NAR typically includes the use of INS, topical antihistamines, intranasal anticholinergics, and nasal saline lavage. INS and antihistamines (ie, azelastine) are recommended for the treatment of persistent NAR.[71] INS have shown improvement in nasal congestion compared with intranasal anticholinergics (ie, ipratropium bromide) in a randomized, controlled trial.[72] Owing to the wide availability of oral antihistamines, many patients with rhinitis symptoms have tried an oral antihistamine at some point during their course of treatment. Because the mechanisms of NAR typically do not involve histamine release, it is intuitive to believe that antihistamines have little impact on NAR. There has been no randomized, controlled study that has examined the use of antihistamines alone in the treatment of NAR.[72] However, 1 study from 1982 used a first-generation antihistamine in combination with a decongestant and found an improvement in NAR symptoms with this regimen.[73] Because the first-generation antihistamines exhibit significant anticholinergic properties, it is likely that the antihistamine improved the rhinorrhea, and the oral decongestant provided more benefit with nasal congestion. Second-generation antihistamines carry no anticholinergic properties, thus explaining the decreased clinical response in NAR.

The topical antihistamines have been shown to be effective in NAR owing to the antiinflammatory and neuroinflammatory blockade properties that azelastine and olopatadine exhibit.[74] Studies that have compared topical antihistamines (azelastine, olopatadine) to INS (fluticasone) found no superiority of either drug in the treatment of NAR.[75,76] Of importance, when the topical antihistamines azelastine is used in conjunction with intranasal fluticasone, patients have obtained greater symptomatic relief than with the use of either drug alone.[77–79]

Although oral decongestants are effective in treating congestion, few studies have examined the use of oral decongestants for the treatment of NAR, especially in the elderly rhinitis population. Two randomized controlled studies using phenylpropanolamine found a decrease in nasal congestion and rhinorrhea, although this drug has since been removed from the market.[72] No studies using pseudoephedrine in NAR have been reported. In general, using oral decongestants in elderly patients is ill advised owing to concomitant medical problems such as hypertension and cardiac disease. Anticholinergics such as ipratroprium bromide have demonstrated efficacy in reducing rhinorrhea in several randomized, controlled trials.[80–82] Despite its potent effect on rhinorrhea, it has little effect on the symptom of nasal congestion. This class of medications is best used when the main rhinitis symptom is rhinorrhea as in cold air–induced rhinitis. Moreover, despite the lack of an allergic component in NAR, environmental controls should be discussed and targeted at irritant triggers such as tobacco smoke, strong odors, and extremes in temperature and humidity.

Mixed Rhinitis

Currently, no treatment is specifically approved by the US Food and Drug Administration for the treatment of mixed rhinitis. The standard approach has been to treat patients with this condition similarly to other patients with allergic or NAR.[62] However, given the effectiveness of azelastine and fluticasone in allergic and NAR, combined use of these agents is likely to address many of the symptoms associated with this condition.

Atrophic Rhinitis

Treatment of primary and secondary atrophic rhinitis involves reducing crusting and alleviating the foul odor by instituting a regimen of nasal hygiene, such as nasal lavage and crust debridement, and the use of topical and/or systemic antibiotics when purulent secretions or an acute infection is present.[83]

UNIQUE MEDICATION AND TREATMENT CONCERNS IN OLDER ADULTS

The selection of medications for the treatment of NAR should take into account that older adults may be more susceptible to adverse effects of many of these medications. Oral first-generation antihistamines dosed at bedtime can be effective in NAR for controlling postnasal drainage in contrast with second-generation antihistamines, which have little to no effect. The adverse effects of first-generation antihistamines include urinary retention, dry mouth, constipation, arrhythmias, and postural hypertension. Therefore, one needs to carefully monitor for these potential side effects if they are required to treat postnasal drainage unresponsive to topical therapy. Typically, intranasal antihistamines are better tolerated than the oral antihistamines, but may not be as effective for drainage.

INS are generally well-tolerated. Although there is theoretical risk of osteoporosis with high-dose INS, studies have failed to show an increase in fractures or bone turnover.[84–86] Health care providers should monitor for glaucoma, especially if the patient is also taking inhaled or systemic corticosteroids. The impact of INSs on cataract formation is less clear than for intraocular pressure; Derby and Maier[87] found no

---

Box 3
Unique issues in treatment of rhinitis among the elderly

- Symptoms of rhinitis are common, and affect approximately 32% of older adults
- Nonallergic (including gustatory) and atrophic rhinitis are more common among older adults than younger populations; determining the rhinitis subtype can help to provide the most appropriate therapy
- Age-related nasal changes and immunosenescence contribute to atrophic rhinitis
- Comorbidities can affect the presentation of rhinitis, cause medication interactions, and impact compliance; the provider needs to be aware of each comorbidity, and how it may affect rhinitis management
- Poverty is common among older adults, and can affect the ability of patients to afford therapeutic recommendations
- Older adults are more likely to use complementary and alternative medication, and rarely tell their physician about it
- Dementia and memory loss are see in 13% older the age of 60, and affect the ability of a patient to manage a chronic disease like rhinitis; screening for memory loss may be appropriate
- Medication side effects are far more common in older adults; the provider should be aware of adverse drug effects for each medication a patient is on

---

increased risk in cataract formation in a large cohort of INS users. Oral decongestants have sympathomimetic effects, which can be of concern in the presence of comorbidities that are known to be more common in older adults, such as hypertension and cardiac disease. Anticholinergic drugs may cause excessive nasal drying and caution should be taken in patients with benign prostatic hypertrophy and narrow-angle glaucoma. In any clinical situation, one must always assess risk of taking a specific drug with benefits and patient preferences.

SUMMARY

Although there remain significant gaps in our knowledge of rhinitis in older adults (ranging from pathophysiology to prevalence to optimal treatments), there has been significant recent progress (**Box 3**). With the increase the in number of older adults in the US population, the magnitude of rhinitis in the elderly will increase. Correct diagnosis of these patients with the appropriate chronic rhinitis subtype is imperative to improve their therapeutic care, minimize rhinitis comorbidities, and improve their overall quality of life.

REFERENCES

1. Mims JW. Epidemiology of allergic rhinitis. Int Forum Allergy Rhinol 2014;4(Suppl 2):S18–20.
2. Enright PL, Kronmal RA, Higgins MW, et al. Prevalence and correlates of respiratory symptoms and disease in the elderly. cardiovascular health study. Chest 1994;106(3):827–34.
3. Slavin RG. Special considerations in treatment of allergic rhinitis in the elderly: role of intranasal corticosteroids. Allergy Asthma Proc 2010;31(3):179–84.
4. Shargorodsky J, Garcia-Esquinas E, Galán I, et al. Allergic sensitization, rhinitis and tobacco smoke exposure in US adults. PLoS One 2015;10(7):e0131957.

5. Georgitis JW. Prevalence and differential diagnosis of chronic rhinitis. Curr Allergy Asthma Rep 2001;1(3):202–6.

6. Warm K, Backman H, Lindberg A, et al. Low incidence and high remission of allergic sensitization among adults. J Allergy Clin Immunol 2012;129(1):136–42.

7. Simola M, Holopainene E, Malmberg H. Changes in skin and nasal sensitivity to allergens and the course of rhinitis; a long-term follow-up study. Ann Allergy Asthma Immunol 1999;82(2):152–6.

8. Busse PJ, Lurslurchachai L, Sampson HA, et al. Perennial allergen-specific immunoglobulin E levels among inner-city elderly asthmatics. J Asthma 2010; 47(7):781–5.

9. Alvares ML, Khan DA. Allergic rhinitis with negative skin tests. Curr Allergy Asthma Rep 2011;11(2):107–14.

10. Rondon C, Canto G, Blanca M. Local allergic rhinitis: a new entity, characterization and further studies. Curr Opin Allergy Clin Immunol 2010;10(1):1–7.

11. Dykewicz MS, Fineman S, Skoner DP, et al. Diagnosis and management of rhinitis: complete guidelines of the joint task force on practice parameters in allergy, asthma and immunology. Ann Allergy Asthma Immunol 1998;81(5): 478–518.

12. Georgalas C, Jovancevic L. Gustatory rhinitis. Curr Opin Otolaryngol Head Neck Surg 2012;20(1):9–14.

13. Settipane RA. Other causes of rhinitis: mixed rhinitis, rhinitis medicamentosa, hormonal rhinitis, rhinitis of the elderly, and gustatory rhinitis. Immunol Allergy Clin North Am 2011;31(3):457–67.

14. Moore EJ, Kern EB. Atrophic rhinitis: a review of 242 cases. Am J Rhinol 2001; 15(6):355–61.

15. Reiss M, Reiss G. Rhinitis in old age. Praxis (Bern 1994) 2002;91(9):353–8 [in German].

16. Patterson CN. The aging nose: characteristics and correction. Otolaryngol Clin North Am 1980;13(2):275–88.

17. Bende M. Blood flow with 133Xe in human nasal mucosa in relation to age, sex and body position. Acta Otolaryngol 1983;96(1–2):175–9.

18. Edelstein DR. Aging of the normal nose in adults. Laryngoscope 1996;106(9 Pt 2):1–25.

19. Dumas JA, Newhouse PA. The cholinergic hypothesis of cognitive aging revisited again: cholinergic functional compensation. Pharmacol Biochem Behav 2011; 99(2):254–61.

20. Seiberling KA, Conley DB. Aging and olfactory and taste function. Otolaryngol Clin North Am 2004;37(6):1209–28, vii.

21. Apter AJ, Mott AE, Frank ME, et al. Allergic rhinitis and olfactory loss. Ann Allergy Asthma Immunol 1995;75(4):311–6.

22. Sivam A, Jeswani S, Reder L, et al. Olfactory cleft inflammation is present in seasonal allergic rhinitis and is reduced with intranasal steroids. Am J Rhinol Allergy 2010;24(4):286–90.

23. Flurkey K, Stadecker M, Miller RA. Memory T lymphocyte hyporesponsiveness to non-cognate stimuli: a key factor in age-related immunodeficiency. Eur J Immunol 1992;22(4):931–5.

24. Murasko DM, Nelson BJ, Silver R, et al. Immunologic response in an elderly population with a mean age of 85. Am J Med 1986;81(4):612–8.

25. Naylor K, Li G, Vallejo AN, et al. The influence of age on T cell generation and TCR diversity. J Immunol 2005;174(11):7446–52.

26. Lages CS, Suffia I, Velilla PA, et al. Functional regulatory T cells accumulate in aged hosts and promote chronic infectious disease reactivation. J Immunol 2008;181(3):1835–48.

27. Sandmand M, Bruunsgaard H, Kemp K, et al. Is ageing associated with a shift in the balance between type 1 and type 2 cytokines in humans? Clin Exp Immunol 2002;127(1):107–14.

28. Bellanti JA, Azem M, MacDowell-Carneiro AL, et al. Possible mechanisms of late-life-onset allergic diseases and asthma in the senior citizen. Allergy Asthma Proc 2000;21(5):267–70.

29. Gruver AL, Hudson LL, Sennpowski GD. Immunosenescence of ageing. J Pathol 2007;211(2):144–56.

30. National Center for Health Statistics. Health, United States, 2012: with special feature on emergency care. Hyattsville (MD): 2013. Library of Congress Catalog Number 76-641496. Available at: http://www.cdc.gov/nchs/data/hus/hus12.pdf.

31. Bayliss EA, Steiner JF, Fernald DH, et al. Descriptions of barriers to self-care by persons with comorbid chronic diseases. Ann Fam Med 2003;1(1):15–21.

32. Schoenberg NE, Leach C, Edwards W. "It's a toss up between my hearing, my heart, and my hip": prioritizing and accommodating multiple morbidities by vulnerable older adults. J Health Care Poor Underserved 2009;20(1):134–51.

33. Nolte H, Nepper-Christensen S, Backer V. Unawareness and undertreatment of asthma and allergic rhinitis in a general population. Respir Med 2006;100(2):354–62.

34. Ozdoganoglu T, Songu M, Inancli HM. Quality of life in allergic rhinitis. Ther Adv Respir Dis 2012;6(1):25–39.

35. Katotomichelakis M, Simopoulos E, Tzikos A, et al. Demographic correlates of anxiety and depression symptoms in chronic sinonasal diseases. Int J Psychiatry Med 2014;48(2):83–94.

36. Audino P, La Grutta S, Cibella F, et al. Rhinitis as a risk factor for depressive mood in pre-adolescents: a new approach to this relationship. Pediatr Allergy Immunol 2014;25(4):360–5.

37. Nanayakkara JP, Igwe C, Roberts D, et al. The impact of mental health on chronic rhinosinusitis symptom scores. Eur Arch Otorhinolaryngol 2013;270(4):1361–4.

38. Wasan A, Fernandez E, Jamison RN, et al. Association of anxiety and depression with reported disease severity in patients undergoing evaluation for chronic rhinosinusitis. Ann Otol Rhinol Laryngol 2007;116(7):491–7.

39. Barry LC, Allore HG, Guo Z, et al. Higher burden of depression among older women: the effect of onset, persistence, and mortality over time. Arch Gen Psychiatry 2008;65(2):172–8.

40. Beekman AT, Copeland JR, Prince MJ. Review of community prevalence of depression in later life. Br J Psychiatry 1999;174:307–11.

41. Erkul E, Cingi C, Özçelik Korkmaz M, et al. Effects of escitalopram on symptoms and quality of life in patients with allergic rhinitis. Am J Rhinol Allergy 2012;26(5):e142–6.

42. Becher A, Dent J. Systematic review: ageing and gastro-oesophageal reflux disease symptoms, oesophageal function and reflux oesophagitis. Aliment Pharmacol Ther 2011;33(4):442–54.

43. Achem SR, DeVault KR. Gastroesophageal reflux disease and the elderly. Gastroenterol Clin North Am 2014;43(1):147–60.

44. Schioler L, Ruth M, Jõgi R, et al. Nocturnal GERD - a risk factor for rhinitis/rhinosinusitis: the RHINE study. Allergy 2015;70(6):697–702.

45. Hellgren J, Olin AC, Toren K. Increased risk of rhinitis symptoms in subjects with gastroesophageal reflux. Acta Otolaryngol 2014;134(6):615–9.

46. Duran J, Esnaola S, Rubio R, et al. Obstructive sleep apnea-hypopnea and related clinical features in a population-based sample of subjects aged 30 to 70 yr. Am J Respir Crit Care Med 2001;163(3 Pt 1):685–9.

47. Acar M, Cingi C, Sakallioglu O, et al. The effects of mometasone furoate and desloratadine in obstructive sleep apnea syndrome patients with allergic rhinitis. Am J Rhinol Allergy 2013;27(4):e113–6.

48. Lavigne F, Petrof BJ, Johnson JR, et al. Effect of topical corticosteroids on allergic airway inflammation and disease severity in obstructive sleep apnoea. Clin Exp Allergy 2013;43(10):1124–33.

49. DeNavas-Walt C, Proctor BD, Smith JC. Income, poverty, and health insurance coverage in the United States: 2012. Washington, DC: U.S. Census Bureau; U.S. Government Printing Office; 2013. p. 60–245.

50. Banerjee S. Time trends in poverty for older Americans between 2001-2009. Washington, DC: Employee Benefit Research Institute; 2012. p. 20.

51. Andrade SE, Gurwitz JH, Fish LS. The effect of an Rx-to-OTC switch on medication prescribing patterns and utilization of physician services: the case of H2-receptor antagonists. Med Care 1999;37(4):424–30.

52. Mainardi T, Kapoor S, Bielory L. Complementary and alternative medicine: herbs, phytochemicals and vitamins and their immunologic effects. J Allergy Clin Immunol 2009;123(2):283–94 [quiz: 295–6].

53. Barnes PM, Bloom B, Nahin RL. Complementary and alternative medicine use among adults and children: United States, 2007. Natl Health Stat Report 2008;(12):1–23.

54. Kemper KJ, Vohra S, Walls R, et al. American academy of pediatrics. The use of complementary and alternative medicine in pediatrics. Pediatrics 2008;122(6):1374–86.

55. Kapoor S, Bielory L. Allergic rhinoconjunctivitis: complementary treatments for the 21st century. Curr Allergy Asthma Rep 2009;9(2):121–7.

56. McFadden KL, Hernandez TD, Ito TA. Attitudes toward complementary and alternative medicine influence its use. Explore (NY) 2010;6(6):380–8.

57. Baptist AP, Deol BB, Reddy RC, et al. Age-specific factors influencing asthma management by older adults. Qual Health Res 2010;20(1):117–24.

58. Centers for Disease Control and Prevention (CDC). Self-reported increased confusion or memory loss and associated functional difficulties among adults aged >/= 60 years - 21 states, 2011. MMWR Morb Mortal Wkly Rep 2013; 62(18):347–50.

59. Mathillas J, Lovheim H, Gustafson Y. Increasing prevalence of dementia among very old people. Age Ageing 2011;40(2):243–9.

60. Hebert LE, Weuve J, Scherr PA, et al. Alzheimer disease in the United States (2010-2050) estimated using the 2010 census. Neurology 2013;80(19):1778–83.

61. Arlt S, Lindner R, Rösler A, et al. Adherence to medication in patients with dementia: predictors and strategies for improvement. Drugs Aging 2008;25(12):1033–47.

62. Dykewicz MS, Fineman S, Skoner DP. Joint task force algorithm and annotations for diagnosis and management of rhinitis. Ann Allergy Asthma Immunol 1998; 81(5):474–7.

63. McCue JD. Safety of antihistamines in the treatment of allergic rhinitis in elderly patients. Arch Fam Med 1996;5(8):464–8.

64. Holgate ST, Canonica GW, Simons FE, et al. Consensus group on new-generation antihistamines (CONGA): present status and recommendations. Clin Exp Allergy 2003;33(9):1305–24.

65. Golden SJ, Craig TJ. Efficacy and safety of azelastine nasal spray for the treatment of allergic rhinitis. J Am Osteopath Assoc 1999;99(7 Suppl):S7–12.

66. Peter G, Romeis P, Borbe HO, et al. Tolerability and pharmacokinetics of single and multiple doses of azelastine hydrochloride in elderly volunteers. Arzneimittelforschung 1995;45(5):576–81.

67. Grossman J, Gopalan G. Efficacy and safety of mometasone furoate nasal spray in elderly subjects with perennial allergic rhinitis. J Allergy Clin Immunol 2009; 123(2):S271.

68. Armentia A, Fernández A, Tapias JA, et al. Immunotherapy with allergenic extracts in geriatric patients: evaluation of effectiveness and safety. Allergol Immunopathol (Madr) 1993;21(5):193–6.

69. Asero R. Efficacy of injection immunotherapy with ragweed and birch pollen in elderly patients. Int Arch Allergy Immunol 2004;135(4):332–5.

70. Marogna M, Bruno ME, Massolo A, et al. Sublingual immunotherapy for allergic respiratory disease in elderly patients: a retrospective study. Eur Ann Allergy Clin Immunol 2008;40(1):22–9.

71. Banov CH, Lieberman P, Vasomotor Rhinitis Study Groups. Efficacy of azelastine nasal spray in the treatment of vasomotor (perennial nonallergic) rhinitis. Ann Allergy Asthma Immunol 2001;86(1):28–35.

72. Long A, McFadden C, DeVine D, et al. Management of allergic and nonallergic rhinitis. Evid Rep Technol Assess (Summ) 2002;54:1–6.

73. Broms P, Malm L. Oral vasoconstrictors in perennial non-allergic rhinitis. Allergy 1982;37(2):67–74.

74. Kaliner MA. Nonallergic rhinopathy (formerly known as vasomotor rhinitis). Immunol Allergy Clin North Am 2011;31(3):441–55.

75. Kaliner MA. Azelastine and olopatadine in the treatment of allergic rhinitis. Ann Allergy Asthma Immunol 2009;103(5):373–80.

76. Kaliner MA, Storms W, Tilles S, et al. Comparison of olopatadine 0.6% nasal spray versus fluticasone propionate 50 microg in the treatment of seasonal allergic rhinitis. Allergy Asthma Proc 2009;30(3):255–62.

77. Ratner PH, Hampel F, Van Bavel J, et al. Combination therapy with azelastine hydrochloride nasal spray and fluticasone propionate nasal spray in the treatment of patients with seasonal allergic rhinitis. Ann Allergy Asthma Immunol 2008; 100(1):74–81.

78. Hampel F, Ratner P, Haeusler JM. Safety and tolerability of levocetirizine dihydrochloride in infants and children with allergic rhinitis or chronic urticaria. Allergy Asthma Proc 2010;31(4):290–5.

79. LaForce CF, Carr W, Tilles SA, et al. Evaluation of olopatadine hydrochloride nasal spray, 0.6%, used in combination with an intranasal corticosteroid in seasonal allergic rhinitis. Allergy Asthma Proc 2010;31(2):132–40.

80. Georgitis JW, Banov C, Boggs PB, et al. Ipratropium bromide nasal spray in nonallergic rhinitis: efficacy, nasal cytological response and patient evaluation on quality of life. Clin Exp Allergy 1994;24(11):1049–55.

81. Becker B, Borum S, Nielsen K, et al. A time-dose study of the effect of topical ipratropium bromide on methacholine-induced rhinorrhoea in patients with perennial non-allergic rhinitis. Clin Otolaryngol Allied Sci 1997;22(2):132–4.

82. Bronsky EA, Druce H, Findlay SR, et al. A clinical trial of ipratropium bromide nasal spray in patients with perennial nonallergic rhinitis. J Allergy Clin Immunol 1995;95(5 Pt 2):1117–22.
83. Mishra A, Kawatra R, Gola M. Interventions for atrophic rhinitis. Cochrane Database Syst Rev 2012 Feb 15;2:CD008280.
84. Wilson AM, McFarlane LC, Lipworth BJ. Effects of repeated once daily dosing of three intranasal corticosteroids on basal and dynamic measures of hypothalamic-pituitary-adrenal-axis activity. J Allergy Clin Immunol 1998;101(4 Pt 1):470–4.
85. Wilson AM, Sims EJ, McFarlane LC, et al. Effects of intranasal corticosteroids on adrenal, bone, and blood markers of systemic activity in allergic rhinitis. J Allergy Clin Immunol 1998;102(4 Pt 1):598–604.
86. Cave A, Arlett P, Lee E. Inhaled and nasal corticosteroids: factors affecting the risks of systemic adverse effects. Pharmacol Ther 1999;83(3):153–79.
87. Derby L, Maier WC. Risk of cataract among users of intranasal corticosteroids. J Allergy Clin Immunol 2000;105(5):912–6.

Complications of Rhinitis

Anjeni Keswani, MD, MS[a],*, Anju T. Peters, MD[b]

KEYWORDS

- Complications • Rhinitis • Asthma and COPD • Sleep disturbance
- Learning impairment • Quality of life

KEY POINTS

- Individuals with chronic rhinitis should be screened for comorbid conditions, including asthma, chronic obstructive pulmonary disease (COPD), and rhinosinusitis to aid in treatment of these disorders.
- Rhinitis can lead to behavioral complications, such as learning impairment and sleep disturbances.
- The multiple complications of rhinitis lead to decreased quality of life (QOL).

INTRODUCTION

Chronic rhinitis involves inflammation of the upper airways and complications and comorbid conditions often arise. As the prevalence rises, there needs to be greater recognition of the influence of rhinitis on other disorders, such as asthma, COPD, and rhinosinusitis, as well as QOL issues, including sleep disturbances and learning impairment (**Fig. 1**).

RHINOSINUSITIS

Rhinosinusitis is often noted as one of the most common complications or comorbidities of rhinitis. A large volume of literature discusses the relationship between allergic rhinitis (AR) and rhinosinusitis, especially chronic rhinosinusitis (CRS). Non-AR (NAR) and its association to rhinosinusitis however, have not been well studied.

Observational studies support the association of AR and acute rhinosinusitis (ARS) in both pediatric and adult studies. In a cross-sectional study of 1008 atopic and nonatopic adults, atopic individuals had significantly increased risk of upper respiratory tract infections, suggesting that atopy may be a risk factor for ARS.[1] Similarly, a large

Disclosure Statement: The authors have nothing to disclose.
[a] Division of Pulmonary, Allergy, and Critical Care, Department of Medicine, Duke University Medical Center, 1821 Hillandale Road, Durham, NC 27705, USA; [b] Division of Allergy and Immunology, Department of Medicine, Northwestern University Feinberg School of Medicine, 251 E Huron St, Chicago, IL 60611, USA
* Corresponding author. Duke Asthma, Allergy, and Airway Center, 1821 Hillandale Avenue, Suite 25A, Durham, NC 27705.
E-mail address: anjeni.keswani@duke.edu

Immunol Allergy Clin N Am 36 (2016) 359–366
http://dx.doi.org/10.1016/j.iac.2015.12.011
0889-8561/16/$ – see front matter © 2016 Elsevier Inc. All rights reserved.

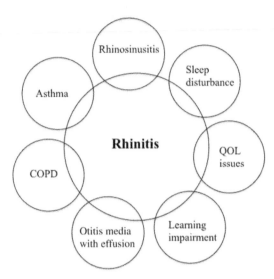

Fig. 1. Complications of rhinitis.

study from Taiwan determined that the prevalence of rhinosinusitis was higher in children with AR than in children without AR.[2] Moreover, Holzmann and colleagues[3] reported that orbital complications of ARS were more likely to occur in patients with AR during their pollen season. The role of AR in ARS is also suggested by a radiologic study that reported sinus mucosal thickening on CT scans of 60% of ragweed allergic subjects during ragweed season.[4] The radiographic abnormalities persisted in many of these subjects despite improvement in symptoms with medical treatment. Persistence of radiographic disease despite clinical improvement suggests a lack of etiologic connection between AR and ARS.

There are also numerous studies showing that atopy is more prevalent in populations with CRS. The prevalence of positive skin prick testing ranges from 50% to 84%.[5–7] Given the high prevalence of atopy in patients with CRS, it has been postulated that atopy and AR contribute to the severity of CRS. In pediatric patients undergoing functional endoscopic sinus surgery, children with AR had a significantly longer recovery time after surgery compared with nonatopic children, suggesting that atopy was a risk factor for protracted sinus disease.[8] When measuring CRS severity by sinus CT scan, there have been mixed results related to atopy. In studies looking at severe CRS, the extent of disease radiographically was significantly correlated with peripheral eosinophilia and the presence of atopy.[9,10] In patients undergoing revision sinus surgery, Batra and colleagues[11] found that patients with AR had worse endoscopic sinus severity and a higher mean Lund-Mackay score than those without allergies. Ramadan and colleagues[12] noted similar findings and found that allergic patients with CRS had higher CT scan scores (mean score = 12) compared with nonallergic patients with CRS (mean score = 6). Pearlman and colleagues[13] found no significant difference between mean Lund-Mackay score and presence of atopy in patients with CRS evaluated at a tertiary care otolaryngology clinic. Similarly, Tan and colleagues[7] found that there was no difference in Lund-Mackay scores among atopic and nonatopic patients with CRS undergoing sinus surgery. Finally, data linking AR and CRS are suggested by an observational study from a large group of primary care patients, which demonstrated that AR and chronic rhinitis were premorbid conditions associated with a diagnosis of CRS.[14] These studies suggest evidence of an association between allergy and CRS but there is no direct evidence of causality between the 2 conditions.

There are also studies that suggest an association between NAR and rhinosinusitis. Comorbidities associated with AR and NAR were studied in a group of Asian children and it was observed that sinusitis was more common in children with NAR compared with children with AR.[15] This study, however, did not distinguish between acute and chronic sinusitis. Finally, according to a retrospective review of a large database of both adults and children, rhinitis was significantly associated with both ARS and CRS.[16] In this group, patients with NAR were more likely to have sinusitis, including sinus radiography and procedures, compared with patients with AR.

ASTHMA AND CHRONIC OBSTRUCTIVE PULMONARY DISEASE

Within the framework of the unified airway concept, there is evidence that asthma and COPD are frequent complications of chronic rhinitis. Epidemiologic data demonstrate that rhinitis and asthma frequently coexist. Asthma is present in 78% of patients with rhinitis, both allergic and nonallergic subtypes.[17] Asthma and bronchial hyperreactivity are more often associated with perennial AR than with seasonal AR (SAR).[18–20] In a study by Guerra and colleagues,[21] subjects with rhinitis, both AR and NAR, had a 3-fold increase in the development of asthma compared with individuals without rhinitis. In a European survey, a strong association was found between asthma development and the presence of AR and CRS in individuals (adjusted odds ratio 11.85).[22] The presence of childhood AR has been associated with an increased likelihood of childhood asthma persisting into adult asthma.[23] Nasal symptoms have been reported in 40% to 75% of patients with COPD.[24] Nasal symptoms were associated with daily sputum production in a cohort of patients with COPD.[25] The presence of AR in individuals with COPD has been associated with an increased risk of COPD exacerbations and increased respiratory symptoms, such as wheeze, cough, and phlegm production.[26] These findings highlight the importance of recognizing and appropriately treating rhinitis in patients with COPD.

There have been many pivotal studies linking AR to bronchial hyper-responsiveness. Patients with AR demonstrate increased bronchial hypersensitivity to methacholine and histamine.[27] Individuals with SAR demonstrate seasonal bronchoconstriction.[28] Furthermore, in individuals with grass or birch pollen allergy, seasonal increases in methacholine-induced bronchial hyper-responsiveness and exercise-induced bronchoconstriction have been commonly observed.[29,30] Additionally, 46% of patients with NAR with eosinophilia syndrome without a history of respiratory symptoms demonstrated bronchial hyper-responsiveness.[31]

The unified airway concept postulates that the respiratory tract functions in a unified manner, with inflammation in the upper airways acting as a predisposing factor to inflammation in the lower airways. Because the mucosa of the upper and lower respiratory airways are structurally similar, there is a similar inflammatory response in rhinitis, rhinosinusitis, and asthma. Cytokines, such as interleukin (IL)-4, IL-5, and IL-13, are released in both rhinitis and asthma, and eosinophils may be elevated in both disorders.[32,33] Stimulation of the nasal passages with antigen has been shown to induce bronchial inflammation.[34,35] Inflammation in the upper and lower airways can be triggered by similar irritants, including allergens and pollutants. Additionally, allergen exposure can induce the expression of intercellular adhesion molecule 1, which is the receptor for 90% of human rhinovirus, and may increase the susceptibility of atopic individuals to rhinovirus infections and consequent asthma and COPD exacerbations.[36] Rhinitis and asthma are similar in their underlying pathophysiology and may represent a continuum of reactive airway disease.

SLEEP DISTURBANCE

Sleep disturbance, in the form of sleep-disordered breathing, obstructive sleep apnea (OSA), and snoring, can be a significant complication of rhinitis. In a 2005 survey of patients with AR by Blaiss and colleagues,[37] 68% of respondents with perennial AR and 51% of respondents with SAR reported that their rhinitis interfered with sleep, A study of approximately 5000 subjects with nasal congestion demonstrated that individuals who experienced nighttime rhinitis symptoms at least 5 or more nights per month were significantly more likely to report habitual snoring, excessive daytime sleepiness, or chronic nonrestorative sleep compared with those with rare or no nighttime rhinitis symptoms.[38] Chronic rhinitis has been demonstrated to be an independent variable for sleep-disordered breathing in children.[39] McColley and colleagues[40] demonstrated that there is a high prevalence of allergic sensitization in children with OSA and snoring.

Several inflammatory mediators and cytokines, which are up-regulated in AR, have also been shown to contribute to sleep disturbances and fatigue. Histamine and H_1 histamine receptors are involved in maintaining arousal and are thought to play a role in the sleep-wake cycle.[41] Cysteinyl leukotrienes may also mediate sleep disturbance through their role in the allergic inflammatory cascade,[42] In a study by Krouse and colleagues,[43] the cytokines IL-1beta, IL-4, and IL-10 were found higher in AR patients than in nonallergic patients. The presence of these 3 cytokines in AR patients correlated with an increased latency to rapid eye movement (REM) sleep, decreased time in REM sleep, and decreased latency to sleep onset.[43] The decrease in REM sleep in the subjects with AR may have contributed to daytime sleepiness and fatigue.

Nasal congestion from AR has been associated with a 1.8-fold increase in the risk of developing moderate to severe OSA.[38] Nasal congestion, irrespective of the allergic or nonallergic etiology, can lead to reduction in the internal nasal diameter and increases in nasal airway resistance,[44] which may lead to OSA. Nasal congestion is frequently accompanied by mouth breathing. In mouth breathing, the tongue is displaced downward, thereby reducing the pharyngeal diameter, which is a risk factor for OSA.[45] OSA can cause frequent arousals and lead to daytime somnolence. NAR has also been shown to be a risk factor for an elevated apnea-hypopnea index.[46]

OTITIS MEDIA

Otitis media with effusion (OME) is characterized by the presence of fluid in the middle ear cavity behind an intact eardrum without evidence of infection. Although OME is considered multifactorial in its etiology, eustachian tube dysfunction is thought to be central in its pathogenesis.[47] OME can lead to a reduction in the compliance of the eardrum and ossicles, leading to conductive hearing loss.[48,49] OME is the most common cause of hearing loss in children in developed countries and can lead to language and speech deficits.[50]

According to Stenstrom and Ingvarsson[51] allergic and atopic children had a 2-fold to 4.5-fold increase in the incidence of OME compared with nonallergic children. In a 2013 study by Kwon and colleagues[52] of 370 children with OME, 33.8% had concomitant AR compared with a prevalence of AR of 16% in the control group without OME. Tomanaga and colleagues[53] demonstrated comorbid AR in 50% of their cohort of 259 children with OME. Finally, in a study single-center study of 291 children by Kreiner-Moller and colleagues,[54] there was an association between OME and AR with an adjusted odds ratio of 3.36. There was no association with NAR or nasal mucosal swelling.[54]

Allergic inflammation may contribute to the pathogenesis of OME by swelling and blockage of the entrance to the eustachian tube, causing dysfunction and secondary inflammation of the middle ear.[55,56] Additionally, a reduction in the lumen size of the inflamed eustachian tube may impede mucociliary clearance, leading to delayed clearance of middle ear effusions and resultant OME.[57] Allergic inflammation may also contribute to OME through increased susceptibility to viral infections.[55] The potential association of NAR and OME is still unclear and requires further study.

LEARNING IMPAIRMENT AND QUALITY OF LIFE

AR can significantly affect cognition, fatigue, and memory in children, which can, therefore, have an impact on learning and school performance.[58] There is increased school absenteeism and decreased productivity at school when present.[59] In 1994, AR accounted for 824,000 missed school days in the United Sates.[60] Rhinosinusitis, eustachian tube dysfunction, and hearing loss from OME, which are complications of rhinitis, may also contribute to decreased learning and school performance.[58] Vuurman and colleagues[61] demonstrated that AR was associated with impairment in academic performance and treatment with a sedating antihistamine led to a further decline. Treatment with a nonsedating antihistamine did not lead to resolution of the impairment demonstrating that AR, independent of treatment, affects learning ability.[61] Adults with allergic sensitization to ragweed have been shown to have impaired working memory and decreased cognitive processing time during ragweed pollen season.[62] Furthermore, a study in adults estimated work productivity decreased by an average of 20% on days when AR symptoms were at their worst.[63]

Chronic rhinitis has also been associated with reduced QOL. Meltzer and colleagues[63] demonstrated that adults with AR rate their overall health significantly lower than those without AR. More than 50% of individuals with AR surveyed described their symptoms as having at least a moderate impact on their daily lives.[63] In a pediatric study of patients with SAR, asthma, and/or cutaneous allergic disease sensitized to grass pollen, health-related QOL measures negatively correlated with the average pollen count in the previous week.[64] Additionally, recreational activities of children with AR are often limited by the disease and can lead to diminished social interactions.[58,65]

SUMMARY

The impact of chronic rhinitis as well as its complications and comorbidities should not be underestimated. The diagnosis and treatment of rhinitis are important both to improve related upper respiratory symptoms and to reduce or prevent associated comorbid disorders.

REFERENCES

1. Rantala A, Jaakkola JJ, Jaakkola MS. Respiratory infections in adults with atopic disease and IgE antibodies to common aeroallergens. PLoS One 2013;8:e68582.
2. Chen CF, Wu KG, Hsu MC, et al. Prevalence and relationship between allergic diseases and infectious diseases. J Microbiol Immunol Infect 2001;34:57–62.
3. Holzmann D, Willi U, Nadal D. Allergic rhinitis as a risk factor for orbital complication of acute rhinosinusitis in children. Am J Rhinol 2001;15:387–90.

4. Naclerio RM, deTineo ML, Baroody FM. Ragweed allergic rhinitis and the paranasal sinuses. A computed tomographic study. Arch Otolaryngol Head Neck Surg 1997;123:193–6.

5. Sedaghat AR, Phipatanakul W, Cunningham MJ. Characterization of aeroallergen sensitivities in children with allergic rhinitis and chronic rhinosinusitis. Allergy Rhinol (Providence) 2014;5:143–5.

6. Gutman M, Torres A, Keen KJ, et al. Prevalence of allergy in patients with chronic rhinosinusitis. Otolaryngol Head Neck Surg 2004;130:545–52.

7. Tan BK, Zirkle W, Chandra RK, et al. Atopic profile of patients failing medical therapy for chronic rhinosinusitis. Int Forum Allergy Rhinol 2011;1:88–94.

8. Lee TJ, Liang CW, Chang PH, et al. Risk factors for protracted sinusitis in pediatrics after endoscopic sinus surgery. Auris Nasus Larynx 2009;36:655–60.

9. Hoover GE, Newman LJ, Platts-Mills TA, et al. Chronic sinusitis: risk factors for extensive disease. J Allergy Clin Immunol 1997;100:185–91.

10. Newman LJ, Platts-Mills TA, Phillips CD, et al. Chronic sinusitis. Relationship of computed tomographic findings to allergy, asthma, and eosinophilia. JAMA 1994;271:363–7.

11. Batra PS, Tong L, Citardi MJ. Analysis of comorbidities and objective parameters in refractory chronic rhinosinusitis. Laryngoscope 2013;123(Suppl 7):S1–11.

12. Ramadan HH, Fornelli R, Ortiz AO, et al. Correlation of allergy and severity of sinus disease. Am J Rhinol 1999;13:345–7.

13. Pearlman AN, Chandra RK, Chang D, et al. Relationships between severity of chronic rhinosinusitis and nasal polyposis, asthma, and atopy. Am J Rhinol Allergy 2009;23:145–8.

14. Tan BK, Chandra RK, Pollak J, et al. Incidence and associated premorbid diagnoses of patients with chronic rhinosinusitis. J Allergy Clin Immunol 2013;131: 1350–60.

15. Vichyanond P, Suratannon C, Lertbunnaphong P, et al. Clinical characteristics of children with non-allergic rhinitis vs with allergic rhinitis. Asian Pac J Allergy Immunol 2010;28:270–4.

16. Schatz M, Zeiger RS, Chen W, et al. The burden of rhinitis in a managed care organization. Ann Allergy Asthma Immunol 2008;101:240–7.

17. Corren J. Allergic rhinitis and asthma: how important is the link? J Allergy Clin Immunol 1997;99:S781–6.

18. Leynaert B, Bousquet J, Neukirch C, et al. Perennial rhinitis: an independent risk factor for asthma in nonatopic subjects: results from the European community respiratory health survey. J Allergy Clin Immunol 1999;104:301–4.

19. Leynaert B, Bousquet J, Henry C, et al. Is bronchial hyperresponsiveness more frequent in women than in men? A population-based study. Am J Respir Crit Care Med 1997;156:1413–20.

20. Sibbald B, Rink E. Epidemiology of seasonal and perennial rhinitis: clinical presentation and medical history. Thorax 1991;46:895–901.

21. Guerra S, Sherrill DL, Martinez FD, et al. Rhinitis as an independent risk factor for adult- onset asthma. J Allergy Clin Immunol 2002;109:419–25.

22. Jarvis D, Newson R, Lovtall J, et al. Asthma in adults and its association with chronic rhinosinusitis: the GA2LEN survey in Europe. Allergy 2012;67(1):91–8.

23. Burgess JA, Walters EH, Byrnes GB, et al. Childhood allergic rhinitis predicts asthma incidence and persistence to middle age: a longitudinal study. J Allergy Clin Immunol 2007;120(4):863–9.

24. Montnemery P, Svensson C, Adelroth E, et al. Prevalence of nasal symptoms and their relation to self-reported asthma and chronic bronchitis/emphysema. Eur Respir J 2001;17(4):596–603.
25. Roberts NJ, Lloyd-Owen SJ, Rapado F, et al. Relationship between chronic nasal and respiratory symptoms in patients with COPD. Respir Med 2003;97(8):909–14.
26. Jamieson DB, Matsui EC, Belli A, et al. Effects of allergic phenotype on respiratory symptoms and exacerbations in patients with chronic obstructive pulmonary disease. Am J Respir Crit Care Med 2013;188(2):187–92.
27. Townley RG, Ryo UY, Kolotkin BM, et al. Bronchial sensitivity to methacholine in current and former asthmatic and allergic rhinitis patients and control subjects. J Allergy Clin Immunol 1975;56:429–42.
28. Gerblich AA, Schwartz HJ, Chester EH. Seasonal variation of airway function in allergic rhinitis. J Allergy Clin Immunol 1986;77:676–81.
29. Madonini E, Briatico-Vangosa G, Pappacoda A, et al. Seasonal increase of bronchial reactivity in allergic rhinitis. J Allergy Clin Immunol 1987;79:358–63.
30. Karjalainen J, Lindqvist A, Laitinen LA. Seasonal variability of exercise-induced asthma especially outdoors. Effect of birch pollen allergy. Clin Exp Allergy 1989;19:273–8.
31. Leone C, Teodoro C, Pelucchi A, et al. Bronchial responsiveness and airway inflammation in patients with nonallergic rhinitis with eosinophilia syndrome. J Allergy Clin Immunol 1997;100:775–80.
32. Bachert C, Vignola M, Gavaert P, et al. Allergic rhinitis, rhinosinusitis, and asthma: one airway disease. Immunol Allergy Clin North Am 2004;24:19–43.
33. Lemanske RF, Busse WW. Asthma. J Allergy Clin Immunol 2003;111:S502–19.
34. Braunstahl GJ, Overbeek SE, Kleinjan A, et al. Nasal allergy provocation induces adhesion molecule expression and tissue eosinophilia in upper and lower airways. J Allergy Clin Immunol 2001;107:469–76.
35. Braunstahl GJ, Hellings PW. Nasobronchial interaction mechanisms in allergic airway disease. Curr Opin Otolaryngol Head Neck Surg 2006;14:176–82.
36. Bianco A, Whiteman SC, Sethi SK, et al. Expression of intercellular adhesion molecule-1 (ICAM-1) in nasal epithelial cells of atopic subjects: a mechanism for increased rhinovirus infection. Clin Exp Immunol 2000;121(2):339–45.
37. Blaiss M, Reigel T, Philpot E. A study to determine the impact of rhinitis on sufferers' sleep and daily routine [abstract]. J Allergy Clin Immunol 2005;115:S197.
38. Young T, Finn L, Kim H. Nasal obstruction as a risk factor for sleep-disordered breathing. The University of Wisconsin Sleep and Respiratory Research Group. J Allergy Clin Immunol 1997;99:S757–62.
39. Bixler EO, Vgontzas AN, Lin HM, et al. Sleep disordered breathing in children in a general population sample: prevalence and risk factors. Sleep 2009;32(6):731–6.
40. McColley SA, Carroll JL, Curtis S, et al. High prevalence of allergic sensitization in children with habitual snoring and obstructive sleep apnea. Chest 1997;111:170–3.
41. Tashiro M, Mochizuki H, Iwabuchi K, et al. Roles of histamine in regulation of arousal and cognition: functional neuroimaging of histamine H1 receptors in human brain. Life Sci 2002;72:409–14.
42. Ferguson BJ. Influences of allergic rhinitis on sleep. Otolaryngol Head Neck Surg 2004;130:617–29.
43. Krouse HJ, Davis JE, Krouse JH. Immune mediators in allergic rhinitis and sleep. Otolaryngol Head Neck Surg 2002;126:607–13.
44. Corey JP, Houser SM, Ng BA. Nasal congestion: a review of its etiology, evaluation, and treatment. Ear Nose Throat J 2000;79:690–3.

45. McNicholas WT, Coffey M, Boyle T. Effects of nasal airflow on breathing during sleep in normal humans. Am Rev Respir Dis 1993;147:620–3.

46. Kalpaklioglu AF, Kavut AB, Ekici M. Allergic and nonallergic rhinitis: the threat for obstructive sleep apnea. Ann Allergy Asthma Immunol 2009;103:20–5.

47. Rosenfeld RM, Culpepper L, Doyle KJ, et al. Clinical practice guideline: otitis media with effusion. Otolaryngol Head Neck Surg 2004;130(Suppl 5):95–118.

48. Rovers MM, Stratman H, Ingels K, et al. The effect of short term ventilation tubes versus watchful waiting on heating in young children with persistent otitis media with effusion: a randomized trial. Ear Hear 2001;22(3):191–9.

49. Gultekin E, Develioglu ON, Yener M, et al. Prevalence and risk factors for persistent otitis media with effusion in primary school children in Istanbul, Turkey. Int J Pediatr Otorhinolaryngol 2004;68(8):1069–74.

50. Klein JO. The burden of otitis media. Vaccine 2000;19(Suppl 1):2–8.

51. Stenstorm C, Ingvarsson L. General illness and need of medical care in otitis prone chidren. Int J Pediatr Otorhinolaryngol 1994;29(1):23–32.

52. Kwon C, Lee HY, Kim MG, et al. Allergic diseases in children with otitis media with effusion. Int J Pediatr Otorhinolaryngol 2013;77(2):158–61.

53. Tomonaga K, Kurona Y, Mogi G. The role of nasal allergy in otitis media with effusion. A clinical study. Acta Otolaryngol Suppl 1988;458:41–7.

54. Kreiner-Moller E, Chawes BL, Caye-Thomasen P, et al. Allergic rhinitis is associated with otitis media with effusion: a birth cohort study. Clin Exp Allergy 2012;42(11):1615–20.

55. Simpson SA, Thomas CL, van der Linden MK, et al. Identification of children in the first four years of life for early treatment for otitis media with effusion. Cochrane Database Syst Rev 2007;(1):CD004163.

56. Lack G, Caulfield H, Penagos M. The ling between otitis media with effusion and allergy: a potential role for intranasal corticosteroids. Pediatr Allergy Immunol 2011;22(3):258–66.

57. Alles R, Parikh A, Hawk L. The prevalence of atopic disorders in children with chronic otitis media with effusion. Pediatr Allergy Immunol 2001;12(2):102–6.

58. Jauregui I, Mullol J, Davilla I, et al. Allergic rhinitis and school performance. J Investig Allergol Clin Immunol 2009;19(Suppl 1):32–9.

59. Mir E, Panjabi C, Shah A. Impact of allergic rhinitis in school going children. Asia Pac Allergy 2012;2:93–100.

60. Malone DC, Lawson KA, Smith DH, et al. A cost of illness study of allergic rhinitis in the United States. J Allergy Clin Immunol 1997;99:22–7.

61. Vuurman EF, van Veggel LM, Uiterwijk MM, et al. Seasonal allergic rhinitis and antihistamine effects on children's learning. Ann Allergy 1993;71:121–6.

62. Marshall PS, O'Hara C, Steinberg P. Effects of seasonal allergic rhinitis on selected cognitive abilities. Ann Allergy Asthma Immunol 2000;84:403–10.

63. Meltzer EO, Gross GN, Katial R, et al. Allergic rhinitis substantially impacts patient quality of life: findings from the nasal allergy survey assessing limitations. J Fam Pract 2012;61(2 Suppl):S5–10.

64. Roberts G, Mylonopoulou M, Hurley C, et al. Impairment in quality of life is directly related to the level of allergen exposure and allergic airway inflammation. Clin Exp Allergy 2005;35:1295–300.

65. Meltzer EO. Quality of life in adults and children with allergic rhinitis. J Allergy Clin Immunol 2001;108:S45–53.

Allergic Rhinitis
Environmental Determinants

Joan Dunlop, MD[a], Elizabeth Matsui, MD, MHS[b], Hemant P. Sharma, MD, MHS[c],*

KEYWORDS

- Allergic rhinitis • Environment • Allergen • Sensitization • Risk

KEY POINTS

- The prevalence of allergic rhinitis (AR) has risen in developed countries, and the rate of this change suggests environmental, more so than genetic, factors may be responsible.
- Multiple environmental influences significantly impact the prevalence of AR.
- Allergen exposure is an important determinant of AR. There is strong evidence that allergen exposure triggers symptoms in those with established AR. However, the relationship between allergen exposure and the initial development of AR is highly complex and incompletely understood, because some studies suggest allergen exposure in early childhood increases risk of AR, whereas others suggest a protective effect.
- There are several additional environmental factors that may influence the development of AR, including bacterial exposures (hygiene, farm residence, exposure to other children, endotoxin), air pollution, and environmental toxicants.

INTRODUCTION

The prevalence of allergic rhinitis (AR) has been rising globally, and seems to be associated with a Western lifestyle.[1] In Westernized countries, the prevalence of AR increased from the 1870s to the 1950s, whereas it began rising in developing countries in the late 1980s to early 1990s.[2,3] AR is now estimated to affect approximately 15% of the general population in Westernized countries,[3] and accounts for children in the United States missing about 2 million school days each year.[4]

Certain intrinsic host factors seem to be linked to the development of AR. For example, children with comorbid atopic diseases, such as atopic dermatitis, food allergy, and asthma, have a much greater risk of AR, likely as part of the atopic march of childhood.[5] Family history of AR and other allergic diseases also is significantly

[a] Division of Emergency Medicine, Children's National Health System, 111 Michigan Avenue NW, Washington, DC 20010, USA; [b] Division of Pediatric Allergy and Immunology, Johns Hopkins School of Medicine, 600 N. Wolfe Street, CMSC 1102, Baltimore, MD 21287, USA; [c] Division of Allergy and Immunology, Children's National Health System, George Washington University School of Medicine and Health Sciences, 111 Michigan Avenue, Northwest, Suite W-100A, Washington, DC 20010, USA
* Corresponding author.
E-mail address: hsharma@childrensnational.org

Immunol Allergy Clin N Am 36 (2016) 367–377
http://dx.doi.org/10.1016/j.iac.2015.12.012
0889-8561/16/$ – see front matter © 2016 Elsevier Inc. All rights reserved.
immunology.theclinics.com

associated with the development of AR. For instance, a 2015 German birth cohort study found that only parental AR and comorbid early eczema predicted AR up to age 20 years.[6] The environmental factors assessed in this study did not predict AR; however, other data strongly suggest an environmental link.

Although there is evidence for a strong genetic component to AR and other atopic disorders, these are complex genetic traits, and their inheritance patterns are incompletely understood.[7] Furthermore, the rapid increase in prevalence of AR during the twentieth century suggests environmental determinants, instead of or perhaps in association with genetic changes, may be the underlying cause. Several of these environmental changes took effect gradually between the late-1800s and mid-1900s in Westernized countries, and are now taking place, often more rapidly and simultaneously, in developing countries.

The manner in which environmental factors interact with underlying genes to lead to atopic disease is complex.[8] In the case of asthma, more than 100 genes have been implicated, and multiple environmental factors likely interact with each of those gene products. Also, there is growing evidence that specific epigenetic changes associated with environmental exposures may contribute to the risk of allergic disease.[9,10] As an example, in mouse studies, a maternal diet rich in methyl donors has been linked to increased allergic inflammation in offspring, mediated through DNA methylation.[10] Additional human studies are needed to further explore the role of epigenetic modifications in atopic disorders.

Because environmental changes may underlie much of the rise in AR prevalence, this article examines the evidence underlying key environmental determinants of AR. The role of hygiene as an AR determinant is first examined, then the contributions of allergen exposure, air pollution, climate change, and environmental toxicants to the development of AR are discussed (**Box 1**). Although some of these factors are known to induce symptoms in those with established AR, the primary focus of this article is to examine the evidence for these environmental exposures as risk factors for the development of AR.

IMPROVED HYGIENE AND BACTERIAL EXPOSURE

The "hygiene hypothesis" posits that improvements in hygiene have resulted in decreased exposure to microbes in early life and thereby an increase in the prevalence of allergic disease.[11] The sharp increase in AR prevalence in Westernized countries during the late-1800s to mid-1900s did coincide with important improvements in hygiene, including the separation of drinking water from sewage, which led to reductions in enteric diseases.[12] Other hygiene changes during that time included decreased exposure to farm animals and horses as transportation, chlorination of water, and eradication of malaria and helminth infections.

Aside from these hygiene improvements simply coinciding with the rise of AR, several epidemiologic studies have shown an association between AR prevalence and environmental factors that impact bacterial exposure. For example, early childhood exposures to farms and other children have been demonstrated to protect against AR. A 2013 European study demonstrated a combined effect of family size and farm exposure on childhood AR. The prevalence of AR ranged from 2% among farmers' children with more than two siblings to 12% among children with no farm exposure and no siblings. No effect modification was found between family size and farm exposure, suggesting different biologic mechanisms underlie the protective effects of each.[13] Additionally, farm exposure in early childhood is associated with lifelong protection against AR. In a large-scale Swedish study, living on a farm during the

---

Box 1
Potential environmental determinants of allergic rhinitis

Improvements in hygiene

Bacterial exposures
  Farm exposure
  Family size/exposure to other children
  Mode of dishwashing
  Cesarean section birth
  Early antibiotic exposure
  Endotoxin exposure, level and bioactivity

Indoor allergen exposures
  Cat, dog, and furry animals
  House dust mites
  Rodents (mouse and rat)
  Mold and indoor dampness
  Occupational allergens
    Rodents (laboratory workers)
    Latex (health care workers)
    Guar gum (carpet workers)

Air pollution
  Ozone
  Traffic pollutants

Climate change

Environmental toxicants
  Antimicrobial products
    Triclosan
    Parabens

---

first 5 years of life was associated with lower prevalence of AR in all age groups, even the oldest (up to age 75 years). Increasing degree of urbanization was associated with increased prevalence of AR, independent of childhood farm living, suggesting both childhood and adult exposures may affect AR risk.[14] Cleaning practices of pacifiers and dishes have also been linked to risk of allergic disease. Hand dishwashing, compared with machine dishwashing, has been associated in one study with lower prevalence of AR, asthma, and atopic dermatitis at 7 to 8 years of age.[15] In a Swedish birth cohort study, children whose parents cleaned their pacifier by sucking it were less likely to have asthma, eczema, and sensitization (to airborne and food allergens) at age 18 months. Furthermore, the salivary microbiota differed in those children whose parents sucked the pacifier, suggesting the observed clinical effect was driven by altered bacterial exposures.[16]

There is growing evidence that the effect of these altered bacterial exposures is mediated through changes in the gut microbiome during infancy. Cesarean section birth and early life antibiotic exposure have been shown to affect the microbiome composition, and are both also associated with increased risk of atopic disease.[17] In a large European birth cohort study, an increase in certain bacteria in fecal samples from 3-week-old infants was associated with heightened risk of allergic disease later in childhood.[18]

Multiple studies have examined the role of endotoxin environmental exposure in modulating allergic response to environmental allergens. Endotoxin may represent a specific bacterial product that affects AR risk. This is supported by findings of polymorphisms in the endotoxin signaling pathway, such as in toll-like receptor 4, which are associated with greater risk of allergic disease.[19] Alternatively, endotoxin may be a marker more generally of certain types of bacterial exposure. Endotoxin is the best studied, but a variety of microbial products serve as innate immune stimulants and may affect risk of allergic disease, such as peptidoglycans, CpGs, and flagellin.[20]

The relationship between endotoxin exposure and development of allergic disease seems to be complex. Some studies have found correlations between house dust endotoxin level in infancy and the development of AR in high-risk patients.[21] An inner-city birth cohort study in New York found that endotoxin levels were positively associated with wheeze, but inversely associated with eczema. No relationship was found with development of AR.[22] Another birth cohort in Boston similarly found an inverse relationship between endotoxin level and early eczema.[23] More research is needed regarding the elements of endotoxin exposure that modulate risk. For example, a nested case control study of infants at high risk for allergy in Cincinnati demonstrated that higher house dust bioactivity was significantly associated with lower numbers of positive skin prick test results to aeroallergens. There was no relationship of house dust endotoxin level and aeroallergen sensitization, suggesting the immunostimulatory activity of house dust may better predict risk of aeroallergen sensitization than endotoxin levels.[24] Finally, there may be a link between endotoxin and respiratory symptoms independent of allergic sensitization. In an occupational mouse allergen exposure study, allergic-type symptoms among workers who were not sensitized to mouse were associated with endotoxin exposure.[25]

ALLERGEN EXPOSURE

The rise in AR prevalence in Westernized countries coincided with several housing and lifestyle changes that increased indoor allergen exposure. Allergen exposure in susceptible hosts has been implicated in the development of AR; however, data regarding a protective effect of allergen exposure are conflicting. For certain allergens, such as those derived from dust mites, cockroach, mold, and pollens, a linear relationship between exposure and disease seems to exist, but the same is not necessarily true for pet allergens, such as cat and dog. The timing of allergen and bacterial exposures may be the key factor responsible for discrepancies between study findings. In an urban birth cohort at high risk for asthma, cumulative allergen exposure over the first 3 years to cockroach, mouse, and dust mite was associated with sensitization to those allergens at age 3 years.[26] In contrast, exposure to these allergens in the first year of life was negatively associated with recurrent wheeze at age 3. Furthermore, the combination of bacterial exposures in dust and higher allergen levels in the first year was the most protective against later wheeze. These findings, although not specifically related to AR, have important implications for the interpretation of conflicting studies of a link between allergen exposure and AR development. Because the first year seems so crucial, cross-sectional studies or even prospective studies in which allergen exposure is captured after the first year of life would be expected to give different results than those that collected exposure in infancy.

Cat/Dog Allergen Exposure

Despite the prevailing theory regarding the natural history of allergen exposure leading to sensitization and disease, several studies have found that early exposure to furry household pets, such as cats and dogs, may decrease the risk of sensitization and atopic disease, thus having a protective effect against allergic disease. A systematic review of recent birth cohort, cross-sectional, and case-control studies concluded that early life cat exposure is likely to protect against allergic disease. However, findings are inconsistent because a meta-analysis from 11 prospective European birth cohorts found no clear evidence for either a protective or detrimental effect of cat exposure on sensitization.[27,28]

The relationship between cat allergen exposure and allergic sensitization is complex. Very high levels of cat allergen in homes do not seem to increase the risk of sensitization, and many children who become sensitized to cat do not live in a house with a cat.[29] There are many determinants that may contribute to whether an individual exposed to pet allergen becomes sensitized. Some factors are related to the allergen itself, such as its biologic activity, and the timing, variability, and intensity of the exposure.[29] With regard to intensity, very high levels of exposure to pet allergen (unlike other allergens) may be tolerogenic. Community prevalence of pets is also important; particularly if there is no pet exposure at home and community prevalence is low, sensitization will unlikely occur. Furthermore, concomitant exposures to other allergens may influence sensitization, but the complexities of these relationships are poorly understood. For example, in New Zealand, where exposure to dust mites and cat in the home is common, cat exposure has little effect on dust mite sensitization. Meanwhile, in Sweden, where dust mites are rare, cat exposure at home is associated with decreased sensitization to other allergens.[29]

Concomitant exposure to microorganisms may additionally determine whether pet exposure leads to allergic sensitization. Animals carry endotoxin, pollens, or fungal spores, in addition to pet-derived proteins. Dog ownership is linked to increased airborne endotoxin, but cat exposure is not.[30] Cats, however, can serve as vectors for other antigens, such as *Staphylococcus aureus*. Dog exposure also alters the house dust microbiome and the fecal microbiome of children. Further studies are needed to determine whether similar effects can occur with other pets, but collectively these findings raise the possibility that animal allergen exposure and sensitization in itself may not be the mechanism by which animal exposure potentiates or prevents AR.

House Dust Mite Exposure

Increasing house dust mite allergen concentrations are associated with risk of allergic sensitization. Some hypothesize that the changes in homes, making them more airtight, warmer, and more humid, and development of an indoor-centric lifestyle have led to increased indoor allergen exposure, particularly dust mites, and associated allergic disease.[31] Specific changes, such as increased indoor temperature and wall-to-wall carpeting, may have contributed to enhanced dust mite allergen levels because mites thrive in warm, humid environments and are distributed not only in beds, but also carpet and upholstery. Several studies have demonstrated that increased dust mite exposure in young children is associated with sensitization and increased later risk for development of AR.[4]

Rodent Allergen Exposure

The role of rodent allergen in occupational rhinitis and asthma has long been described (discussed later). However, within the past decade, the importance of rodent allergen exposure in inner-city allergic disease has been uncovered. Mouse allergen is present in much greater concentrations in inner-city homes compared with suburban homes, and exposure to mouse allergen in homes has been associated with sensitization. Inner-city children with asthma who are both exposed and sensitized to mouse have significantly worse asthma morbidity.[32] In addition, mouse sensitization in early life has been linked with an increased risk of wheeze, rhinitis, and eczema by age 3 years in an inner-city birth cohort, suggesting that it is a risk factor not only for asthma, but other allergic diseases including AR and eczema.[33]

Mold Exposure

Both indoor dampness and mold exposure have been explored as potential determinants of AR. Several studies have found an association between mold exposure and asthma in childhood.[1] A 2013 systematic review and meta-analysis examined the association between mold exposure and risk of rhinitis. Prior studies were inconclusive, and this was the first meta-analysis. It concluded that exposure to dampness and mold at home are associated with increased odds of all rhinitis types, including AR. The association was strongest for mold exposure as measured by mold odor, a surrogate marker for microbial volatile organic acids. These findings suggest that interventions to prevent and remediate indoor dampness and mold may reduce risk of rhinitis.[34] A longitudinal study of Finnish children also demonstrated that water damage and moisture on household surfaces were consistent determinants of physician-diagnosed AR to a variety of allergens, again suggesting that indoor dampness and mold exposure play a significant role in the development of AR.[35]

Allergic Occupational Rhinitis

The natural history of occupational rhinitis argues for a disease model of allergen exposure leading to sensitization and then disease. High-molecular-weight allergens or low-molecular-weight allergens bound to proteins (hapten-protein conjugates) can elicit an allergic response.[36] Regular exposure to the allergen in occupational settings leads to sensitization and then development of allergic disease, usually within 1 to 3 years of employment. Occupational AR may be associated with ocular symptoms of allergic conjunctivitis, such as itching, tearing, and redness. The same mechanisms are responsible for occupational allergic asthma.

A well-studied example of occupational AR involves exposure to mice among laboratory workers who then progress to develop sensitization and rhinitis. In an observational study, it was noted that by 2 years almost 25% of workers in a mouse facility developed sensitization (positive skin prick test response to mouse).[37] Both the level and variability of mouse allergen exposure were found to influence immune responses. Sensitization increased as exposure levels increased until the peak, beyond which the incidence of sensitization declined. In addition, the more variable mouse exposure was over time, the less likely workers were to develop allergic sensitization.

Other examples of allergens that can induce occupational AR include latex in health care workers, guar gum in carpet workers, and psyllium used in laxatives in nurses.[38] Occupational rhinitis is covered in more detail elsewhere (See Grammer LC: Occupational Rhinitis, in this issue).

AIR POLLUTION

Individuals with AR have nasal hyperreactivity, rendering them more responsive to airborne irritants. These irritants likely therefore play some role in exacerbating symptoms of AR. Air pollution is known to have an impact on allergic diseases. Some studies suggest that the irritant effect of pollutants potentiates the allergic immune response.[39] Pollution may damage the nasal mucosa and impair mucociliary clearance, thereby facilitating the access of inhaled allergens to the cells of the immune system.[40] Airborne particles, including diesel fuel exhaust, are also able to carry allergens, thus potentially increasing their spread, or the duration of exposure. However, studies have not demonstrated a consistent link between living in regions with higher air pollution and a higher prevalence of AR.[41] The relationships of ozone and traffic pollution to AR are reviewed next.

Ozone

Ground-level ozone is created by chemical reactions between nitrogen oxides and volatile organic compounds in the presence of sunlight. The major sources of nitrogen oxides and volatile organic compounds include emissions from industrial facilities and electric utilities, motor vehicle exhaust, gasoline vapors, and chemical solvents. In challenge studies, ozone has been noted to directly induce inflammation in the nasal mucosa.[42] It also has been implicated in increasing allergenicity of tree pollens, such as birch.[43] In a Korean study, ozone exposure was associated with AR prevalence in children who resided in industrial areas. In addition, ozone exposure was significantly associated with the rate of newly developed sensitization to outdoor allergens, which may explain the mechanism for the related increase in AR prevalance.[44]

Traffic Pollution

Studies of components of traffic pollution have demonstrated varying degrees of association with AR. It is thought that diesel particles and other irritant gases, such as ozone, exert aggravating effects on allergenicity in AR.[1] These particles may potentiate allergenicity through multiple mechanisms including modification of the nasal epithelium, influencing immune response, and increasing the allergenicity of particular antigens. For example, nasal provocation studies in dust mite–sensitive individuals showed that combined challenge with dust mite allergen and diesel exhaust particles led to enhanced mast cell degranulation and increased severity of clinical rhinitis symptoms.[45] Increased air pollution has also been associated with increased IgE production against common outdoor allergens, such as tree pollen.[39]

In a Swedish birth cohort study of 2500 children, air pollution exposure was assessed by outdoor concentration of nitrous oxides (a marker of exhaust particles) and particles of less than 10 μm diameter (a marker of road dust). Pollution exposure during infancy was associated with increased risk of pollen sensitization at age 4 years, but exposures after the first year of life were not associated with later aeroallergen sensitization.[46] Therefore, the timing of pollutant exposure (during infancy) may be a key determinant in the observed increase in allergic sensitization. However, it is unclear if this sensitization leads to later AR. In a recent prospective study of more than 600 children, diesel exhaust particles exposure during infancy was associated with aeroallergen sensitization at ages 2 and 3 years, but not with AR at age 4 years.[47]

CLIMATE CHANGE

There is some evidence that climate factors may indirectly contribute to increased AR symptom severity (through its effects on the previously mentioned factors, such as pollution and pollen allergens), but not necessarily an increase in AR prevalence. A recent analysis found that regional differences in AR prevalence in the United States were related to a variety of climate factors, including humidity, drought, heat, and precipitation.[48] The highest prevalence was found in Southeastern and Southern states. No association between changes in climate over time and AR prevalence trends has been found. Therefore, more studies are needed to determine what role, if any, climate factors play in development of AR.

Some studies have suggested that global temperature changes may impact AR disease severity through effects on pollens and air pollutants. For example, temperature changes have been linked to longer duration of pollen seasons (such as ragweed), and a resultant increase in pollen allergen levels.[1] Temperature changes may also increase ozone levels, which as discussed previously are associated with enhanced allergenicity of birch tree pollen.[43] There is also some thought that increased temperature potentiates the effect of air pollution as an irritant.

ENVIRONMENTAL TOXICANTS

Environmental toxicants have increasingly been linked to allergic disease. These include antimicrobial agents, such as triclosan and parabens. Using data from the 2003 to 2006 US National Health and Nutrition Examination Survey, one study found that higher urinary levels of triclosan, but not bisphenol A (an endocrine-disrupting compound used in plastics), were associated with significantly greater odds of AR diagnosis in children younger than 18 years.[49] In another study that used 2005 to 2006 National Health and Nutrition Examination Survey data, urinary levels of triclosan and parabens were associated with increased odds of aeroallergen sensitization.[50] Similar associations between urinary triclosan and aeroallergen sensitization, and current AR diagnosis, were found in a study of Norwegian children.[51] The mechanisms of the effects of antimicrobials, such as triclosan, on the immune and respiratory systems remain unknown. In a mouse model of asthma, triclosan exposure alone was not observed to be allergenic; however, coexposure with a known allergen (ovalbumin) resulted in enhanced allergic response to that allergen.[52] Given how commonly antimicrobials are used in Westernized countries, more research is warranted to further examine their potential role in allergic disease.

SUMMARY

Increases in prevalence of AR may be related to a host of environmental factors that interact with underlying genetic predisposition. There is significant evidence that early life bacterial and allergen exposures serve as important environmental determinants of later AR. However, the exact mechanisms by which these exposures modulate AR risk are poorly understood, as evidenced, for example, by the complex relationship between pet allergen exposure and subsequent AR. Less is known about the role, if any, that air pollutants and climate change may play in the prevalence of AR. Further research is needed to delineate the most important environmental determinants of AR and their mechanisms of action, so that future prevention strategies may be devised targeting these environmental factors.

REFERENCES

1. Moussu L, Saint-Pierre P, Panayotopoulos V, et al. Determinants of allergic rhinitis in young children with asthma. PLoS One 2014;9(5):e97236.
2. Ratner B, Silberman DE. Critical analysis of the hereditary concept of allergy. J Allergy 1953;24(4):371–8.
3. Bjorksten B, Clayton T, Ellwood P, et al. Worldwide time trends for symptoms of rhinitis and conjunctivitis: Phase III of the International Study of Asthma and Allergies in Childhood. Pediatr Allergy Immunol 2008;19(2):110–24.
4. Greiner AN, Hellings PW, Rotiroti G, et al. Allergic rhinitis. Lancet 2011;378(9809): 2112–22.
5. Bantz SK, Zhu Z, Zheng T. The atopic march: progression from atopic dermatitis to allergic rhinitis and asthma. J Clin Cell Immunol 2014;5(2):202–10.
6. Grabenhenrich LB, Keil T, Reich A, et al. Prediction and prevention of allergic rhinitis: a birth cohort study of 20 years. J Allergy Clin Immunol 2015;136(4): 932–40.e12.

7. Wang DY. Risk factors of allergic rhinitis: genetic or environmental? Ther Clin Risk Manag 2005;1(2):115–23.

8. Schwartz DA. Gene-environment interactions and airway disease in children. Pediatrics 2009;123(Suppl 3):S151–9.

9. Begin P, Nadeau KC. Epigenetic regulation of asthma and allergic disease. Allergy Asthma Clin Immunol 2014;10(1):27.

10. North ML, Ellis AK. The role of epigenetics in the developmental origins of allergic disease. Ann Allergy Asthma Immunol 2011;106(5):355–61 [quiz: 362].

11. Fishbein AB, Fuleihan RL. The hygiene hypothesis revisited: does exposure to infectious agents protect us from allergy? Curr Opin Pediatr 2012;24(1):98–102.

12. Emanuel MB. Hay fever, a post industrial revolution epidemic: a history of its growth during the 19th century. Clin Allergy 1988;18(3):295–304.

13. Genuneit J, Strachan DP, Buchele G, et al. The combined effects of family size and farm exposure on childhood hay fever and atopy. Pediatr Allergy Immunol 2013;24(3):293–8.

14. Eriksson J, Ekerljung L, Lotvall J, et al. Growing up on a farm leads to lifelong protection against allergic rhinitis. Allergy 2010;65(11):1397–403.

15. Hesselmar B, Hicke-Roberts A, Wennergren G. Allergy in children in hand versus machine dishwashing. Pediatrics 2015;135(3):e590–7.

16. Hesselmar B, Sjoberg F, Saalman R, et al. Pacifier cleaning practices and risk of allergy development. Pediatrics 2013;131(6):e1829–37.

17. Johnson CC, Ownby DR, Alford SH, et al. Antibiotic exposure in early infancy and risk for childhood atopy. J Allergy Clin Immunol 2005;115(6):1218–24.

18. Penders J, Thijs C, van den Brandt PA, et al. Gut microbiota composition and development of atopic manifestations in infancy: the KOALA Birth Cohort Study. Gut 2007;56(5):661–7.

19. Sahiner UM, Semic-Jusufagic A, Curtin JA, et al. Polymorphisms of endotoxin pathway and endotoxin exposure: in vitro IgE synthesis and replication in a birth cohort. Allergy 2014;69(12):1648–58.

20. Shim JU, Lee SE, Hwang W, et al. Flagellin suppresses experimental asthma by generating regulatory dendritic cells and T cells. J Allergy Clin Immunol 2015. [Epub ahead of print].

21. Codispoti CD, Levin L, LeMasters GK, et al. Breast-feeding, aeroallergen sensitization, and environmental exposures during infancy are determinants of childhood allergic rhinitis. J Allergy Clin Immunol 2010;125(5):1054–60.e1051.

22. Perzanowski MS, Miller RL, Thorne PS, et al. Endotoxin in inner-city homes: associations with wheeze and eczema in early childhood. J Allergy Clin Immunol 2006;117(5):1082–9.

23. Phipatanakul W, Celedon JC, Raby BA, et al. Endotoxin exposure and eczema in the first year of life. Pediatrics 2004;114(1):13–8.

24. Kim H, Tse K, Levin L, et al. House dust bioactivities predict skin prick test reactivity for children with high risk of allergy. J Allergy Clin Immunol 2012;129(6):1529–37.e1522.

25. Pacheco KA, McCammon C, Liu AH, et al. Airborne endotoxin predicts symptoms in non-mouse-sensitized technicians and research scientists exposed to laboratory mice. Am J Respir Crit Care Med 2003;167(7):983–90.

26. Lynch SV, Wood RA, Boushey H, et al. Effects of early-life exposure to allergens and bacteria on recurrent wheeze and atopy in urban children. J Allergy Clin Immunol 2014;134(3):593–601.e512.

27. Dharmage SC, Lodge CL, Matheson MC, et al. Exposure to cats: update on risks for sensitization and allergic diseases. Curr Allergy Asthma Rep 2012;12(5): 413–23.

28. Lodge CJ, Allen KJ, Lowe AJ, et al. Perinatal cat and dog exposure and the risk of asthma and allergy in the urban environment: a systematic review of longitudinal studies. Clin Dev Immunol 2012;2012:176484.

29. Konradsen JR, Fujisawa T, van Hage M, et al. Allergy to furry animals: new insights, diagnostic approaches, and challenges. J Allergy Clin Immunol 2015;135(3): 616–25.

30. Platts-Mills JA, Custis NJ, Woodfolk JA, et al. Airborne endotoxin in homes with domestic animals: implications for cat-specific tolerance. J Allergy Clin Immunol 2005;116(2):384–9.

31. Platts-Mills TA. How environment affects patients with allergic disease: indoor allergens and asthma. Ann Allergy 1994;72(4):381–4.

32. Matsui EC. Management of rodent exposure and allergy in the pediatric population. Curr Allergy Asthma Rep 2013;13(6):681–6.

33. Donohue KM, Al-alem U, Perzanowski MS, et al. Anti-cockroach and anti-mouse IgE are associated with early wheeze and atopy in an inner-city birth cohort. J Allergy Clin Immunol 2008;122(5):914–20.

34. Jaakkola MS, Quansah R, Hugg TT, et al. Association of indoor dampness and molds with rhinitis risk: a systematic review and meta-analysis. J Allergy Clin Immunol 2013;132(5):1099–110.e1018.

35. Jaakkola JJ, Hwang BF, Jaakkola MS. Home dampness and molds as determinants of allergic rhinitis in childhood: a 6-year, population-based cohort study. Am J Epidemiol 2010;172(4):451–9.

36. Slavin RG. Occupational rhinitis. Ann Allergy Asthma Immunol 2003; 90(5 Suppl 2):2–6.

37. Peng RD, Paigen B, Eggleston PA, et al. Both the variability and level of mouse allergen exposure influence the phenotype of the immune response in workers at a mouse facility. J Allergy Clin Immunol 2011;128(2):390–6.e397.

38. Moscato G, Vandenplas O, Gerth Van Wijk R, et al. Occupational rhinitis. Allergy 2008;63(8):969–80.

39. Diaz-Sanchez D. Pollution and the immune response: atopic diseases–are we too dirty or too clean? Immunology 2000;101(1):11–8.

40. D'Amato G, Liccardi G, D'Amato M, et al. The role of outdoor air pollution and climatic changes on the rising trends in respiratory allergy. Respir Med 2001; 95(7):606–11.

41. Dockery DW, Speizer FE, Stram DO, et al. Effects of inhalable particles on respiratory health of children. Am Rev Respir Dis 1989;139(3):587–94.

42. Dokic D, Trajkovska-Dokic E. Ozone exaggerates nasal allergic inflammation. Prilozi 2013;34(1):131–41.

43. Beck I, Jochner S, Gilles S, et al. High environmental ozone levels lead to enhanced allergenicity of birch pollen. PLoS One 2013;8(11):e80147.

44. Kim BJ, Kwon JW, Seo JH, et al. Association of ozone exposure with asthma, allergic rhinitis, and allergic sensitization. Ann Allergy Asthma Immunol 2011; 107(3):214–9.e211.

45. Diaz-Sanchez D, Penichet-Garcia M, Saxon A. Diesel exhaust particles directly induce activated mast cells to degranulate and increase histamine levels and symptom severity. J Allergy Clin Immunol 2000;106(6):1140–6.

46. Gruzieva O, Bellander T, Eneroth K, et al. Traffic-related air pollution and development of allergic sensitization in children during the first 8 years of life. J Allergy Clin Immunol 2012;129(1):240–6.

47. Codispoti CD, LeMasters GK, Levin L, et al. Traffic pollution is associated with early childhood aeroallergen sensitization. Ann Allergy Asthma Immunol 2015; 114(2):126–33.

48. Silverberg JI, Braunstein M, Lee-Wong M. Association between climate factors, pollen counts, and childhood hay fever prevalence in the United States. J Allergy Clin Immunol 2015;135(2):463–9.

49. Clayton EM, Todd M, Dowd JB, et al. The impact of bisphenol A and triclosan on immune parameters in the U.S. population, NHANES 2003-2006. Environ Health Perspect 2011;119(3):390–6.

50. Savage JH, Matsui EC, Wood RA, et al. Urinary levels of triclosan and parabens are associated with aeroallergen and food sensitization. J Allergy Clin Immunol 2012;130(2):453–60.e457.

51. Bertelsen RJ, Longnecker MP, Lovik M, et al. Triclosan exposure and allergic sensitization in Norwegian children. Allergy 2013;68(1):84–91.

52. Anderson SE, Franko J, Kashon ML, et al. Exposure to triclosan augments the allergic response to ovalbumin in a mouse model of asthma. Toxicol Sci 2013; 132(1):96–106.

Nonallergic Rhinitis
Environmental Determinants

Dennis Shusterman, MD, MPH

KEYWORDS

- Nonallergic rhinitis • Environment • Air pollution • Chemical irritants
- Ambient temperature • Ambient humidity

KEY POINTS

- Nonallergic rhinitis (NAR) is a broad term, including conditions of known etiology, as well as a residual group whose main phenotypic characteristic is nonspecific nasal hyperreactivity.
- This hyperreactive subgroup has been variously labeled as having vasomotor rhinitis, idiopathic NAR, noninfectious NAR, and nonallergic, noninfectious, perennial rhinitis; nonallergic rhinopathy has also been proposed.
- Nonspecific nasal hyperreactivity is found, not only in idiopathic NAR, but also in a subset of allergic rhinitis patients.
- Common nonallergic environmental triggers include cold and dry air, second-hand tobacco smoke, wood smoke, fragrances and cleaning products, and industrial chemicals.
- A subset of individuals with apparent NAR may instead have local allergic rhinitis, characterized by mucosal-only production of relevant antigen-specific IgE. Nasal antigen challenge is necessary to identify this subset of patients.

INTRODUCTION

From the perspective of the environment, the nose serves as the portal of entry to the respiratory tract, filtering and conditioning inspired air, as well as signaling the quality of the surrounding atmosphere.[1–4] In this exposed position, the nose is vulnerable to the effects of physical or chemical agents, and may manifest acute, subacute, or chronic pathophysiologic changes.

Individuals who experience acute and reversible nasal symptoms (obstruction and/or hypersecretion) triggered by ambient physical or chemical exposures, and who do so without evidence of a typical allergic (immunoglobulin [Ig]E-mediated) mechanism, can be considered to have "environmental nonallergic rhinitis" ("environmental NAR").

Author Disclosure: No support was received for the writing of this article. The author has no commercial conflicts regarding the subject matter of this article.

Division of Occupational & Environmental Medicine, University of California, San Francisco, Campus Box 0843, San Francisco, CA 94143, USA

E-mail address: Dennis.Shusterman@ucsf.edu

Immunol Allergy Clin N Am 36 (2016) 379–399
http://dx.doi.org/10.1016/j.iac.2015.12.013
0889-8561/16/$ – see front matter © 2016 Elsevier Inc. All rights reserved.

The state of exaggerated nasal reflexes underlying this condition is referred to as nonspecific nasal hyperreactivity.[5] Such hyperreactivity is also reported by a significant subset of allergic rhinitis (AR) patients, rendering the condition more a phenotypic trait than a specific response mechanism.[6,7]

This article deals with the topic of environmental NAR. The objective of this article is to review the epidemiology, clinical manifestations, and unique mechanistic features of environmental NAR, and in particular to catalog the range of environmental exposures that may prove problematic to individuals with idiopathic NAR.

BACKGROUND: ANATOMY, PHYSIOLOGY, AND REGIONAL DEPOSITION OF AIR POLLUTANTS

The functional anatomy of the nose includes the extensive mucosal area of the turbinates, providing for warming and humidification of inspired air, as well as for removal of particulate and gaseous phase air pollutants. In the process, physical and chemical stimuli can elicit specific nasal sensations, including olfaction, warming or cooling, irritation and, less typically, nasal pruritus. Conveying these sensations, the nasal cavity is innervated by 2 main structures: the olfactory nerve (cranial nerve I, providing for the sense of smell), and the trigeminal nerve (cranial nerve V, providing for the sense of temperature and irritation; **Fig. 1**). Just as our appreciation of foods involves a combination of the senses of taste and smell, our appreciation of many inhaled compounds involves both olfaction and trigeminal stimulation. The latter carries sensations ranging from "freshness" or "cooling" (eg, in response to menthol) to burning or stinging (as elicited by ammonia or chlorine).[8]

Of relevance, our understanding of the peripheral neurobiology of trigeminal chemoreception has benefitted from significant molecular biologic developments over the last 2 decades. We have learned that the small diameter nociceptive neurons (C- and Aδ-fibers) constituting the terminal branches of the trigeminal nerve are invested with wide variety of nociceptive ion channels with both thermal and chemical responsiveness.[9–12] The C-fiber population also elaborates vasoactive neuropeptides, which in turn can be released locally as part of nociceptive reflexes.[13] More recently,

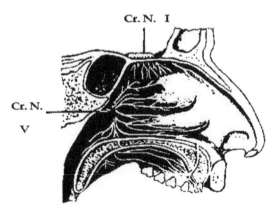

Fig. 1. Innervation of the nasal cavity. Cr. N. I, olfactory nerve; Cr. N. V, trigeminal nerve. (*From* Shusterman D. The upper airway, including olfaction, as mediator of symptoms. Environ Health Perspect 2002;110(Suppl 4):649–53.)

solitary chemosensory cells, with the capacity to sense both airborne irritants and bitter tastants, have also been documented in the human nasal mucosa.[14] Central and peripheral reflexes arising from nasal mucosal nerve stimulation include sneezing, rhinorrhea, nasal obstruction ("congestion"), cough, bronchospasm, and laryngospasm.[15,16] Although the vast majority of these reflexes are thought to be neurogenic in nature, the mechanism(s) underlying reflex nasal obstruction are less clear cut, as noted elsewhere in this paper.

The term "sensory irritation" is used by environmental scientists to describe trigeminally mediated mucous membrane (eye, nose, and throat) irritation, a symptom constellation common in so-called problem buildings.[17] Although rhinorrhea and nasal congestion are typical presenting complaints in environmental NAR, nasal hyperesthesia may, in fact, constitute the primary symptom in some patients, along with the related phenomenon of odor intolerance. Although odor intolerance is beyond the scope of this review,[18,19] irritation and nasal hyperesthesia are relevant to an understanding of environmental NAR. Neurobiological terms that have been invoked to explain nasal hyperesthesia and/or hyperreactivity after allergic or irritant stimulation include "neuromodulation," "phenotypic switching," and "central sensitization."[20,21]

Both physical and chemical stimuli can trigger nasal reflexes, including nasal secretion and obstruction. Classic examples include rhinorrhea occurring in response to consumption of spicy foods ("gustatory rhinitis") and cold air–induced rhinorrhea ("skier's nose"), both of which can be blocked symptomatically by the topical application of a cholinergic antagonist.[22,23] This clinical response, as well as the results of numerous nasal provocation experiments, have implicated a central parasympathetic reflex in most reflex rhinorrhea.[16,24] Nonallergically triggered nasal obstruction, on the other hand, ultimately reflecting vasodilation and/or plasma extravasation, has less clear reflex mechanisms.

In addition to acute and reversible symptom triggering (as in neurogenic inflammation), the rubric of environmental NAR can also encompass irritant-induced pathologic changes. For example, nasal mucosal swelling, whether from allergy, infection, or nonallergic reflexes, can potentially interfere with Eustachian tube and sinus ostial patency, thereby producing pressure disequilibrium in the middle ear and paranasal sinuses, and associated signs and symptoms otitis media or sinusitis.[25,26] Furthermore, exposures to photochemical oxidant air pollutants can produce actual histologic changes in the nasal mucosa, as reviewed elsewhere in this paper. In terms of exposures, irritant air pollutants include, in addition to "criteria air pollutants" (ozone, nitrogen oxides, sulfur dioxide, and particulate matter), a variety of industrial chemicals, combustion products (smokes and fumes), cleaning chemicals, and volatiles evolved by building materials and/or microbial growth (**Tables 1** and **2**).

When considering the impact of air pollutants on the upper airway, whether from vapors, gases, smokes, or fumes, regional dosimetry is an important consideration. With reference to particulate matter, the upper airway is disproportionately affected by large particles (ie, those >5–10 μm in diameter; **Fig. 2**). The regional deposition of gases and vapors, on the other hand, is dominated by the property of water solubility, with highly water-soluble compounds readily dissolving in mucus and thence activating upper airway mucosal irritant receptors (**Fig. 3**). Clearance of highly water-soluble gases and vapors in the upper airway ("scrubbing") can also be significant. For chlorine gas, for example, more than 90% of an inhaled bolus at concentrations up to 3 ppm is cleared above the larynx (ie, before entering the large conductive airways of the lower respiratory tract).[27]

Table 1
Environmental irritants

Source or Class	Specific Pollutant	Comment
Combustion Products	Second-hand tobacco smoke	Complex mixture of vapors, gases, and particulates
	NOx	Unvented stoves and heaters Vehicular exhaust
	SOx	Oil refineries; coal- and oil-burning power plants
	Ozone + PAN	Photochemical reaction products of VOCs + NOx from vehicular exhaust
	Particulate matter	Fireplaces and wood-burning stoves; power plants; diesel engines
Cleaning products	Hypochlorite, ammonia	—
	Chloramines, chlorine gas	Reaction products of inappropriate mixing
VOCs	Formaldehyde,[a] glycol ethers, various others	Off-gassing construction materials and furnishings
	Various	Stationery and art materials; polishes and waxes
	MVOCs	Microbial VOCs (byproducts of mold growth)

Abbreviations: MVOCs, volatile organic compounds of microbial origin; NOx, nitrogen oxides; PAN, peroxyacetyl nitrite; SOx, sulfur oxides; VOCs, volatile organic compounds.
[a] The formaldehyde content of pressed-board products is regulated by the US Consumer Products Safety Commission.
Modified from Shusterman D. Upper respiratory tract disorders. In: LaDou J, Harrison R, editors. Current occupational and environmental medicine. 5th edition. New York: McGraw-Hill; 2014. p. 348–61.

Table 2
Selected occupational irritants

Occupation	Irritant
Agricultural workers	Ammonia, nitrogen dioxide, hydrogen sulfide
Custodians	Ammonia, bleach (hypochlorite), chloramines
Firefighters	Smoke, hazardous materials releases
Food service workers	Cooking vapors, cigarette smoke
Health professionals	Glutaraldehyde, formaldehyde
Laboratory workers	Solvent vapors, inorganic acid vapors/mists
Military personnel	Zinc chloride smoke
Power plant and oil refinery workers	Sulfur dioxide
Printers, painters	Solvent vapors
Pulp mill workers	Chlorine, chlorine dioxide, hydrogen sulfide
Railroad personnel, miners, truck drivers	Diesel exhaust
Refrigeration workers (commercial)	Ammonia
Roofers, pavers	Asphalt vapors, PAHs[a]
Swimming pool service workers	Chlorine, hydrogen chloride, nitrogen trichloride
Waste water treatment workers	Chlorine, hydrogen sulfide
Welders	Metallic oxide fumes, nitrogen oxides, ozone
Woodworkers	Wood dust

[a] Polycyclic aromatic hydrocarbons (also skin and lung carcinogen).
From Zhao YA, Shusterman D. Work-related upper respiratory tract conditions. Clin Chest Med 2012;33:637–47.

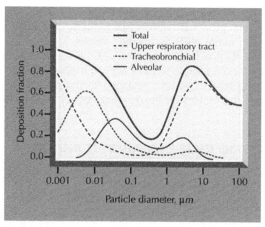

Fig. 2. Regional deposition of particles within the respiratory tract, by particle diameter. (*Data from* Zhao YA, Shusterman D. Work-related upper respiratory tract conditions. Clin Chest Med 2012;33:637–47.)

EPIDEMIOLOGY OF NONALLERGIC RHINITIS

Estimates of the prevalence of NAR in industrialized countries vary considerably. A population-based study of adults conducted in Sweden, for example, found the self-reported prevalence of NAR to be 19%, approaching the prevalence of 24% for allergic rhinoconjunctivitis.[28] Analysis of data across age groups in the United States,

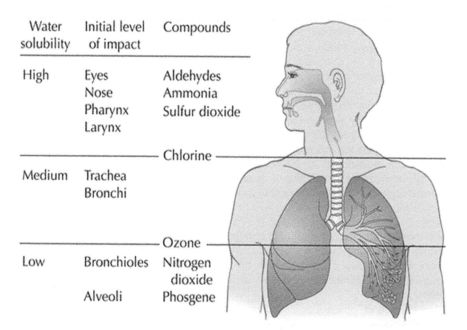

Fig. 3. Water solubility and site of initial impact of airborne irritants. (*From* Zhao YA, Shusterman D. Occupational rhinitis and other work-related upper respiratory tract conditions. Clin Chest Med 2012;33:637–47.)

on the other hand, points to a population prevalence of AR of 20%, NAR of 7%, and "mixed" rhinitis (AR with prominent nonallergic triggers) of 9%, with a total of 16% of the population having either NAR or "mixed" rhinitis.[29] Looked at from a different perspective, AR patients (the largest subgroup of rhinitis patients) are between 40% to 67% likely to report both allergic and nonallergic triggers, making the identification of a single underlying mechanism for nonspecific nasal hyperreactivity an elusive task.[6,7] Demographic risk factors for the development of NAR include female gender and advancing age.[30]

SYMPTOM TRIGGERS AND OTHER ENVIRONMENTAL INCITANTS

Symptom triggering (and other nonallergic upper airway health effects) have been addressed in NAR using 3 main study designs:

1. Symptom surveys of patients;
2. Observational studies correlating symptoms or biomarkers with environmental measurements; and
3. Controlled human exposure studies.

These 3 study types are considered individually in the following subsections.

Symptom Surveys of Patients

Shusterman and Murphy[7] ascertained the prevalence of nonallergic symptom triggers among 60 adults, including 31 with seasonal AR (SAR) and 29 nonrhinitis (NR), nonatopic controls. All subjects were nonsmokers without a history of occupational exposure to irritants. Overall, the number of self-reported nonallergic triggers was bimodal, with peaks at 1 and 5 (of a possible 8). Forty-two percent of SAR subjects reported more than 3 nonallergic triggers, compared with only 3% of NR controls ($P<.01$). The relative order of trigger reporting for SAR and NR subjects was identical (spicy foods > changes in temperature and humidity > environmental tobacco smoke ≃ exercise > household cleaning products ≃ perfumes and colognes > alcohol consumption > bright lights), with all triggers except spicy food and bright lights being significantly more prevalent among SAR subjects than controls. Subjects over 35 years of age were more likely to report one or more nonallergic triggers, particularly second-hand tobacco smoke ($P<.05$).[7]

Segboer and colleagues[6] administered a symptom (trigger) questionnaire to 585 consecutively referred AR and 408 NAR patients. The 2 groups showed no difference in the prevalence of nonspecific symptom triggering, with greater than 60% of both groups reporting a response to at least one nonallergic trigger. The relative importance of various triggers was also indistinguishable between the 2 subgroups (ie, temperature changes > smoke or smells > exercise > emotional stress > humidity). In a substudy of 18 AR, 21 NAR, and 17 healthy control patients, both rhinitis subgroups reported significant increases in subjective rhinorrhea, burning, and nasal secretion after cold, dry air (CDA) exposure, with a significant increase in self-reported congestion in the AR group only. However, neither rhinitis group showed significant changes in nasal peak inspiratory flow post-CDA challenge.

Bernstein and colleagues[31] compared the characteristics 404 patients with physician-diagnosed chronic AR, 123 NAR, and 129 mixed rhinitis before and after stratifying patients using an "irritant index questionnaire" in conjunction with a skin prick test. Principle component analysis was performed to determine discriminating cut points between allergic and NAR. They found that a significant number of rhinitis patients were reclassified based on having a high or low irritant index score, resulting in 4 groups: AR without and with a high irritant index score (ie, AR and mixed rhinitis) and NAR with and without a high irritant index score. In contrast with correlations for the consensus diagnoses, the reclassified AR and NAR patients with high irritant index scores had more severe and more frequent rhinitis symptoms and a greater likelihood of physician-diagnosed asthma.

Observational Studies

Numerous observational (epidemiologic) studies have addressed the nasal effects of physical and/or chemical aspects of ambient or indoor air quality. In some studies, individual factors (age, gender, or rhinitis status) were examined as potential markers of differential susceptibility. Although many of these studies have focused on single aspects of the inspired atmosphere (eg, meteorology, ozone [O_3] levels, presence of wet and/or moldy indoor conditions), potential confounding is always a concern in epidemiologic investigations. We have presented herein a selective sample of these studies (**Table 3**).

Ambient air quality

Hoshino and colleagues[32] performed a retrospective chart review of outpatients in a general medicine clinic over a 1-year period, examining unscheduled visits for NAR. A time-series analysis was conducted comparing visit incidence with air temperature, humidity ("vapor pressure"), and various air pollution indices. Significantly more visits occurred during periods with exaggerated diurnal temperature variation, during cold, dry weather, high winds, and with high concentrations of photochemical oxidants.

Braat and colleagues[33] performed a time-series analysis of nasal symptoms recorded on a daily basis over a 7-month period among 16 NAR patients and 7 normal controls, correlating symptoms with daily measurements of temperature, humidity, and air pollutant levels. After correcting for autocorrelation and introducing optimal lag times, NAR patients' symptoms were predicted by minimum daytime temperature, average daytime relative humidity (%), O_3 levels, and particulate matter of 10 microns in diameter or smaller.

In a series of related studies, Calderon-Garciduenas and colleagues[34] have examined the upper airway impact of air pollutants in Mexico City (including O_3, particulate matter, and aldehydes). One such study compared urban residents with residents of an unpolluted locale, revealing squamous metaplasia, loss of normal cilia, vascular congestion, and glandular atrophy on nasal biopsy of the urban residents. Another study examined visitors to the city who came from a more rural areas; such short-term visitors developed epithelial desquamation and neutrophilic inflammation that took more than 2 weeks to resolve after returning to their home towns.[35] Additional studies identified ultrastructural abnormalities of both cellular maturation and ciliary morphology, as well as evidence p53 tumor suppressor protein activation among Mexico City residents versus controls.[36,37]

Kopp and colleagues[38] studied the effects of varying atmospheric O_3 levels on the upper airway by examining serial nasal lavage specimens collected over a 7-month period from nonatopic school children in Germany. The investigators found an initial increase in nasal leukocytes and eosinophilic cationic protein with the initial seasonal increase in O_3 levels, but an apparent adaptation effect with continued high O_3 exposures.

Pacini and co-workers[39] compared nasal mucosal cells taken by brushing from residents of Florence, Italy (a high O_3 area) versus rural residents of Sardinia.

Table 3
Observational studies of air quality and the upper airway

Exposure:	Endpoint	Observation	Reference
Meteorologic conditions	Nasal symptoms	Symptoms in nonallergic rhintic subjects varied with minimum daytime temperature, relative humidity, and air pollutant levels	Braat et al,[33] 2002
	Clinic visits for NAR	Unscheduled clinic visits for NAR increased with diurnal temperature variation, cold/dry weather, and with photochemical oxidants	Hoshino et al,[32] 2015
Ambient air pollutants	Nasal biopsy	Squamous metaplasia comparing Mexico City versus rural residents	Calderon–Garciduenas et al,[34] 1992
	Nasal biopsy	Short-term visitors to Mexico City developed nasal neutrophilia	Calderon–Garciduenas et al,[35] 1994
	Nasal biopsy	Children from Mexico City versus unpolluted area showed squamous metaplasia, ciliary disorientation, intraepithelial exudate	Calderon–Garciduenas et al,[36] 2001
	Nasal symptoms and biopsy	Children from Mexico City versus unpolluted area reported greater nasal symptoms and showed squamous metaplasia, neutrophilia, $\pm$ p53 expression	Calderon–Garciduenas et al,[37] 2001
	Nasal lavage	Austrian school children underwent serial nasal lavage during air pollution season. An increase in WBC count and ECP concentration was apparent with increasing O_3 (early season only)	Kopp et al,[38] 1999
	Nasal brushings	Adults from Florence, Italy (high O_3) versus Sardinia (low O_3) showed more DNA damage	Pacini et al,[39] 2003
Indoor air pollutants	Acoustic rhinometry; nasal lavage	Cross-sectional study of school personnel in which nasal patency, nasal ECP and lysozyme levels varied by building characteristic	Walinder et al,[40] 2000
	Nasal symptoms	Individuals living in houses with elevated levels of the MVOC, 1-octen-3-ol, had higher rates of eye, nose and throat irritation	Araki et al,[41] 2010

Abbreviations: ECP, eosinophilic cationic protein; IL, interleukin; MVOC, volatile organic compounds of microbial origin; NAR, nonallergic rhinitis; NO, nitrous oxide; TNF, tumor necrosis factor; WBC, white blood cell.

Modified from Shusterman D. Environmental nonallergic rhinitis. In: Baraniuk JN, Shusterman D, editors. Nonallergic rhinitis. New York: Informa Healthcare; 2007. p. 249–66.

They found greater levels of DNA damage and more inflammatory changes among cytologic specimens from the Florence residents than from the rural Sardinians.

Indoor air quality

Studies of indoor air quality documenting nonallergic upper airway responses are quite numerous. We discuss a few representative studies.

Walinder and colleagues[40] studied 234 primary school employees from 12 randomly selected Swedish schools. Health history was obtained by structured interview, and nasal symptoms documented using a self-administered questionnaire. Environmental measures included indoor temperature and concentrations of carbon dioxide, nitrogen dioxide, formaldehyde and other volatile organic compounds (VOCs), and dust. Acoustic rhinometry was performed after at least 1 hour of building occupancy. Nasal lavage fluid was analyzed for eosinophilic cationic protein, lysozyme, myeloperoxidase, and albumin. Symptomatically, self-reported nasal obstruction was related to ventilation type (mechanical vs natural), as well as dust concentrations. On acoustic rhinometry, nasal cross-sectional area was reduced as a function of dust concentrations, formaldehyde levels, the presence of polyvinyl chloride flooring, and the use of mechanical (vs natural) ventilation. On nasal lavage, lysozyme levels were higher with mechanical ventilation and wet mopping of floors whereas eosinophilic cationic protein levels were higher with decrease frequency of floor cleaning and with increasing levels of formaldehyde and nitrogen dioxide.

Araki and colleagues[41] studied the occupants of 182 single family dwellings in Japan, performing indoor air analyses for VOCs, including those of microbial origin. Among the approximately 5% of respondents who reported home-related mucous membrane symptoms (eye, nose, and throat irritation), a significant relationship emerged between mucous membrane symptoms and indoor air concentrations of the VOCs of microbial origin [1-octen-3-ol] and [2-pentanol].

Intervention studies

Two studies were identified in which the effects of various interventions were evaluated on nonallergic mediated nasal symptoms or pathology. In one, atopic asthmatic children in Mexico City exposed to urban air pollution (as discussed) were given either antioxidant dietary supplements (vitamins C and E) or placebo, and concentrations of cytokines (interleukin [IL]-6 and IL-8) and antioxidants (glutathione and uric acid) in nasal lavage fluid were evaluated. The antioxidant-treated group showed significantly lower levels of IL-6 (and borderline lower levels of IL-8) during high-O_3 days compared with placebo-treated children.[42]

The second interventional study involved office workers who reported mucous membrane irritation at work. Their offices were subjected to either comprehensive or superficial (sham) cleaning on a blinded basis, resulting in significant reductions in airborne dust levels in the former group. Both subjective irritation and objective airway patency (by acoustic rhinometry) were recorded. The active intervention group reported a significant reduction in upper airway irritation symptoms after the intervention, as well as an increase in nasal patency.[43]

Controlled Human Exposure Studies

A number of studies have examined subjective and/or objective nasal responses to environmental incitants in controlled human exposure protocols (**Table 4**). Although CDA provocation constitutes the dominant provocation paradigm for experimental

Table 4
Controlled human exposure studies of nonallergic stimuli in the upper airway

Pollutant	Nasal Patency	Nasal Lavage	Mucociliary Clearance	Reference
Acetic acid	↑ R_{nasal}[a]	—	—	Shusterman et al,[72] 2005
Ammonia	↑ R_{nasal}	—	—	McLean et al,[61] 1979
Barometric pressure	↓ PIFn vs PIFo	—	—	Barry et al,[48] 2002
Carbonless copy paper	↑ R_{nasal}[b]	—	—	Morgan & Camp,[73] 1986
Chlorine gas	↑ R_{nasal}[a]	—	—	Shusterman et al,[62] 1998; Shusterman,[18] 2002; Shusterman et al,[63] 2003; Shusterman et al,[65] 2003; Shusterman et al,[66] 2004
Environmental tobacco smoke	↑ R_{nasal}[b]	NC histamine, albumin, kinins	—	Bascom et al,[49] 1991
	↑ R_{nasal}	NC PMNs	↓ Clearance[b]	Bascom et al,[50] 1995; Nowak et al,[51] 1997; Schick et al,[53] 2013
Ozone		↑ PMNs	—	Graham et al,[69] 1988
	NC R_{nasal}	↑ PMNs	—	Graham and Koren,[70] 1990
		↑ PMNs, IL-8	—	McBride et al,[71] 1994
Sulfur dioxide	↑ R_{nasal}	—	↓ Clearance	Andersen et al,[68] 1974
	NC R_{nasal}	—	—	Tam et al,[67] 1988
VOCs	↓ NV	↑ PMNs	—	Kjaergaard et al,[54] 1995; Koren et al,[56] 1992
		↑ Cytokines	NC Clearance	Muttray et al,[57] 1999
		NC Cytokines	↓ Clearance	Muttray et al,[58] 2002
		↑ Cytokines	NC clearance	Mann et al,[59] 2002

Abbreviations: ↑, increased; ↓, decreased; NC, no change; NV, nasal volume (by acoustic rhinometry); PIFn, nasal peak inspiratory flow; PIFo, oral peak inspiratory flow; PMNs, polymorphonuclear leukocytes; R_{nasal}, nasal airway resistance (by rhinomanometry); VOC, volatile organic compounds.

a Allergic rhinitic subjects only.
b Historically sensitive subjects only.

Modified from Shusterman D. Environmental nonallergic rhinitis. In: Baraniuk JN, Shusterman D, editors. Nonallergic rhinitis. New York: Informa Healthcare; 2007. p. 249–66.

physical triggering in NAR, inhaled chemical irritants have also been used to document nonspecific nasal hyperreactivity in both NAR and AR patients/research subjects.

PHYSICAL INCITANTS
Cold, Dry Air

The CDA challenge has been used as the sine qua non of provocation agents in idiopathic NAR, and has been applied in a variety of study designs. These include clinical diagnosis/classification (including comparisons with methacholine or histamine challenge), pathophysiologic studies, and to monitor the therapeutic response to pharmacologic or surgical interventions. Typical endpoints include symptom ratings, weight of nasal secretions, and nasal patency. Because the volume of literature on this topic could justify a separate review article, only a few representative CDA studies are reviewed herein.

Braat and colleagues[44] compared CDA challenge with histamine challenge with respect to their ability discriminate NAR subjects (n = 16) from NR controls (n = 7). Study endpoints included decreased nasal patency (by anterior rhinomanometry), weight of secretions, and number of sneezes. In a progressive challenge protocol, the investigators found both methods to be highly sensitive in identifying NAR subjects, but only CDA specific for NAR.

In an attempt to identify phenotypic subsets of NAR patients, Shusterman and Tilles[45] compared the response to CDA challenge in 10 subjects who reported predominantly physical symptom triggers, 4 NAR subjects with predominantly chemical triggers, and 10 NR, nonatopic controls (NR). In the initial protocol, as few as 1 of 5 self-identified physical triggers classified a subject as NAR with physical symptom triggers, whereas at least 2 of 5 chemical triggers were required to qualify as NAR with predominantly chemical triggers. The 2 NAR subgroups combined showed significantly greater nasal obstruction after the CDA challenge than did the NR controls, but only after the definition of NAR with physical symptom triggers was modified, on a post hoc basis, to require 2 reported physical triggers ($P<.05$). Across subjects, a positive trend was observed in degree of post-CDA nasal obstruction as a function of the number of self-reported physical triggers ($P<.05$). Subjectively, self-reported nasal congestion after exposure was significantly greater in subjects with NAR with physical symptom triggers than in the other 2 subgroups.[45]

Kim and colleagues[46] compared the response to CDA challenge between 21 normal controls, 24 AR patients, and 32 NAR patients. Subjects were stratified, before the challenge, into "hyperreactive" and "nonhyperreactive" subgroups based on their self-reported reactivity to cold air. Symptom scores by visual analog scales and nasal volumes by acoustic rhinometry were evaluated before and after the CDA challenge, and the degree of CDA-induced rhinorrhea assessed by weight of nasal secretions after the exposure. Both AR and NAR groups exhibited significantly greater increases in symptoms and nasal secretions—and decreases in nasal volume—after the CDA challenge than did normal controls. In addition, objective findings (ie, nasal patency and secretions) were more prominent among subjects with a self-reported history of nasal hyperreactivity.

Bernstein and colleagues[47] evaluated 37 NAR subjects with CDA challenge (and with temperature change alone) in a multiseat environmental chamber. Acoustic rhinometry was used to evaluate nasal patency, weight of nasal secretions was the index of rhinorrhea, and subjective congestion, rhinorrhea, and postnasal drip were self-rated. With CDA challenge, 25 of 37 subjects met preset criteria for a symptomatic response, and 20 of 37 met rhinometric criteria (ie, demonstrated a $\geq$10% decrease in nasal patency). The observed increase in rhinorrhea was highest for CDA and the cold air phase of the temperature change protocol. The study was interpreted as a proof-of-concept for the feasibility of using a multi-seat environmental challenge chamber to simultaneously elicit weather-induced symptoms and physiologic changes in multiple NAR patients.

Barometric Pressure and Altitude

Using a hypobaric chamber, Barry and colleagues[48] simulated ascent to more than 8000 m while maintaining constant temperature and humidity, measuring both nasal and oral peak inspiratory flow at the equivalent of 0, 5000, and 8000 m altitude. Although both peak inspiratory flows increased with decreasing barometric pressure, the increase in nasal peak inspiratory flow was considerably less than that of oral peak inspiratory flow, which was interpreted as showing a relative airflow limitation in the upper versus lower airway.

CHEMICAL INCITANTS
Environmental Tobacco Smoke

Bascom and colleagues[49] exposed 21 adult subjects to sidestream tobacco smoke (STS) for 15 minutes, asking subjects to rate symptoms before and after exposure. The surrogate measure of exposure was a carbon monoxide concentration of 45 ppm (equivalent to a smoky bar). The subjects were subdivided into 10 who previously reported being sensitive to environmental tobacco smoke (ETS-S) and 11 historically nonsensitive (ETS-NS), with the majority of the ETS-S subjects being atopic and the majority of the ETS-NS subjects being nonatopic. ETS-S subjects reported significantly more nose and throat irritation than ETS-NS subjects. Furthermore, on posterior rhinomanometry the ETS-S group showed significant increases in nasal airway resistance when compared with the ETS-NS group. The exposures were repeated subsequently and followed by nasal lavage rather than rhinomanometry. Neither subgroup showed evidence of an IgE-mediated reaction, as evidenced by a lack of significant alterations in nasal lavage fluid histamine, kinins, TAME-esterase, or albumin after exposure.

The same group examined the endpoint of nasal mucociliary clearance after STS exposure. 99mTc-sulfur colloid was aerosolized into the nose after STS and clean air exposures, and clearance was measured by scintillation counter and compared between the 2 exposure conditions. One-half of the subjects showed increased clearance, 25% showed no change, and 25% showed decreased clearance after STS exposure. The group with decreased clearance all gave a history of ETS–related rhinitis symptoms.[50]

Nowak and colleagues[51] performed nasal lavage on 10 mild asthmatics before and after exposure to STS at 22 ppm carbon monoxide, analyzing for histamine, albumin, eosinophil cationic protein, myeloperoxidase, hyaluraonic acid, and tryptase. Bronchoscopy was also performed the morning after exposure. Although there was an increase in respiratory symptoms after exposure, no systematic changes were observed in spirometry, nasal lavage fluid, or bronchoalveolar lavage fluid.

Junker and colleagues[52] exposed 24 subjects to STS at variable concentrations. They found a dose–response for self-rated odor intensity, eye irritation, and annoyance as a function of airborne particle, polycyclic aromatic hydrocarbon, and VOC concentrations. Subjective nasal irritation, on the other hand, was related only to particle concentration. Neither breathing pattern nor eye blink rate (a measure of eye irritation) varied significantly with STS concentration. The mean threshold for

STS odor detection among these subjects corresponded with a PM (Particulate Matter)$_{2.25}$ concentration of approximately 0.6 to 1.4 $\mu g/m^3$.

Schick and colleagues[53] studied 26 healthy nonsmokers (10 nonatopic without rhinitis, 7 atopic without rhinitis, 7 atopic with rhinitis, and 2 nonatopic with rhinitis) in a STS provocation study. Subjective nasal symptoms were assessed by questionnaire, objective nasal congestion by active anterior rhinomanometry, and nasal nitric oxide concentrations were determined before and after exposure. Exposure to experimentally aged cigarette smoke (at 1 mg/m^3 particulate concentration/14 ppm carbon monoxide) for 30 minutes was compared with exposure to clean air on a separate day. Overall, exposure to SHS increased nasal resistance in healthy nonsmokers ($P<.05$). The increase in nasal resistance was most pronounced in rhinitis subjects. No systematic changes in nasal nitric oxide were observed as a function of exposure in any of the subgroups.

Volatile Organic Compounds

Kjaergaard and colleagues[54] exposed 18 each "hay fever" and normal subjects to a mixture of 22 different VOCs at a total concentration of 20 mg/m^3 for 4 hours. Exposure to the clean air control condition occurred on a separate day. Hayfever subjects showed more pronounced increases in self-reported eye, nose, and throat irritation over the course of the exposure than did nonallergic subjects. However, rhinitis and NR subjects showed equivalent exposure-related decreases in nasal volume on AR.

Hudnell and colleagues[55] compared the response of adult male volunteers exposed to the same mixture of 22 VOCs at a total concentration of 20 mg/m^3 over a 2.75-hour period, and found increasing self-reported eye and throat irritation, headache, and drowsiness, whereas odor ratings decreased during exposure (consistent with odor adaptation). In the same laboratory, Koren and colleagues[56] conducted identical VOC exposures over 4 hours, obtaining nasal lavage fluid before and after exposure. Investigators found increases in polymorphonuclear leukocytes (PMNs) in nasal lavage fluid both immediately after exposure and at 18 hours after exposure.

Muttray and colleagues[57] exposed 12 healthy subjects to 1,1,1-trichloroethane (TCA) at 20 and 200 ppm for 4 hours, assessing nasal mucociliary function (by saccharine transit time) and sampling nasal secretions 20 minutes after exposure. Cytokines, including IL-B1, IL-6, and IL-8 were analyzed in nasal secretions, and ciliary beat frequency determined on sampled cells studied ex vivo. Although neither measure of mucociliary function was significantly altered, all 3 cytokines were elevated in concentration after exposure.

The same laboratory group studied 19 healthy volunteers exposed to 0 and 200 ppm methyl ethyl ketone, again analyzing secretions for cytokines and documenting mucociliary function (saccharine transit time). In this study, mucociliary transport time was increased significantly after exposure, but cytokines showed no changes (the inverse of the pattern observed in their TCA study).[58] Also from this group, Mann and colleagues,[59] studied the response of 12 healthy subjects to 20 and 200 ppm of methanol, examining cytokines, mucociliary clearance, and ciliary beat frequency of sampled nasal epithelial cells. Both IL1B and IL-8 concentrations were increased after exposure, whereas IL-6 and prostaglandin E2 were unchanged. However, neither measure of mucociliary function was altered by the exposure.

Andersen and colleagues[60] studied nasal airway resistance and mucociliary clearance during 6-hour exposures to 10, 40, or 100 ppm of toluene vapor. No significant exposure-related changes were noted in either physiologic parameter.

Ammonia

McLean and colleagues[61] measured nasal airway resistance among 33 SAR and NR subjects before and after exposure to ammonia (100 ppm times 5 seconds per nostril). Exposures were repeated at 15-minute intervals, with successively longer durations of exposure (10, 15, and 20 seconds). The mean nasal airway resistance increased after NH_3 exposures, and a dose–response was evident for exposure duration; however, no difference was apparent between subgroups by rhinitis status. Pretreatment with topical atropine, but not chlorpheniramine, inhibited ammonia-induced nasal airflow obstruction.

Chlorine

Shusterman and colleagues[62] compared the response of 8 SAR and 8 NR subjects, exposed for 15 minutes to chlorine (Cl_2) at 0.5 ppm, with control (clean air) exposures occurring either a week before or after the irritant exposure (in counterbalanced order). SAR subjects were tested out of season. Endpoints included self-rated nasal symptoms and nasal airway resistance by active posterior rhinomanometry. After chlorine provocation, significant increases in self-rated nasal irritation and increases in nasal airway resistance were documented in SAR subjects only. In a larger (n = 60) sample of subjects stratified by age, sex, and allergy status, the same group found that both AR and age (older subjects) predicted an augmented congestive response to 1.0 ppm Cl_2 gas.[63]

This Cl_2 exposure paradigm was applied by Shusterman and colleagues[64] to explore underlying mechanism(s) of irritant-induced nasal airway obstruction. In the first pathophysiologic study, subjects were pretreated with iptratropium bromide nasal spray on a double-blinded, placebo-controlled basis before Cl_2 or fresh air exposure. Differential Cl_2-induced nasal obstruction by rhinitis status was not affected by iptratropium bromide pretreatment, suggesting that cholinergic reflexes were not responsible for the observed response. In a separate experiment, nasal lavage fluid was analyzed for evidence of mast cell degranulation (tryptase) and neuropeptide release (SP, calcitonin gene-related peptide, VIP, and NPY), but neither set of markers were systematically affected by exposure. Thus, in this series of experiments no evidence was found that mast cell degranulation, neuropeptide release, or cholinergic reflexes were responsible for chlorine's effect on nasal patency.[65,66]

Sulfur Dioxide

Tam and colleagues[67] studied 22 AR subjects exposed by nasal mask to 4 ppm of sulfur dioxide (SO_2) for 10 minutes, as well as 8 subjects with combined asthma and rhinitis exposed to 1 to 2 ppm SO_2 by mouthpiece. There were no exposure-related changes in either nasal airway resistance or nasal symptoms. These results are in contrast with an earlier study by Andersen and colleagues,[68] which documented SO_2-induced nasal airflow obstruction, as well as alterations in nasal mucociliary clearance.

Ozone

Graham and colleagues[69] exposed 20 subjects to filtered air and 19 subjects to 0.5 ppm O_3 for 4 hours on 2 successive days. Subjects underwent nasal lavage before exposure on both days, as well as immediately after exposure on day 1 and 22 hours after exposure on day 2. The O_3-exposed group showed increased numbers of PMNs in nasal lavage fluid in all postexposure samples, including an elevated baseline before the second day's exposure.

Graham and Koren[70] compared the upper and lower respiratory tract responses of 10 nonsmoking subjects without asthma exposed to 0.4 ppm O_3 for 2 hours with exercise. Parallel increases in PMNs and albumin were apparent in nasal lavage and bronchoalveolar lavage fluids at 18 hours after exposure, in addition to an early increase in PMNs documented on nasal lavage.[70]

McBride and colleagues[71] exposed 10 atopic asthmatic subjects to 0, 0.12, and 0.24 ppm O_3 for 90 minutes during intermittent exercise. Nasal lavage and nasal work of breathing were obtained before exposure, immediately after exposure, and at 6 and 24 hours after exposure. At the higher exposure level (0.24 ppm), a significant increase in nasal lavage white blood cell count was observed at the earliest and latest postexposure sampling time, but not at 6 hours. In addition, a significant correlation was found between nasal lavage white blood cell count and IL-8 levels. However, no changes in either nasal work of breathing or pulmonary function were observed after exposure.

Acetic Acid

Shusterman and colleagues[72] compared the responses of 8 SAR and 8 NR subjects exposed to acetic acid vapor (at 15 ppm) versus filtered air for 15 minutes on separate days. The AR subjects showed significant increases in nasal airway resistance compared with NR, with responses evident both immediately after exposure and at 15 minutes after exposure.

Carbonless Copy Paper

Morgan and Camp[73] studied 30 workers with self-reported skin and/or respiratory sensitivity to carbonless copy paper. Air was passed through shredded carbonless copy paper or bond paper and supplied to the breathing zone of subjects. Mean nasal airway resistance by rhinomanometry increased by 34% after carbonless copy paper exposure compared with 8% after bond paper exposure. However, symptoms did not correlate with the magnitude of nasal airway resistance changes.[73]

Paper Dust

Theander and Bender[74] studied 15 NAR subjects who reported nasal symptoms to newspapers, and compared them with 6 healthy controls. Subjects inhaled either vapors from printing ink or paper dust, and then rated nasal symptoms on visual analog scales, as well as having their nasal airway resistance measured by anterior rhinomanometry. The NAR subjects reported significantly greater symptoms than did controls after paper dust, but not ink vapor, exposure. However, neither group showed significant changes in nasal airway resistance.[74]

Dry Powder Mannitol

Although more properly classified as a pharmacologic than an environmental exposure study, Koskela and colleagues[75] study of dry powder mannitol exposure (a noxious, hyperosmolar stimulus) is relevant in the context of this discussion. Ten healthy controls, 11 with SAR (studied out of season while asymptomatic), and 9 symptomatic rhinitis patients (all but one with perennial AR) underwent nasal challenge. Nasal symptoms, nasal peak inspiratory flow, and nasal lavage was performed before and after dry powder mannitol or sham exposure, with the order of exposure randomized on separate days. All patients reported an immediate burning sensation of varying severity, and both AR subgroups showed increases in nasal lavage 15-hydroxyeicosatetraenoic acid (15-HETE; a marker of epithelial cell activation). However, only the AR patients with active symptoms experienced a decrease in nasal peak inspiratory flow (ie, nasally congested). No increases in nasal lavage substance P were observed, although a third of the AR patients showed exposure-related increases in mast cell tryptase (a marker of mast cell degranulation that, however, did not predict the severity of nasal blockage).

MECHANISM(S) UNDERLYING CHEMICAL IRRITANT-INDUCED NASAL REFLEXES

Potential reflex mechanisms for irritant-induced rhinorrhea and nasal obstruction are diagrammed in **Fig. 4**. Reading from "right to left," rhinorrhea generally reflects a glandular response, although some contribution may come from plasma extravasation. Nasal "congestion" (obstruction), on the other hand, involves primarily vasodilation of large capacitance vessels, again with a secondary contribution by extravasated plasma.

Moving "upstream" with respect to reflex mechanisms, rhinorrhea induced by both cold air and capsaicin can occur contralaterally after unilateral nasal stimulation, and can be inhibited by topical cholinergic blockers, thereby implicating a central (parasympathetic) reflex mechanism affecting submucosal glands.[24,76] Of note, nasal lavage biomarkers can provide insight into reaction mechanisms. Neurogenic secretions (ie, in cold air– or capsaicin–induced rhinorrhea) are characterized by the predominant nasal lavage proteins being glandular products (ie, lactoferrin and lysozyme). By contrast, in nasal lavage fluids obtained after mast cell degranulation (ie, after an allergic reaction), the predominant proteins are derived from plasma (ie, albumin and various Igs) along with histamine and/or tryptase.[24] This matrix of physiologic endpoints, biochemical markers, and pharmacologic blockers has been applied, to a limited extent, to the question of chemical irritant-induced nasal congestion, for which the results of relevant provocation experiments appear in **Table 4**.

A brief summary of biochemical marker/pharmacologic blocker studies is as follows.

- In 3 separate experiments, irritant-induced nasal obstruction (provoked by STS, chlorine gas, or dry powder mannitol) occurred in susceptible individuals without consistent evidence in nasal lavage fluid of mast cell degranulation.[49,65,75]

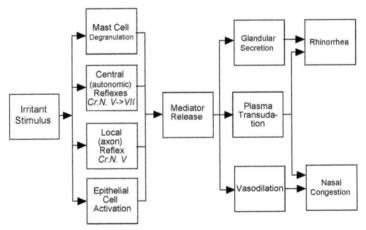

Fig. 4. Potential mechanisms involved in the reflex response to inhaled irritants. Cr.N. V, trigeminal nerve; Cr.N. VII, facial nerve. (*Adapted from* Shusterman D. Upper respiratory tract disorders. In: LaDou J, editor. Current occupational and environmental medicine. 4th edition. New York: McGraw-Hill; 2007. p. 298–309.)

- In 1 double-blinded, placebo-controlled, crossover study, pretreatment with a cholinergic blocker did not diminish the degree of Cl_2-induced nasal obstruction in susceptible individuals. However, in another (noncrossover) study, pretreatment with atropine did diminish ammonia-induced nasal obstruction.[61]
- In 2 different studies (using either Cl_2 gas or dry powder mannitol as provocation agents), neither nasal lavage substance P nor other nasal lavage neuropeptides (calcitonin gene-related peptide, NPY, or VIP) were systematically altered in individuals who experienced irritant-induced nasal obstruction.[66,75]
- One study (using dry powder mannitol provocation) examined 15-HETE, a biochemical marker of epithelial cell activation, and found significant increases in nasal lavage fluid concentrations among AR subjects, a subset of whom experienced objective irritant-induced nasal obstruction.[75]

Summary of mechanistic studies

- Acute irritant-induced nasal obstruction could potentially occur through mast cell degranulation, central neurogenic (eg, parasympathetic) reflexes, peripheral neurogenic (ie, "axon") reflexes, or epithelial cell activation (see **Fig. 4**). Human studies evaluating these potential mechanisms have generally been either negative or have produced contradictory results. Early indications that epithelial cell activation may be an operative mechanism should be replicated using a wider range of provocation agents and in various subsets of susceptible individuals (ie, NAR; AR with nasal hyperreactivity).
- NAR patients, in general, have yet to be studied with chemical irritant provocation (other than with capsaicin or hypertonic saline). This constitutes a gap in the research literature.

SUMMARY

Idiopathic NAR, because of its inconsistent association with mucosal inflammation, has been renamed by some as "nonallergic rhinopathy." This condition has a slight female predominance, and tends to have its onset in adulthood. The clinical hallmark of this condition is nonspecific nasal hyperreactivity (ie, hyperresponsiveness to physical and chemical agents), although this phenotypic trait is also shared by many patients with AR. Cardinal symptoms of NAR—nasal hypersecretion and obstruction—have been explored mechanistically, but with varying degrees of success. Common triggers of NAR of environmental concern include cold/dry air, fragrance products, household cleaners, tobacco and wood smoke, vehicular exhaust, and industrial chemicals (vapors, gases, and particulate matter). Avoidance of these triggers can be challenging for some individuals, and as a consequence the condition has attracted significant attention in pharmaceutical circles.

Current controversies in idiopathic NAR include the role of sensory nerves, as nociceptive ion channel (eg, TRPV1, TRPA1) blockers increasingly become available, and as capsaicin desensitization trials continue to be conducted. Importantly, the advent of the competing diagnosis "local AR" calls into question the very classification of many patients labeled as having NAR, absent their having shown negative results on nasal allergen provocation testing and/or having proved refractory to conventional allergy medications.[77] Amid all this uncertainty, what seems clear is that our clinical practice and mechanistic understanding regarding idiopathic NAR (or nonallergic rhinopathy) is likely to undergo dramatic changes over the next few decades.

REFERENCES

1. Settipane RA. Epidemiology of vasomotor rhinitis. World Allergy Organ J 2009; 2(6):115–8.
2. Kaliner MA, Baraniuk JN, Benninger M, et al. Consensus definition of nonallergic rhinopathy, previously referred to as vasomotor rhinitis, nonallergic rhinitis, and/or idiopathic rhinitis. World Allergy Organ J 2009;2(6):119–20.
3. Leroyer C, Malo JL, Girard D, et al. Chronic rhinitis in workers at risk of reactive airways dysfunction syndrome due to exposure to chlorine. Occup Environ Med 1999;56(5):334–8.
4. Meggs WJ, Elsheik T, Metzger WJ, et al. Nasal pathology and ultrastructure in patients with chronic airway inflammation (RADS and RUDS) following an irritant exposure. J Toxicol Clin Toxicol 1996;34(4):383–96.
5. Gerth van Wijk RG, de Graaf-in 't Veld C, Garrelds IM. Nasal hyperreactivity. Rhinology 1999;37(2):50–5.
6. Segboer CL, Holland CT, Reinartz SM, et al. Nasal hyper-reactivity is a common feature in both allergic and nonallergic rhinitis. Allergy 2013;68(11):1427–34.
7. Shusterman D, Murphy MA. Nasal hyperreactivity in allergic and non-allergic rhinitis: a potential risk factor for non-specific building-related illness. Indoor Air 2007;17(4):328–33.
8. Shusterman D. Qualitative effects in nasal trigeminal chemoreception. Ann N Y Acad Sci 2009;1170:196–201.
9. Silver WL, Finger TE. The anatomical and electrophysiological basis of peripheral nasal trigeminal chemoreception. Ann NY Acad Sci 2009;1170:202–5.
10. Bessac BF, Jordt SE. Sensory detection and responses to toxic gases: mechanisms, health effects, and countermeasures. Proc Am Thorac Soc 2010;7(4): 269–77.
11. Silver WL, Clapp TR, Stone LM, et al. TRPV1 receptors and nasal trigeminal chemesthesis. Chem Senses 2006;31(9):807–12.
12. Viana F. Chemosensory properties of the trigeminal system. ACS Chem Neurosci 2011;2(1):38–50.
13. Tai CF, Baraniuk JN. Upper airway neurogenic mechanisms. Curr Opin Allergy Clin Immunol 2002;2(1):11–9.
14. Barham HP, Cooper SE, Anderson CB, et al. Solitary chemosensory cells and bitter taste receptor signaling in human sinonasal mucosa. Int Forum Allergy Rhinol 2013;3(6):450–7.
15. Widdicombe J. Nasal and pharyngeal reflexes: Protective and respiratory functions. In: Mathew OP, Sant'Ambrogio G, editors. Respiratory function of the upper airway. New York: Marcel Dekker; 1988. p. 233–58.
16. van Rijswijk JB, Blom HM, Fokkens WJ. Idiopathic rhinitis, the ongoing quest. Allergy 2005;60(12):1471–81.
17. Cometto-Muñiz JE, Cain WS. Sensory irritation. Relation to indoor air pollution. Ann N Y Acad Sci 1992;30(641):137–51.
18. Shusterman D. Review of the upper airway, including olfaction, as mediator of symptoms. Environ Health Perspect 2002;110(Suppl 4):649–53.
19. Tarlo SM, Poonai N, Binkley K, et al. Responses to panic induction procedures in subjects with multiple chemical sensitivity/idiopathic environmental intolerance: Understanding the relationship with panic disorder. Environ Health Perspect 2002;110(Suppl 4):669–71.
20. Sarin S, Undem B, Sanico A, et al. The role of the nervous system in rhinitis. J Allergy Clin Immunol 2006;118(5):999–1016.

21. Undem BJ, Taylor-Clark T. Mechanisms underlying the neuronal-based symptoms of allergy. J Allergy Clin Immunol 2014;133(6):1521–34.

22. Silvers WS. The skier's nose: a model of cold-induced rhinorrhea. Ann Allergy 1991;67(1):32–6.

23. Raphael G, Raphael MH, Kaliner M. Gustatory rhinitis: a syndrome of food-induced rhinorrhea. J Allergy Clin Immunol 1989;83(1):110–5.

24. Raphael GD, Baraniuk JN, Kaliner MA. How and why the nose runs. J Allergy Clin Immunol 1991;87:457–67.

25. Fireman P. Otitis media and Eustachian tube dysfunction: connection to allergic rhinitis. J Allergy Clin Immunol 1997;99(2):S787–97.

26. Chandra RK, Pearlman A, Conley DB, et al. Significance of ostiomeatal complex obstruction. J Otolaryngol Head Neck Surg 2010;39(2):171–4.

27. Nodelman V, Ultman JS. Longitudinal distribution of chlorine absorption in human airways: comparison of nasal and oral quiet breathing. J Appl Physiol (1985) 1999;86(6):1984–93.

28. Olsson P, Berglind N, Bellander T, et al. Prevalence of self-reported allergic and non-allergic rhinitis symptoms in Stockholm: relation to age, gender, olfactory sense and smoking. Acta Otolaryngol 2003;123(1):75–80.

29. Settipane RA. Demographics and epidemiology of allergic and nonallergic rhinitis. Allergy Asthma Proc 2001;22(4):185–9.

30. Settipane RA. Rhinitis: a dose of epidemiological reality. Allergy Asthma Proc 2003;24(3):147–54.

31. Bernstein JA, Levin LS, Al-Shuik E, et al. Clinical characteristics of chronic rhinitis patients with high vs low irritant trigger burdens. Ann Allergy Asthma Immunol 2012;109(3):173–8.

32. Hoshino T, Hoshino A, Nishino J. Relationship between environment factors and the number of outpatient visits at a clinic for nonallergic rhinitis in Japan, extracted from electronic medical records. Eur J Med Res 2015;20:60–76.

33. Braat JP, Mulder PG, Duivenvoorden HJ, et al. Pollutional and meteorological factors are closely related to complaints of non-allergic, non-infectious perennial rhinitis patients: a time series model. Clin Exp Allergy 2002;32(5):690–7.

34. Calderon-Garciduenas L, Osorno-Velazquez A, Bravo-Alvarez H, et al. Histopathologic changes of the nasal mucosa in southwest Metropolitan Mexico City inhabitants. Am J Pathol 1992;140(1):225–32.

35. Calderon-Garciduenas L, Rodriguez-Alcaraz A, Garcia R, et al. Human nasal mucosal changes after exposure to urban pollution. Environ Health Perspect 1994;102(12):1074–80.

36. Calderon-Garciduenas L, Valencia-Salazar G, Rodriguez-Alcaraz A, et al. Ultrastructural nasal pathology in children chronically and sequentially exposed to air pollutants. Am J Respir Cell Mol Biol 2001;24(2):132–8.

37. Calderon-Garciduenas L, Rodriguez-Alcaraz A, Valencia-Salazar G, et al. Nasal biopsies of children exposed to air pollutants. Toxicol Pathol 2001;29(5):558–64.

38. Kopp MV, Ulmer C, Ihorst G, et al. Upper airway inflammation in children exposed to ambient ozone and potential signs of adaptation. Eur Respir J 1999;14(4):854–61.

39. Pacini S, Giovannelli L, Gulisano M, et al. Association between atmospheric ozone levels and damage to human nasal mucosa in Florence, Italy. Environ Mol Mutagen 2003;42(3):127–35.

40. Walinder R, Norback D, Wieslander G, et al. Acoustic rhinometry in epidemiological studies–nasal reactions in Swedish schools. Rhinol Suppl 2000;16:59–64.

41. Araki A, Kawai T, Eitaki Y, et al. Relationship between selected indoor volatile organic compounds, so-called microbial VOC, and the prevalence of mucous membrane symptoms in single family homes. Sci Total Environ 2010;408(10): 2208–15.

42. Sienra-Monge JJ, Ramirez-Aguilar M, Moreno-Macias H, et al. Antioxidant supplementation and nasal inflammatory responses among young asthmatics exposed to high levels of ozone. Clin Exp Immunol 2004;138(2):317–22.

43. Skulberg KR, Skyberg K, Kruse K, et al. The effect of cleaning on dust and the health of office workers: an intervention study. Epidemiology 2004;15(1):71–8.

44. Braat JP, Mulder PG, Fokkens WJ, et al. Intranasal cold dry air is superior to histamine challenge in determining the presence and degree of nasal hyperreactivity in nonallergic noninfectious perennial rhinitis. Am J Respir Crit Care Med 1998;157(6 Pt 1):1748–55.

45. Shusterman DJ, Tilles SA. Nasal physiological reactivity of subjects with nonallergic rhinitis to cold air provocation: a pilot comparison of subgroups. Am J Rhinol Allergy 2009;23(5):475–9.

46. Kim YH, Oh YS, Kim KJ, et al. Use of cold dry air provocation with acoustic rhinometry in detecting nonspecific nasal hyperreactivity. Am J Rhinol Allergy 2010; 24(4):260–2.

47. Bernstein JA, Salapatek AM, Lee JS, et al. Provocation of nonallergic rhinitis subjects in response to simulated weather conditions using an environmental exposure chamber model. Allergy Asthma Proc 2012;33(4):333–40.

48. Barry PW, Mason NP, Richalet JP. Nasal peak inspiratory flow at altitude. Eur Respir J 2002;19:16–9.

49. Bascom R, Kulle T, Kagey-Sobotka A, et al. Upper respiratory tract environmental tobacco smoke sensitivity. Am Rev Respir Dis 1991;143(6):1304–11.

50. Bascom R, Kesavanathan J, Fitzgerald TK, et al. Sidestream tobacco smoke exposure acutely alters human nasal mucociliary clearance. Environ Health Perspect 1995;103(11):1026–30.

51. Nowak D, Jorres R, Martinez-Muller L, et al. Effect of 3 hours of passive smoke exposure in the evening on inflammatory markers in bronchoalveolar and nasal lavage fluid in subjects with mild asthma. Int Arch Occup Environ Health 1997; 70(2):85–93.

52. Junker MH, Danuser B, Monn C, et al. Acute sensory responses of nonsmokers at very low environmental tobacco smoke concentrations in controlled laboratory settings. Environ Health Perspect 2001;109(10):1045–52.

53. Schick SF, van den Vossenberg G, Luo A, et al. Thirty minute-exposure to aged cigarette smoke increases nasal congestion in nonsmokers. J Toxicol Environ Health A 2013;76(10):601–13.

54. Kjaergaard S, Rasmussen TR, Molhave L, et al. An experimental comparison of indoor air VOC effects on hay fever and healthy subjects. Proceedings of Healthy Buildings '95. Milan (Italy): STET; 1995.

55. Hudnell HK, Otto DA, House DE, et al. Exposure of humans to a volatile organic mixture: II. Sensory. Arch Environ Health 1992;47(1):31–8.

56. Koren HS, Graham DE, Devlin RB. Exposure of humans to a volatile organic mixture: III. Inflammatory response. Arch Environ Health 1992;47(1):39–44.

57. Muttray A, Klimek L, Faas M, et al. The exposure of healthy volunteers to 200 ppm 1,1,1-trichloroethane increases the concentration of proinflammatory cytokines in nasal secretions. Int Arch Occup Environ Health 1999;72(7):485–8.

58. Muttray A, Jung D, Klimek L, et al. Effects of an external exposure to 200 ppm methyl ethyl ketone on nasal mucosa in healthy volunteers. Int Arch Occup Environ Health 2002;75(3):197–200.
59. Mann WJ, Muttray A, Schaefer D, et al. Exposure to 200 ppm of methanol increases the concentrations of interleukin-1beta and interleukin-8 in nasal secretions of healthy volunteers. Ann Otol Rhinol Laryngol 2002;111(7 Pt 1):633–8.
60. Andersen I, Lundqvist GR, Molhave L, et al. Human response to controlled levels of toluene in six-hour exposures. Scand J Work Environ Health 1983;9(5):405–18.
61. McLean JA, Mathews KP, Solomon WR, et al. Effect of ammonia on nasal resistance in atopic and nonatopic subjects. Ann Otol Rhinol Laryngol 1979;88(2 Pt 1):228–34.
62. Shusterman DJ, Murphy MA, Balmes JR. Subjects with seasonal allergic rhinitis and nonrhinitic subjects react differentially to nasal provocation with chlorine gas. J Allergy Clin Immunol 1998;101(6 Pt 1):732–40.
63. Shusterman D, Murphy MA, Balmes J. Influence of age, gender, and allergy status on nasal reactivity to inhaled chlorine. Inhal Toxicol 2003;15(12):1179–89.
64. Shusterman D, Murphy MA, Walsh P, et al. Cholinergic blockade does not alter the nasal congestive response to irritant provocation. Rhinology 2002;40(3): 141–6.
65. Shusterman D, Balmes J, Avila PC, et al. Chlorine inhalation produces nasal congestion in allergic rhinitics without mast cell degranulation. Eur Respir J 2003;21(4):652–7.
66. Shusterman D, Balmes J, Murphy MA, et al. Chlorine inhalation produces nasal airflow limitation in allergic rhinitic subjects without evidence of neuropeptide release. Neuropeptides 2004;38(6):351–8.
67. Tam EK, Liu J, Bigby BG, et al. Sulfur dioxide does not acutely increase nasal symptoms or nasal resistance in subjects with rhinitis or in subjects with bronchial responsiveness to sulfur dioxide. Am Rev Respir Dis 1988;138(6):1559–64.
68. Andersen IB, Lundqvist GR, Jensen PL, et al. Human response to controlled levels of sulfur dioxide. Arch Environ Health 1974;28(1):31–9.
69. Graham D, Henderson F, House D. Neutrophil influx measured in nasal lavages of humans exposed to ozone. Arch Environ Health 1988;43(3):228–33.
70. Graham DE, Koren HS. Biomarkers of inflammation in ozone-exposed humans. Comparison of the nasal and bronchoalveolar lavage. Am Rev Respir Dis 1990; 142(1):152–6.
71. McBride DE, Koenig JQ, Luchtel DL, et al. Inflammatory effects of ozone in the upper airways of subjects with asthma. Am J Respir Crit Care Med 1994; 149(5):1192–7.
72. Shusterman D, Tarun A, Murphy MA, et al. Seasonal allergic rhinitic and normal subjects respond differentially to nasal provocation with acetic acid vapor. Inhal Toxicol 2005;17(3):147–52.
73. Morgan MS, Camp JE. Upper respiratory irritation from controlled exposure to vapor from carbonless copy forms. J Occup Med 1986;28(6):415–9.
74. Theander C, Bende M. Nasal hyperreactivity to newspapers. Clin Exp Allergy 1989;19(1):57–8.
75. Koskela H, Di Sciascio MB, Anderson SD, et al. Nasal hyperosmolar challenge with a dry powder of mannitol in patients with allergic rhinitis. Evidence for epithelial cell involvement. Clin Exp Allergy 2000;30(11):1627–36.
76. Philip G, Jankowski R, Baroody FM, et al. Reflex activation of nasal secretion by unilateral inhalation of cold dry air. Am Rev Respir Dis 1993;148(6 Pt 1):1616–22.
77. Rondon C, Campo P, Togias A, et al. Local allergic rhinitis: concept, pathophysiology, and management. J Allergy Clin Immunol 2012;129:1460–7.

Novel, Alternative, and Controversial Therapies of Rhinitis

 CrossMark

Pavol Surda, MD, Wytske J. Fokkens, MD, PhD*

KEYWORDS

- Allergic rhinitis • Nonallergic rhinitis • Novel therapies • Alternative • Controversial
- Immunotherapy • Neurogenic pathway modulators

KEY POINTS

- The current treatments for rhinitis are generally effective and well-tolerated in mild-to-moderate patients, but a significant group, with so-called severe chronic upper airway disease, continues to experience bothersome symptoms despite adequate treatment.
- Local corticosteroids remain the mainstay in the management of rhinitis; research has focused on the improvement of the efficacy, side-effect profile, and possible combinations with the other known agents.
- The new combination of local corticosteroid and azelastine seems to be a major improvement for allergic rhinitis patients failing local corticosteroid treatment alone.
- Substantial advances in the understanding of the allergic rhinitis immunologic response cascade resulted in finding treatment modalities that are geared toward being curative in nature rather than palliative in terms of symptom relief, which include new drugs that target immunoglobulin E and the molecules involved in the type 2 helper T—mediated pathways of allergic inflammation and subcutaneous or sublingual therapy.
- Although the heterogeneous nature of nonallergic rhinitis poses a therapeutic challenge, newer agents such as neurogenic pathway modulators have shown promising results.

INTRODUCTION

Rhinitis is a multifactorial disease characterized by symptoms of sneezing, rhinorrhea, postnasal drip, and nasal congestion. Rhinitis affects 10% to 40% of the population in industrialized countries, which is responsible for billions of spent health care dollars and impairment in quality of life for those affected.[1] Direct costs relate to medications to treat the primary disease and associated comorbidities, whereas the indirect costs derive from missed work, missed school, and decreased productivity. Classification of rhinitis entities on the basis of phenotypes has facilitated their characterization and

Department of Otorhinolaryngology, Academic Medical Center, Meibergdreef 29, Amsterdam 1105 AZ, The Netherlands
* Corresponding author. Academic Medical Center, Room A2-234, Amsterdam 1100 DD, The Netherlands.
E-mail address: w.j.fokkens@amc.nl

Immunol Allergy Clin N Am 36 (2016) 401–423
http://dx.doi.org/10.1016/j.iac.2015.12.014
0889-8561/16/$ – see front matter © 2016 Elsevier Inc. All rights reserved.

helped practicing clinicians to efficiently diagnose and manage these patients.[2] The current treatments for rhinitis are generally effective and well-tolerated in most patients, but in real life, a significant percentage of patients with chronic rhinitis are uncontrolled and continue to experience bothersome symptoms despite adequate treatment.[3] This group of allergic rhinitis (AR) patients with so-called severe chronic upper airway disease represents a therapeutic challenge because they remain poorly controlled.[4–6]

In addition, some treatment options have side effects that may limit their long-term use in some patients. A recent survey performed among rhinitis patients undergoing skin prick testing revealed that up to 50% feared adverse events of the medication prescribed for AR.[7] In the past 10 years, there have been substantial advances in the understanding of rhinitis, airway biology, and immune cell signaling. Ongoing clinical trials are aimed at improving the side-effect profile of these treatments and determining safe combinations of medicines for clinical use. It is hoped that a better understanding of phenotypes and endotypes will lead to more personalized medicine to further clinically benefit patient outcomes.[2] New drugs targeting other molecules involved in the immunologic response cascade are being studied in an effort to improve clinical benefit in these patients (**Fig. 1**). Last, there has been a shift in focus toward finding treatment modalities that are geared toward being curative, rather than palliative, in terms of symptom relief. For example, recent research in AR has focused on finding new routes for immunotherapy and developing new drugs that target immunoglobulin E (IgE) and the molecules involved in the type 2 helper T (Th2)-mediated pathways of allergic inflammation. This finding is emphasized by a recent survey, which demonstrated that up to 40% of patients with a new diagnosis of AR want to be cured from their allergies rather than simply achieving symptomatic relief.[7] In this article, novel, alternative, and controversial therapies in allergic and non-allergic rhinitis (NAR) are discussed. For the sake of clarity, the treatment options are divided into the following: advances in known intranasal treatment, treatments targeting a single mediator or receptor, neurogenic pathway modulators, treatments with widespread effects like immunotherapy, surgical treatment, and finally, alternative and controversial treatments. Of course, determination of what is considered alternative and controversial may be considered arbitrary by some. However, the more important objective was to provide a broad overview of nonmainstream therapies to the reader. Emerging drugs and those already commercially available are summarized in **Tables 1** and **2**.

ADVANCES IN THE KNOWN INTRANASAL TREATMENT

State-of-the-art guidelines like Allergic Rhinitis and its Impact on Asthma provide clinicians with evidence-based treatment algorithms for chronic rhinitis. These algorithms consist of a stepwise approach based on symptom duration and severity. Primary treatments are divided into several categories: decongestants, antihistamines, chromones, antileukotrienes, anticholinergics, corticosteroids, and immunotherapy. Nowadays, the most effective treatment modalities are topical corticosteroids (intranasal corticosteroids [INCs]) or a combination of topical corticosteroids and antihistamines nasal sprays. However, even despite compliance with optimal therapy, there is a fraction of patients whose symptoms are inadequately controlled despite adherence to the recommended treatment guidelines.

As mentioned, INCs are most effective in reducing rhinitis symptoms, especially nasal congestion. The doses used in nasal sprays are low and generally well tolerated with relatively few systemic side effects because of their low bioavailability. Clinical trials continue to study the optimal dose of INCs that is both safe and effective. Recently, the optimal dose of beclomethasone dipropionate was determined to be 320 µg for treatment of

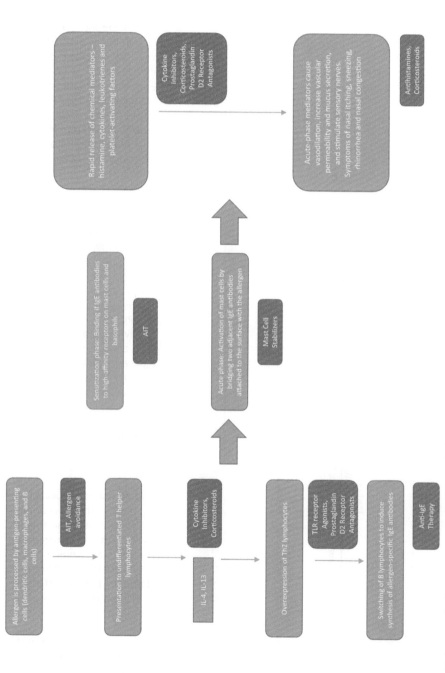

Fig. 1. AR immunologic response cascade (*blue color*) and the mechanism of action of the novel treatment modalities (*orange color*). Green color indicates the sensitization phase of the cascade.

Table 1
Summary of drugs for allergic rhinitis

Classification	Agent	Trade Name (If Already on the Market)	ClinicalTrials.gov Identifier/Clinical Trial/Phase	Mechanism of Action	Efficacy/Safety
Corticosteroid	CIC, nasal aerosol	Zetonna, Omnaris	Already on the market	Higher affinity for the glucocorticoid receptor	The regional deposition of the HFA propellant-based formulation resulted in increased retention of drug product in the nasal cavity[12,13]
Antihistamine/corticosteroid	AZE/FP, nasal spray	Dymista	Already on the market	Histamine H1-receptor antagonist and synthetic corticosteroid	It has shown superior efficacy in AR patients than either commercially available AZE or FP monotherapy for both nasal and ocular symptom relief, regardless of disease severity[14]
Antihistamine	JNJ-39220675, oral solution	Not yet. In the clinical trial phase of the drug development process	NCT00804687/phase 2	H3-antagonist	Relieved allergen-induced nasal congestion compared with placebo, but in contrast with pseudoephedrine, it only showed a trend for increasing nasal patency by using objective measures[20]
Antihistamine	PF-03654764, tablet	Not yet. In the clinical trial phase of the drug development process	NCT01033396 /phase 2	H3 receptor antagonist	Combination of PF-03654764/fexofenadine did not provide superior relief of AR-associated nasal symptoms on exposure to ragweed pollen but improved TNSS compared with placebo. Side effects in the PF-03654764-treated groups were clinically significant compared with the controls[21]
Antihistamine	GSK1004723, nasal spray	Not yet. In the clinical trial phase of the drug development process	NCT00972504/phase 2	H1/H3 receptor antagonist	Combined H1/H3 antagonism did not show differentiation from H1 antagonism in reducing total nasal symptom score or nasal blockage[22]

			Status	Mechanism	Clinical evidence
Anti-IgE therapy	Omalizumab	Xolair	Already on the market	Humanized monoclonal antibody that binds to the Ce3 domain of IgE at the site of FceR1 binding, thus blocking binding of IgE to effector cells	There have been many studies that demonstrated beneficial effects in patients with AR such as decreasing daily symptoms and rescue medication usage as well as decreasing nasal allergen challenge responses[27–30]
TLR agonists	GSK2245035, nasal spray		Not yet. In the clinical trial phase of the drug development process	Selective TLR7 agonist	Clinical trial demonstrated a safe profile of the nasal spray[47]
TLR agonists	AZD8848, nasal spray		Not yet. In the clinical trial phase of the drug development process	Selective TLR7 agonist	Clinical trial demonstrated a safe profile and a sustained reduction in the responsiveness to allergen in AR when compared with placebo[49]
PGD2 receptor antagonists	BI 671800, tablet		Not yet. In the clinical trial phase of the drug development process	PGD2 receptor antagonists inhibit the recruitment and activation of TH2 cells	Clinical trial in 146 patients with AR demonstrated efficacy in reducing total and individual symptoms[54]
PGD2 receptor antagonists	OC000459, tablet		Not yet. In the clinical trial phase of the drug development process	PGD2 receptor antagonists inhibit the recruitment and activation of TH2 cells	Effects of OC000459 on nasal symptoms were at least as good as those of levocetirizine or fexofenadine,[57] and approach those observed with fluticasone furoate

Data from Horak F, Stubner P, Zieglmayer R, et al. Controlled comparison of the efficacy and safety of cetirizine 10 mg o.d. and fexofenadine 120 mg o.d. in reducing symptoms of seasonal allergic rhinitis. Int Arch Allergy Immunol 2001;125(1):73–9.

Table 2
Summary of drugs for nonallergic rhinitis

Classification	Agent	Trade Name (If Already on the Market)	ClinicalTrials.gov Identifier/ Clinical Trial/Phase	Mechanism of Action	Efficacy/Safety
Neurogenic pathway modulators	Ipratropium bromide	Atrovent, Rinatec	Already on the market	Anticholinergic mechanism of action	Clinical studies using this drug as a nasal spray have shown it to be effective in reducing the severity and duration of rhinorrhea in the common cold,[77] and in NAR, especially in rhinitis of the elderly.[78-80] It is therefore the first treatment option in rhinitis of the elderly
Neurogenic pathway modulators	Capsaicin	Not yet. In the clinical trial phase of the drug development process	NCT02493257/Phase 2 In progress	Reduces nasal hyperreactivity and the receptor TRPV1 overexpression	Capsaicin treatment has been shown to be safe: blood pressure, heart rate, olfactory function, and mucosal sensibility are not affected by the treatment. *Cochrane Review* of the effectiveness of capsaicin has been conducted. Four studies were analyzed, and all showed improvement of the nasal symptoms[69]

Data from Refs.[77-80]

AR in adolescents and adults. At this dose, there was a statistically significant change (P<.013) from baseline in total nasal symptom scores over a 2-week treatment period.[8]

Ciclesonide (CIC), a corticosteroid prodrug, is enzymatically converted by esterases to its active metabolite, des-isobutyryl CIC, which displays a substantially higher affinity (120-fold) for the glucocorticoid receptor compared with the parent compound.[9,10] Other INCs prodrugs, such as rofleponide palmitate, have been investigated with comparable efficacy to that of other INCs.[8,11]

Clinical trials analyzing the nasal deposition and activity of CIC using novel forms of delivery such as a nasal metered dose inhaler (NCT01371786) led to the approval of a dry-nose-spray formulation in the United States.[12] The regional deposition of the hydrofluoroalkane (HFA) propellant-based formulation resulted in increased retention of drug product in the nasal cavity and decreased deposition in the back of the throat compared with the 2 aqueous formulations.[13]

Promising results have been achieved with combination therapy using an INC and intranasal antihistamine. MP29-02 (Dymista; Meda, Solna, Sweden) contains azelastine hydrochloride (AZE) and fluticasone propionate (FP), in a novel formulation that is delivered in an improved device as a single nasal spray. It has shown superior efficacy in AR patients compared with either AZE or FP monotherapy for both nasal and ocular symptom relief, regardless of disease severity. MP29-02 also provided more effective and rapid symptom relief compared with either AZE or FP monotherapy when delivered in the same MP29-02 formulation and device.[14] It is indicated for the treatment of moderate-to-severe seasonal AR and perennial AR when monotherapy with either an intranasal antihistamine or an INC is not considered sufficient. Combination therapy using a nasal ICS and a topical antihistamine has not been specifically studied in chronic NAR.

Selective glucocorticoid receptor agonists (SEGRAs) are a new class of drugs designed to have an improved therapeutic index associated with a reduced side-effect profile over classic corticosteroids.[15] In guinea pig, the new SEGRA mapracorat reduced clinical symptoms of allergic conjunctivitis and conjunctival eosinophil inflammation in a manner comparable to that induced by dexamethasone eye drops.[16] In human conjunctival fibroblasts and epithelial cells cultures, mapracorat effectively reduced interleukin (IL)-4 or IL-13 plus tumor necrosis factor-α (TNF-α) induced release of pro-inflammatory and allergy-related cytokines, chemokines, and intercellular adhesion molecule 1 (ICAM-1).[17] It also inhibits the migration of cultured human eosinophils and IL-8 release from eosinophils or the release of IL-6, IL-8, chemokine (C-C motif) ligand 5 (CCL5)/regulated on activation, normal T cell expressed and secreted (RANTES), and TNF-α from a human mast cell line with potency equal to dexamethasone.[16] Although SEGRAs appear to be a promising candidate for topical treatment of rhinitis, no specific study in rhinitis has thus far been conducted.

Conclusion

Advances in the known treatments have brought an important change in the approach to AR. For the first time, there is a treatment that is more effective than a local corticosteroid, MP29-02, which is the combination of fluticasone and azelastine. In addition, the new forms of nasal spray delivery, such as HFA propellant-based formulations, increase drug retention in the nasal cavity.

TARGETING SINGLE MEDIATOR OR RECEPTOR
Mast Cell Stabilizers

Mast-cell stabilizers act by inhibiting mast cell activation, thereby preventing the release of mediators and consequent inhibition of the allergic cascade, this may improve the nasal symptoms because the synthesis and release of mediators, such as histamine, leukotrienes, and tryptase, are reduced.

A currently used mast cell stabilizing agent is cromolyn sodium, but because it has a short duration of action (12 hours), it is not very effective as a long-term controller. The new molecule Syk kinase inhibitor R112 acts as a transducer of signaling through the FcεI receptor of mast cells, blocking mast cell responses to allergic stimuli. Intranasal R112 demonstrated significant improvement when compared with placebo. However, whether its effect persists beyond 4 hours could not be determined from this study.[18]

Antihistamines

New experimental antihistamines that target histamine receptors other than H1 receptors are under clinical investigation. A therapeutic role for histamine H3 receptor antagonism in AR has been proposed and may be complementary to the currently used H1-antihistamines.[19]

Prophylactic treatment with the H3-antagonist JNJ-39220675 relieved allergen-induced nasal congestion by using standard nasal symptom scoring; however, in contrast with pseudoephedrine, it only showed a trend for increasing nasal patency using objective measures.[20]

The new molecule PF-03654764 is a potent and specific H3 receptor antagonist. The combination of PF-03654764/fexofenadine did not provide superior relief of AR-associated nasal symptoms after exposure to ragweed pollen but improved TNSS compared with placebo. The PF-03654764-treated group experienced clinically significantly more side effects compared with controls.[21]

In addition, a combined H1/H3 antagonist has been investigated (GSK1004723). In clinical phase I and II safety and efficacy studies, combined H1/H3 antagonism did not demonstrate a significant difference in reducing total nasal symptom scores or nasal blockage compared with H1 antagonism alone.[22]

Recently, new antihistamine drugs, such as histamine H3/H4R antagonists/inverse agonists, were studied for the treatment of AR, and in general, allergic respiratory diseases. However, the currently published data do not demonstrate an additional benefit compared with H1 antagonism in reducing nasal blockage.[23]

Anti-immunoglobulin E Therapy

The monoclonal antibody, omalizumab, which is a recombinant DNA-derived humanized IgG1k monoclonal antibody that binds circulating IgE, is now currently approved for clinical use in several countries. By blocking IgE from binding to the high-affinity IgE receptor, Fc epsilon RI (FCER1), on mast cells and basophils, it can inactivate soluble and membrane-bound IgE[24] and reduce the overall serum level of IgE after continuous therapy.[25] Omalizumab also prevents IgE interactions with high-affinity IgE receptors (FcεRI) expressed by dendritic cells and eosinophils. As a consequence, IgE-dependent antigen presentation, mast cell and basophil activation, and eosinophil infiltration are inhibited. Anti-IgE therapy with omalizumab also results in decreased FcεRI expression. All of these mechanistic effects are thought to be responsible for the observed reduction of allergic airway inflammation.[26]

There have been multiple clinical studies on the use of omalizumab in AR, which have shown beneficial effects such as decreasing daily symptoms. A randomized controlled clinical trial was able to show that omalizumab pretreatment ameliorated the side effects of subcutaneous rush immunotherapy for ragweed seasonal AR,[27] which was shown to be secondary to inhibition of allergen-specific IgE binding.[28]

Another randomized trial investigated the effect of add-on omalizumab versus placebo for an additional 6 months after 3 months of subcutaneous immunotherapy

(SCIT) in 92 children with seasonal allergic rhinitis (SAR) aged 6 to 17. Both treatments were effective, although patients receiving SCIT with omalizumab had significantly lower symptom scores during pollen season than those treated with SCIT alone.[29]

Omalizumab may provide a new treatment strategy for AR, but there is still a cost issue that needs to be resolved. For example, the benefits of omalizumab for allergic asthma have been calculated to outweigh the cost, but only in severely affected subgroups of patients.[30]

Cytokine Inhibitors

Cytokines play a crucial role in orchestrating acute as well as chronic inflammation, making them potential targets for blockade in AR. Eosinophilic inflammation of the airways with specific Th2 pattern and B-cell release of antigen-specific IgE is promoted through various proinflammatory cytokines, particularly IL-4, IL-13, and IL-5.[31]

Suplatast tosilate (IPD-1151T) is an immunomodulator that suppresses eosinophil infiltration, IgE production, and allergic inflammation by suppressing the production of IL-4 and IL-5.[32] The efficacy of systemic administration of suplatast in nasal allergy has been reported. Nasal symptom scores significantly decreased in 12 subjects with AR after treatment. After treatment, the levels of cytokines (IL-4, IL-5, IL-13, and interferon [IFN]-γ) and the IL-5/IFN-γ ratio were significantly decreased, and the IL-4/IFN-γ ratio was not significantly different from that in normal subjects.[33]

There is more extensive ongoing research of cytokine modulation in patients with asthma. Promising treatments include modulators of IL-4Rα,[34] IL-4Rα/IL-13Rα1 complex,[35] and IL-5.[36] With the successful advent of cytokine modulation therapy in refractory asthma patients, future research may also be warranted in difficult-to-control chronic rhinitis patients.

Toll-like Receptor Agonists

The allergic immune response is a complex process beginning with the activation of allergen-specific Th2 cells by antigen-presenting cells followed by their proliferation, cytokine production, helper functions, and the emergence of memory cells. Numerous experimental models and clinical studies support a central role of allergen-specific Th2 cells in pathophysiologic responses.[37–40]

Attention has been directed toward methods that promote the down-modulation of Th2 responsiveness to allergens by inducing counterbalancing type 1 helper T (Th1)-type cytokines (ie, IFNs and IL-12) through manipulation of elements of host defense, such as the toll-like receptors (TLRs).[41,42]

TLRs are widely expressed on immune and epithelial cells. By recognizing pathogen-associated molecular patterns, the innate and adaptive immune mechanisms are activated to eliminate the "danger" and preserve immune homeostasis and health.[43]

Synthetic TLR4 and TLR9 agonists have been assessed as adjuvants of allergen-specific immunotherapy with the hope that they may boost Th1/T regulatory cell-type antiallergic activity and thus enhance clinical benefit.[37,44–46] GSK2245035, a selective TLR7 agonist with preferential type-1 IFN-stimulating properties, was developed for intranasal application. Animal models showed efficacy in reducing symptoms, and a phase 1 clinical trial demonstrated a good safety profile for this nasal spray.[47]

TLR8 agonist, VTX-1463, seems to be a promising new agent for the treatment of seasonal, and potentially perennial, AR. The first human study demonstrated statistically significant improvement in nasal symptoms.[48]

Repeated intranasal stimulation of TLR7 by AZD8848 was safe and produced a sustained reduction in allergen responsiveness in AR compared with placebo.[49]

Prostaglandin D2 Receptor Antagonists

Prostaglandin D2 (PGD2), an arachidonic acid metabolite, is a key mediator in inflammation after allergen exposure and is released by IgE-activated mast cells and other inflammatory cell types.[50,51] PGD2 might help in recruiting and activating TH2 lymphocytes and eosinophils,[52] and therefore, plays an important role in AR. The proinflammatory effects of PGD2 occur through interactions with the "chemoattractant receptor homologous molecule on TH2 cells" (CRTH2). Activation of CRTH2 triggers the release of chemokines and inflammatory mediators, and as recently discovered, it functions as a survival signal for TH2 lymphocytes.[51,53]

This finding suggests that CRTH2 antagonists might not only inhibit the recruitment and activation of TH2 cells but also accelerate apoptosis and clearance of these cells from inflamed tissue, thereby promoting the resolution of the underlying inflammation in AR.[51,52]

A clinical trial investigating the oral CRTH2 antagonist BI 671800 in 146 patients with AR demonstrated efficacy in reducing total and individual symptoms.[54]

Another CRTH2 antagonist OC000459 has previously been shown to reduce airway inflammation and to improve lung function and quality of life in subjects with moderate persistent asthma.[55] A study by Horak and colleagues[56] compared OC000459 with placebo in subjects with allergic rhinoconjunctivitis. This study showed that the effects of OC000459 on nasal symptoms were at least as good as that of levocetirizine or fexofenadine[57] and approached those observed with fluticasone furoate[58]; however, further study is warranted to confirm these observations.

Conclusion

There has been a shift in focus toward finding treatment modalities that are geared toward being curative, rather than palliative. The novel treatments targeting a single mediator or receptor provide mainly symptomatic treatment, but the combination with subcutaneous or sublingual therapy is promising for the future. The combination of omalizumab and SCIT has already showed significant symptom improvement in AR patients as have an ultrashort treatment course of an allergoid in combination with the TLR4 agonist.[59] Cytokine modulation therapy yields optimistic results in patients with asthma, but further research in AR patients is needed. The data available in the literature on new antihistamines do not demonstrate a clear additional benefit compared with H1 antagonism at improving nasal symptoms.

NEUROGENIC PATHWAY MODULATORS
Nasal Application of Botulinum Toxin A

Botulinum toxin type A (BTA) is a neurotoxin that inhibits the release of acetylcholine (ACH) in synapses. ACH acts as a neurotransmitter for the innervation of muscles and different gland tissues. Blocking the release of ACH leads to a reduction of pathologic muscle movement and gland secretion.[60] The use of BTA injections into the septum or lower or middle turbinates[61,62] or application with a sponge soaked in a solution of BTA have been described.[63,64] Efficacy of BTA injection in a double-blind, placebo-controlled clinical trial on AR patients has demonstrated a reduction in rhinorrhea, nasal obstruction, and sneezing scores.[65] In NAR double-blind, placebo-controlled clinical trials, using BTA injections[66] or BTA administered with soaked sponges[63] has shown efficacy. The effect of the treatment lasted 2 to 3 months. Side effects such as epistaxis or nasal crusting were uncommon.

Capsaicin

Capsaicin, the pungent agent in hot pepper, is known for its degeneration/desensitization effect on peptidergic sensory C-fibers.[67] An imbalance in the nonadrenergic, noncholinergic peptidergic neuronal system has been proposed as the underlying mechanism of idiopathic rhinitis.[68] Treatment with capsaicin may fit in with this hypothesis.[67] In a recent *Cochrane Review*, the effectiveness of capsaicin in the management of NAR compared with no therapy, placebo, or other topical or systemic medications, or 2 or more of the above therapies in combination, or different capsaicin regimens, was assessed.[69] Four studies (5 publications) involving 302 adult patients with moderate to severe idiopathic NAR were analyzed. Studies had follow-up periods ranging from 4 to 38 weeks. Two studies compared capsaicin with placebo.[70,71] One study reported that capsaicin resulted in an improvement of overall nasal symptoms (a primary outcome) measured on a visual analogue scale (VAS) of 0 to 10.[70] There was a mean difference (MD) of −3.34 (95% confidence interval [CI] −5.24 to −1.44), MD −3.73 (95% CI −5.45 to −2.01), and MD −3.52 (95% CI −5.55 to −1.48) at 2, 12, and 36 weeks after treatment, respectively. Another study reported that, compared with placebo, capsaicin (at 4 µg/puff) was more likely to produce overall symptom resolution (reduction in nasal blockage, sneezing/itching/coughing, and nasal secretion measured with a daily record chart) at 4 weeks after treatment (a primary outcome).[71] The risk ratio was 3.17 (95% CI 1.38–7.29). One study compared capsaicin to budesonide.[72] This study found that patients treated with capsaicin had a better overall symptom score compared with those treated with budesonide (MD 2.50, 95% CI 1.06–3.94, VAS of 0–10). The last study compared 2 different regimens of capsaicin administration: 5 treatments in 1 day versus 5 treatments given every 2 to 3 days for 2 weeks.[73] Using daily record charts, the study reported significant improvement of individual symptom scores for rhinorrhea in patients treated 5 times per day; however, numerical data were not presented.

Capsaicin treatment has been shown to be safe: blood pressure, heart rate, olfactory function, and mucosal sensibility are not affected by the treatment.[73] The treatment effect lasts at least 1 year and can easily be repeated.[67]

Recently, a potential working mechanism of capsaicin treatment was proposed. It was demonstrated that capsaicin treatment reduced nasal hyperreactivity and transient receptor potential cation channel subfamily V, receptor 1 (TRPV1) overexpression in patients with idiopathic rhinitis.[74]

New drugs targeting TRPV1 have been developed and may offer the potential to control medical conditions characterized by sensory neuronal hyperresponsiveness, including the nasal hyperreactivity that underlies NAR.[75]

Ipratropium Bromide

Ipratropium bromide is an anticholinergic drug used mainly in the treatment of asthma.[76] Clinical studies using this drug as a nasal spray have shown it to be effective in reducing the severity and duration of rhinorrhea in the common cold[77] and in NAR, especially in rhinitis of the elderly.[78–80] It is therefore the first treatment option in rhinitis of the elderly. Ipratropium bromide is usually administered as a 0.03% spray for common rhinorrhea but comes as a stronger concentration, 0.06%, for anterior or posterior rhinorrhea associated with a viral upper respiratory infection. The dosage necessary to achieve the optimal effect may vary considerably. It is advised to start with 80 to 100 μg twice daily. Some patients require higher dosages, and dosage can usually be safely increased to 400 μg 4 times daily.[81–83]

Conclusion

NAR is a therapeutic challenge because of its heterogeneous nature. However, neurogenic pathway modulators might be the future perspective. *Cochrane Review* demonstrated that capsaicin is an effective treatment for NAR. Nasal application of BTA seems to be safe, and the effect of the treatment lasts 2 to 3 months. The reduction of symptoms has been shown in patients with NAR as well as AR. Ipratropium bromide controls rhinorrhea in rhinitis of the elderly well. Frequent application is usually recommended to achieve the optimal effect.

WIDESPREAD EFFECT
Developments in Immunotherapy

SCIT has been used to treat allergic diseases, such as asthma, AR, and venom allergy, since first described over a century ago. Allergen immunotherapy (AIT) has been shown to prevent asthma in patients with AR.[84] Immunotherapy has been shown to have disease-modifying effects, results in long-term remission of allergic symptoms, and reduces the risk of progression from rhinitis to asthma as well as the chances of developing new sensitizations to allergens.[85]

Immunotherapy with sublingual immunotherapy (SLIT) offers several distinct advantages over SCIT: it can be self-administered at home, it is less painful, and it has a much lower risk of anaphylaxis.[86,87] However, it has to be administered daily by the patient, and it is unclear whether efficacy is as large as SCIT. SLIT tablets are now commercially available for grass and ragweed,[88] and in some European countries, for house dust mites.[89,90] Studies with tree-pollen have been conducted, and the products are expected to be commercially available soon.[91] Because immunotherapy has potential risks especially in patients with asthma, the final decision on the administration of AIT should be based on individual evaluation of any medical condition and a risk/benefit assessment for each patient.[92] Compared with SCIT, SLIT has been shown to be relatively safe for patients with mild asthma.[93]

Modern technology has enabled the synthesis of recombinant proteins, whose main advantages are their fully characterized physical, chemical, and immunologic properties. It has become possible to produce well-defined recombinant and synthetic allergy vaccines that can specifically target the mechanisms of the allergic disease.[94] This approach is considered the promising future of immunotherapy and an important facet of personalized medicine. Clinical use of recombinant allergens can be expected in the near future. Studies investigating the clinical effects of chemically altered allergens (allergoids) and recombinant allergen proteins or peptides have been evaluated with promising results. In addition, adjuvants, such as probiotics,[95] detoxified bacterial toxins,[96] TLR,[97] vitamin D,[98,99] and anti-IgE (see also earlier discussion at anti-IgE treatment),[100] can be added to immunotherapy to amplify the therapeutic effect by modulating the immune response or to further improve its safety profile.

Other methods of administering AIT have been studied, including epicutaneous, intralymphatic, intranasal, and oral immunotherapy with variable results.[98]

SURGICAL TREATMENT

Surgical intervention should only be considered if aggressive medical therapy has failed to control a patient's symptoms. Nowadays, no single modality has evolved as the gold standard for the treatment of rhinitis. The mainstay of surgical intervention targets the inferior turbinate to control prominent nasal congestion. Complications such as atrophic rhinitis or empty nose syndrome have driven practitioners away from radical turbinectomy. Minimally invasive techniques are more favorable because there are fewer complications and they preserve the ciliary anatomy of the nose.

Nasal Passage Widening Procedures

Turbinoplasty (septoplasty with reduction of inferior turbinates),[101] laser, coblation (the shrinkage of tissue using radiofrequency and saline),[102,103] and anterior turbinectomy are the most commonly used techniques to control the nasal obstruction. There is no consensus as to which surgical technique is most effective in decreasing nasal obstruction,[104,105] but when septoplasty is performed, concomitant inferior turbinate reduction may decrease the likelihood of revision nasal surgery.[101] Recently, in a new procedure, pyriform turbinoplasty, the submucosal reduction of the bone of the frontal process of the maxilla and the lacrimal bone has been described, which seems to give an improvement in airflow when compared with inferior turbinate surgery.[106]

Vidian Neurectomy

Recently, endoscopic vidian neurectomy (EVN) became a popular surgical treatment option for selected refractory patients with vasomotor NAR. Traditional transeptal/transantral vidian neurectomy is not a novel technique. It was first described in 1961 but subsequently abandoned because of significant complications.[107] With the advent of endoscopic sinus surgery, this procedure was revitalized because it became easier to delineate the anatomy of the vidian nerve. The literature available on EVN has shown that it is effective at alleviating symptoms of vasomotor rhinitis in most patients and that the benefit is maintained over a period of 2 to 5 years. The effect of this procedure was most pronounced for improving rhinorrhea. The most common complication of EVN is postoperative xerophthalmia (dry eyes), which has been reported to occur in anywhere from 24% to 100% of cases.[77,108–112]

Silver Nitrate

Application of silver nitrate (15%–20%) to the anterior portion of both inferior turbinates and the anterior part of the nasal septum has been reported to be an effective treatment for NAR, especially for the symptoms of rhinorrhea and sneezing.[113,114] A placebo controlled study for which the randomization scheme was unclear compared silver nitrate and flunisolide in patients with NAR and found that silver nitrate seemed to be more effective at improving nasal symptoms as well as at improving physical findings on examination and nasal biopsy changes compared with flunisolide, but both treatments were superior to placebo. Symptoms recurred within 1 to 3 months and within 6 months after completion of flunisolide and silver nitrate treatment, respectively.[115]

Conclusion

Surgical treatment of rhinitis should be performed only when aggressive medical treatment is ineffective. It is still unclear whether inferior turbinate surgery in AR patients has long-term benefits or whether the risks outweigh the benefit.[116] For some patients with refractory vasomotor NAR, EVN might be a promising treatment option.

ALTERNATIVE + CONTROVERSIAL
Acupuncture

Acupuncture had been suggested to have anti-inflammatory effects. It may possibly exert its clinical effect through multiple physiologic pathways at the level of the hypothalamus-pituitary-adrenal axis and/or via the adrenergic (sympathetic) and cholinergic (parasympathetic) autonomic pathways.[117] Other reported anti-inflammatory effects of acupuncture include a histamine antagonist effect, downregulation of proinflammatory cytokines (eg, TNF-α, IL-1β, IL-6, and IL-10), proinflammatory neuropeptides (eg, substance P [SP], calcitonin gene-related peptide [CGRP], and vasoactive intestinal polypeptide [VIP]), and neurotrophins (eg, NGF and BDNF).[117] Acupuncture has also been reported to suppress the expression of cyclooxygenase (COX) -1, COX-2, and inducible nitric oxide synthase during experimentally induced inflammation. Furthermore, downregulation of the expression and sensitivity of the transient receptor potential vallinoid 1 (TRPV1) ion channel after acupuncture has been reported.[117]

A recent systematic review of 13 studies evaluated a total of 2365 participants (1126 treated and 1239 controls)[118] with AR. Compared with the control group, the acupuncture treatment group exerted a significant reduction in nasal symptom scores (weighted mean difference [WMD]: 4.42, 95% CI: 8.42–0.43, $P = 0.03$), and serum IgE (WMD: 75.00, 95% CI: 91.17–58.83, $P<.00001$) as well as improvement in the physical and mental component of the Short Form Survey-36 (SF-36). A nonsignificant trend was found for relief medication scores, and no effect was observed for the rhinitis quality-of-life questionnaire (RQLQ). No serious adverse reaction related to the acupuncture treatment was observed.[118] More recently, one additional trial was published that reported in 175 participants a decrease in sneezing and itching symptom scores and improvement of RQLQ scores.[119]

One study investigating acupuncture for 24 NAR subjects reported improvement in the primary endpoint and nasal sickness scores for the acupuncture-treated group compared with the sham-treated group, but there were no significant differences for any of the secondary endpoints, including patient symptom diaries or quality of life (SF-12). However, because of the significant baseline differences in symptom scores between the actively treated and sham-treated groups as well as the small number of subjects included in the study, these major limitations make it difficult to draw any definitive conclusions regarding use of this therapy for NAR patients.[120]

Moxibustion is a traditional Chinese medicine therapy using moxa made from dried mugwort. Practitioners use moxa to warm regions of meridian points with the intention of stimulating circulation through these points to induce smoother blood flow and qi. However, to the authors' knowledge, there are no randomized trials using Moxibustion in the English literature.[121] In conclusion, acupuncture seems to be a safe and effective treatment for AR, but its use for NAR remains unclear.

Acupressure

Acupressure is a noninvasive alternative to acupuncture. When acupressure is applied on ear acupoints (EAP), semi-self-administration by patients is possible, reducing the frequency and time required for practitioner visits.[122] In an Australian trial, 63 patients with SAR were randomly assigned to real (n = 31) and sham EAP (n = 32) groups. Twenty-five participants discontinued during treatment and 15 participants dropped out during follow-up. Subjects were treated for 8 weeks. After the treatment, total nasal symptoms score, global nasal/nonnasal symptom scores, sneezing, and regular activities at home and work were significantly improved in the real EAP group compared with the sham EAP group.[122] A second study investigated 245 perennial AR patients randomized to receive real or sham EAP treatment once a week for 8 weeks with a 12-week follow-up period. Changes of global quality-of-life score and sneezing were significantly greater in the real EAP group compared with the sham group. Although no differences were observed at the end of treatment period for total nasal symptom scores, runny nose, or eye symptoms, total nasal symptom scores were significantly reduced for the real EAP group at the end of the follow-up period. There was no difference between the 2 groups for change of medication usage at the end of treatment or at the end of follow-up periods.[123] These studies demonstrate a significant effect of ear acupressure on AR. Thus far, this treatment approach has not been investigated for NAR.

Rhinophototherapy

Phototherapy has been demonstrated to have an immunosuppressive effect, which is useful for the treatment of various inflammatory skin diseases, including atopic dermatitis.

A randomized, double-blind placebo-controlled study was conducted to assess the effect of rhinophototherapy in 49 ragweed-allergic SAR patients during the ragweed season, using a combination of ultraviolet (UV) -B (5%), UV-A (25%), and visible light (70%). Rhinophototherapy resulted in a significant improvement of total nasal symptoms score, sneezing, rhinorrhea, and nasal itching, whereas no significant effect was observed in the control group.[124] However, no direct comparisons between treatment and controls were done. Nasal lavage collected for all subjects before and after the study revealed that the active phototherapy group had significantly reduced the number of eosinophils, levels of eosinophil cationic protein, and IL-5.[124] Cytology samples examined 2 months after completion of therapy showed that any UV damage to the nasal mucosa induced by intranasal phototherapy resolved.[125] A randomized uncontrolled study adding phototherapy to mometasone demonstrated significantly improved symptoms scores and RQLQ in the phototherapy add-on group compared with the mometasone-alone group.[126]

In conclusion, there are no direct controlled data available for the effect of phototherapy in AR, but the limited data available point to a possible effect of rhinophototherapy on symptoms and reduction of eosinophils in AR.

Intranasal Carbon Dioxide

Intranasal carbon dioxide (CO_2) has been suggested to inhibit trigeminal neuronal activation and suppress the release of calcitonin gene-related peptide. Two 60-second intranasal treatments with CO_2, evaluated in a randomized, double-blind, placebo-controlled, study, resulted in rapid (10 minutes) and sustained (24 hours) relief of seasonal AR symptoms.[127] No data are currently available for the use of this treatment in NAR.

Kinetic Oscillation Stimulation

Kinetic oscillation stimulation treatment involves applying low-frequency mechanical vibrations to simulate naturally occurring turbulence, which is thought to have an anti-inflammatory effect in rhinitis. One nasal mucosa treatment with kinetic oscillation stimulation demonstrated a significant reduction of rhinitis symptoms compared with placebo in a randomized, double-blind, placebo-controlled, study conducted in NAR patients (idiopathic rhinitis or rhinitis medicamentosa).[128] The authors are not aware of subsequent studies investigating this treatment for AR.

Crenotherapy

Crenotherapy is the application of steam inhalation and/or aerosol with sodium chloride (NaCl) sulfate hyperthermal water rich in mineral salts.[129] Crenotherapy has been suggested to induce down-regulation of nasal mucosal inflammatory mediators in trials of patients with chronic rhinosinusitis (CRS) without polyps.[130,131] In a randomized trial comparing Crenotherapy to NaCl in elderly patients with NAR, a significant reduction in symptoms and VAS observed by nasal endoscopy were observed for the Crenotherapy group compared with the NaCl-treated group. In another study, the same group of investigators reported that Crenotherapy effectively improved olfactory function in elderly patients with CRS.[132] No direct comparison between the groups was made in both studies.[129,132] In another study conducted in children with AR sensitized to Parietaria, thermal water significantly reduced both TSS and fractional exhaled nitric oxide (FeNO) levels, and there was a significant relationship between reduction of nasal symptoms and FeNO values at the end of treatment with thermal water. Although this study included a NaCl control treatment, no direct comparisons between thermal water and NaCl were made.[133]

In conclusion, (hyper)thermal water has been shown to be effective in reducing symptoms in rhinitis and rhinosinusitis. Whether this effect is greater than NaCl alone has to be proven.

REFERENCES

1. Zuberbier T, Lotvall J, Simoens S, et al. Economic burden of inadequate management of allergic diseases in the European Union: a GA(2) LEN review. Allergy 2014;69(10):1275–9.
2. Papadopoulos NG, Bernstein JA, Demoly P, et al. Phenotypes and endotypes of rhinitis and their impact on management: a PRACTALL report. Allergy 2015; 70(5):474–94.
3. Hellings PW, Fokkens WJ, Akdis C, et al. Uncontrolled allergic rhinitis and chronic rhinosinusitis: where do we stand today? Allergy 2013;68(1):1–7.
4. Bousquet J, Addis A, Adcock I, et al. Integrated care pathways for airway diseases (AIRWAYS-ICPs). Eur Respir J 2014;44(2):304–23.
5. Ciprandi G, Incorvaia C, Scurati S, et al. Patient-related factors in rhinitis and asthma: the satisfaction with allergy treatment survey. Curr Med Res Opin 2011;27(5):1005–11.
6. Bousquet J, Schunemann HJ, Fonseca J, et al. MACVIA-ARIA Sentinel NetworK for allergic rhinitis (MASK-rhinitis): the new generation guideline implementation. Allergy 2015;70(11):1372–92.
7. Hellings PW, Dobbels F, Denhaerynck K, et al. Explorative study on patient's perceived knowledge level, expectations, preferences and fear of side effects for treatment for allergic rhinitis. Clin Transl Allergy 2012;2(1):9.
8. Raphael GD, Berger WE, Prenner BM, et al. Efficacy, safety, and optimal dose selection of beclomethasone dipropionate nasal aerosol for seasonal allergic rhinitis in adolescents and adults. Curr Med Res Opin 2013;29(10):1329–40.
9. Nave R, McCracken N. Metabolism of ciclesonide in the upper and lower airways: review of available data. J Asthma Allergy 2008;1:11–8.
10. Mutch E, Nave R, McCracken N, et al. The role of esterases in the metabolism of ciclesonide to desisobutyryl-ciclesonide in human tissue. Biochem Pharmacol 2007;73(10):1657–64.
11. Ahlstrom-Emanuelsson C, Andersson M, Persson C, et al. Topical treatment with aqueous solutions of rofleponide palmitate and budesonide in a pollen-season model of allergic rhinitis. Clin Exp Allergy 2004;34(5):731–5.
12. Meltzer EO, Bensch GW, Storms WW. New intranasal formulations for the treatment of allergic rhinitis. Allergy Asthma Proc 2014;35(Suppl 1):S11–9.
13. Leach CL, Kuehl PJ, Chand R, et al. Nasal deposition of HFA-beclomethasone, aqueous fluticasone propionate and aqueous mometasone furoate in allergic rhinitis patients. J Aerosol Med Pulm Drug Deliv 2015;28(5):334–40.

14. Bousquet J, Bachert C, Bernstein J, et al. Advances in pharmacotherapy for the treatment of allergic rhinitis; MP29-02 (a novel formulation of azelastine hydrochloride and fluticasone propionate in an advanced delivery system) fills the gaps. Expert Opin Pharmacother 2015;16(6):913–28.

15. Schacke H, Berger M, Rehwinkel H, et al. Selective glucocorticoid receptor agonists (SEGRAs): novel ligands with an improved therapeutic index. Mol Cell Endocrinol 2007;275(1–2):109–17.

16. Baiula M, Sparta A, Bedini A, et al. Eosinophil as a cellular target of the ocular anti-allergic action of mapracorat, a novel selective glucocorticoid receptor agonist. Mol Vis 2011;17:3208–23.

17. Cavet ME, Volhejn S, Harrington KL, et al. Anti-allergic effects of mapracorat, a novel selective glucocorticoid receptor agonist, in human conjunctival fibroblasts and epithelial cells. Mol Vis 2013;19:1515–25.

18. Meltzer EO, Berkowitz RB, Grossbard EB. An intranasal Syk-kinase inhibitor (R112) improves the symptoms of seasonal allergic rhinitis in a park environment. J Allergy Clin Immunol 2005;115(4):791–6.

19. Ridolo E, Montagni M, Caminati M, et al. Emerging drugs for allergic conjunctivitis. Expert Opin Emerg Drugs 2014;19(2):291–302.

20. Barchuk WT, Salapatek AM, Ge T, et al. A proof-of-concept study of the effect of a novel H3-receptor antagonist in allergen-induced nasal congestion. J Allergy Clin Immunol 2013;132(4):838–46.e1–e6.

21. North ML, Walker TJ, Steacy LM, et al. Add-on histamine receptor-3 antagonist for allergic rhinitis: a double blind randomized crossover trial using the environmental exposure unit. Allergy Asthma Clin Immunol 2014;10(1):33.

22. Daley-Yates P, Ambery C, Sweeney L, et al. The efficacy and tolerability of two novel H(1)/H(3) receptor antagonists in seasonal allergic rhinitis. Int Arch Allergy Immunol 2012;158(1):84–98.

23. Lazewska D, Kiec-Kononowicz K. Azines as histamine H4 receptor antagonists. Front Biosci (Schol Ed) 2012;4:967–87.

24. Chang TW, Shiung YY. Anti-IgE as a mast cell-stabilizing therapeutic agent. J Allergy Clin Immunol 2006;117(6):1203–12 [quiz: 1213].

25. Lin H, Boesel KM, Griffith DT, et al. Omalizumab rapidly decreases nasal allergic response and FcepsilonRI on basophils. J Allergy Clin Immunol 2004;113(2):297–302.

26. Pelaia G, Gallelli L, Renda T, et al. Update on optimal use of omalizumab in management of asthma. J Asthma Allergy 2011;4:49–59.

27. Casale TB, Busse WW, Kline JN, et al. Omalizumab pretreatment decreases acute reactions after rush immunotherapy for ragweed-induced seasonal allergic rhinitis. J Allergy Clin Immunol 2006;117(1):134–40.

28. Klunker S, Saggar LR, Seyfert-Margolis V, et al. Combination treatment with omalizumab and rush immunotherapy for ragweed-induced allergic rhinitis: inhibition of IgE-facilitated allergen binding. J Allergy Clin Immunol 2007;120(3):688–95.

29. Kopp MV, Brauburger J, Riedinger F, et al. The effect of anti-IgE treatment on in vitro leukotriene release in children with seasonal allergic rhinitis. J Allergy Clin Immunol 2002;110(5):728–35.

30. Faria R, McKenna C, Palmer S. Optimizing the position and use of omalizumab for severe persistent allergic asthma using cost-effectiveness analysis. Value Health 2014;17(8):772–82.

31. Hambly N, Nair P. Monoclonal antibodies for the treatment of refractory asthma. Curr Opin Pulm Med 2014;20(1):87–94.

32. Murakami T, Yamanaka K, Tokime K, et al. Topical suplatast tosilate (IPD) ameliorates Th2 cytokine-mediated dermatitis in caspase-1 transgenic mice by downregulating interleukin-4 and interleukin-5. Br J Dermatol 2006;155(1): 27–32.

33. Furukido K, Takeno S, Ueda T, et al. Suppression of the Th2 pathway by suplatast tosilate in patients with perennial nasal allergies. Am J Rhinol 2002;16(6): 329–36.

34. Borish LC, Nelson HS, Corren J, et al. Efficacy of soluble IL-4 receptor for the treatment of adults with asthma. J Allergy Clin Immunol 2001;107(6):963–70.

35. Wenzel S, Wilbraham D, Fuller R, et al. Effect of an interleukin-4 variant on late phase asthmatic response to allergen challenge in asthmatic patients: results of two phase 2a studies. Lancet 2007;370(9596):1422–31.

36. Haldar P, Brightling CE, Hargadon B, et al. Mepolizumab and exacerbations of refractory eosinophilic asthma. N Engl J Med 2009;360(10):973–84.

37. Garlisi CG, Falcone A, Kung TT, et al. T cells are necessary for Th2 cytokine production and eosinophil accumulation in airways of antigen-challenged allergic mice. Clin Immunol Immunopathol 1995;75(1):75–83.

38. Leigh R, Ellis R, Wattie JN, et al. Type 2 cytokines in the pathogenesis of sustained airway dysfunction and airway remodeling in mice. Am J Respir Crit Care Med 2004;169(7):860–7.

39. Larche M, Robinson DS, Kay AB. The role of T lymphocytes in the pathogenesis of asthma. J Allergy Clin Immunol 2003;111(3):450–63 [quiz: 464].

40. Robinson DS, Hamid Q, Ying S, et al. Predominant TH2-like bronchoalveolar T-lymphocyte population in atopic asthma. N Engl J Med 1992;326(5):298–304.

41. Horner AA. Toll-like receptor ligands and atopy: a coin with at least two sides. J Allergy Clin Immunol 2006;117(5):1133–40.

42. Feleszko W, Jaworska J, Hamelmann E. Toll-like receptors–novel targets in allergic airway disease (probiotics, friends and relatives). Eur J Pharmacol 2006;533(1–3):308–18.

43. Kawai T, Akira S. The role of pattern-recognition receptors in innate immunity: update on Toll-like receptors. Nat Immunol 2010;11(5):373–84.

44. Rosewich M, Lee D, Zielen S. Pollinex quattro: an innovative four injections immunotherapy in allergic rhinitis. Hum Vaccin Immunother 2013;9(7):1523–31.

45. Klimek L, Willers J, Hammann-Haenni A, et al. Assessment of clinical efficacy of CYT003-QbG10 in patients with allergic rhinoconjunctivitis: a phase IIb study. Clin Exp Allergy 2011;41(9):1305–12.

46. Creticos PS, Schroeder JT, Hamilton RG, et al. Immunotherapy with a ragweed-toll-like receptor 9 agonist vaccine for allergic rhinitis. N Engl J Med 2006; 355(14):1445–55.

47. Tsitoura D, Ambery C, Price M, et al. Early clinical evaluation of the intranasal TLR7 agonist GSK2245035: use of translational biomarkers to guide dosing and confirm target engagement. Clin Pharmacol Ther 2015;98(4):369–80.

48. Horak F. VTX-1463, a novel TLR8 agonist for the treatment of allergic rhinitis. Expert Opin Investig Drugs 2011;20(7):981–6.

49. Greiff L, Cervin A, Ahlstrom-Emanuelsson C, et al. Repeated intranasal TLR7 stimulation reduces allergen responsiveness in allergic rhinitis. Respir Res 2012;13:53.

50. Kostenis E, Ulven T. Emerging roles of DP and CRTH2 in allergic inflammation. Trends Mol Med 2006;12(4):148–58.

51. Pettipher R, Whittaker M. Update on the development of antagonists of chemoattractant receptor-homologous molecule expressed on Th2 cells (CRTH2).

From lead optimization to clinical proof-of-concept in asthma and allergic rhinitis. J Med Chem 2012;55(7):2915–31.

52. Pettipher R, Hansel TT, Armer R. Antagonism of the prostaglandin D2 receptors DP1 and CRTH2 as an approach to treat allergic diseases. Nat Rev Drug Discov 2007;6(4):313–25.

53. Xue L, Barrow A, Pettipher R. Novel function of CRTH2 in preventing apoptosis of human Th2 cells through activation of the phosphatidylinositol 3-kinase pathway. J Immunol 2009;182(12):7580–6.

54. Krug N, Gupta A, Badorrek P, et al. Efficacy of the oral chemoattractant receptor homologous molecule on TH2 cells antagonist BI 671800 in patients with seasonal allergic rhinitis. J Allergy Clin Immunol 2014;133(2):414–9.

55. Barnes N, Pavord I, Chuchalin A, et al. A randomized, double-blind, placebo-controlled study of the CRTH2 antagonist OC000459 in moderate persistent asthma. Clin Exp Allergy 2012;42(1):38–48.

56. Horak F, Zieglmayer P, Zieglmayer R, et al. The CRTH2 antagonist OC000459 reduces nasal and ocular symptoms in allergic subjects exposed to grass pollen, a randomised, placebo-controlled, double-blind trial. Allergy 2012;67(12):1572–9.

57. Horak F, Stubner P, Zieglmayer R, et al. Controlled comparison of the efficacy and safety of cetirizine 10 mg o.d. and fexofenadine 120 mg o.d. in reducing symptoms of seasonal allergic rhinitis. Int Arch Allergy Immunol 2001;125(1):73–9.

58. Zieglmayer P, Zieglmayer R, Bareille P, et al. Fluticasone furoate versus placebo in symptoms of grass-pollen allergic rhinitis induced by exposure in the Vienna Challenge Chamber. Curr Med Res Opin 2008;24(6):1833–40.

59. Baldrick P, Richardson D, Woroniecki SR, et al. Pollinex Quattro Ragweed: safety evaluation of a new allergy vaccine adjuvanted with monophosphoryl lipid A (MPL) for the treatment of ragweed pollen allergy. J Appl Toxicol 2007;27(4):399–409.

60. Naumann M, Dressler D, Hallett M, et al. Evidence-based review and assessment of botulinum neurotoxin for the treatment of secretory disorders. Toxicon 2013;67:141–52.

61. Braun T, Gurkov R, Kramer MF, et al. Septal injection of botulinum neurotoxin A for idiopathic rhinitis: a pilot study. Am J Otolaryngol 2012;33(1):64–7.

62. Ozcan C, Vayisoglu Y, Dogu O, et al. The effect of intranasal injection of botulinum toxin A on the symptoms of vasomotor rhinitis. Am J Otolaryngol 2006;27(5):314–8.

63. Rohrbach S, Junghans K, Kohler S, et al. Minimally invasive application of botulinum toxin A in patients with idiopathic rhinitis. Head Face Med 2009;5:18.

64. Rohrbach S, Laskawi R. Minimally invasive application of botulinum toxin type A in nasal hypersecretion. ORL J Otorhinolaryngol Relat Spec 2001;63(6):382–4.

65. Unal M, Sevim S, Dogu O, et al. Effect of botulinum toxin type A on nasal symptoms in patients with allergic rhinitis: a double-blind, placebo-controlled clinical trial. Acta Otolaryngol 2003;123(9):1060–3.

66. Kim KS, Kim SS, Yoon JH, et al. The effect of botulinum toxin type A injection for intrinsic rhinitis. J Laryngol Otol 1998;112(3):248–51.

67. van Rijswijk JB, Blom HM, Fokkens WJ. Idiopathic rhinitis, the ongoing quest. Allergy 2005;60(12):1471–81.

68. Baraniuk JN. Sensory, parasympathetic, and sympathetic neural influences in the nasal mucosa. J Allergy Clin Immunol 1992;90(6 Pt 2):1045–50.

69. Gevorgyan A, Segboer C, Gorissen R, et al. Capsaicin for non-allergic rhinitis. Cochrane Database Syst Rev 2015;(7):CD010591.

70. Blom HM, Van Rijswijk JB, Garrelds IM, et al. Intranasal capsaicin is efficacious in non-allergic, non-infectious perennial rhinitis. A placebo-controlled study. Clin Exp Allergy 1997;27(7):796–801.

71. Ciabatti PG, D'Ascanio L. Intranasal Capsicum spray in idiopathic rhinitis: a randomized prospective application regimen trial. Acta Otolaryngol 2009;129(4): 367–71.

72. Havas TE, Taplin MA. Intranasal neuropeptide depletion using topical capsaicin for the control of symptoms in non-allergic, non-infectious perennial rhinitis (NANIPER). Aust J Oto Laryngol 2002;5(2):107.

73. Van Rijswijk JB, Boeke EL, Keizer JM, et al. Intranasal capsaicin reduces nasal hyperreactivity in idiopathic rhinitis: a double-blind randomized application regimen study. Allergy 2003;58(8):754–61.

74. Van Gerven L, Alpizar YA, Wouters MM, et al. Capsaicin treatment reduces nasal hyperreactivity and transient receptor potential cation channel subfamily V, receptor 1 (TRPV1) overexpression in patients with idiopathic rhinitis. J Allergy Clin Immunol 2014;133(5):1332–9, 1339.e1–3.

75. Holland C, van Drunen C, Denyer J, et al. Inhibition of capsaicin-driven nasal hyper-reactivity by SB-705498, a TRPV1 antagonist. Br J Clin Pharmacol 2014;77(5):777–88.

76. Cheyne L, Irvin-Sellers MJ, White J. Tiotropium versus ipratropium bromide for chronic obstructive pulmonary disease. Cochrane Database Syst Rev 2013;(9):CD009552.

77. AlBalawi ZH, Othman SS, Alfaleh K. Intranasal ipratropium bromide for the common cold. Cochrane Database Syst Rev 2013;(6):CD008231.

78. Jokinen K, Sipila P. Intranasal ipratropium in the treatment of vasomotor rhinitis. Rhinology 1983;21(4):341–5.

79. Malmberg H, Grahne B, Holopainen E, et al. Ipratropium (Atrovent) in the treatment of vasomotor rhinitis of elderly patients. Clin Otolaryngol Allied Sci 1983; 8(4):273–6.

80. Knight A, Kazim F, Salvatori VA. A trial of intranasal atrovent versus placebo in the treatment of vasomotor rhinitis. Ann Allergy 1986;57(5):348–54.

81. Assanasen P, Baroody FM, Rouadi P, et al. Ipratropium bromide increases the ability of the nose to warm and humidify air. Am J Respir Crit Care Med 2000; 162(3 Pt 1):1031–7.

82. Ostberg B, Winther B, Borum P, et al. Common cold and high-dose ipratropium bromide: use of anticholinergic medication as an indicator of reflex-mediated hypersecretion. Rhinology 1997;35(2):58–62.

83. Becker B, Borum S, Nielsen K, et al. A time-dose study of the effect of topical ipratropium bromide on methacholine-induced rhinorrhoea in patients with perennial non-allergic rhinitis. Clin Otolaryngol Allied Sci 1997;22(2):132–4.

84. Schmitt J, Schwarz K, Stadler E, et al. Allergy immunotherapy for allergic rhinitis effectively prevents asthma: results from a large retrospective cohort study. J Allergy Clin Immunol 2015;136(6):1511–6.

85. Petalas K, Durham SR. Allergen immunotherapy for allergic rhinitis. Rhinology 2013;51(2):99–110.

86. Kariyawasam HK, Rotiroti G, Robinson DS. Sublingual immunotherapy in allergic rhinitis: indications, efficacy and safety. Rhinology 2013;51(1):9–17.

87. Cornelis M, Rombaux P, Jorissen M, et al. Nationwide survey on immunotherapy practice by ENT specialists. Rhinology 2014;52(1):72–7.

88. Li JT, Bernstein DI, Calderon MA, et al. Sublingual grass and ragweed immunotherapy: clinical considerations—a PRACTALL consensus report. J Allergy Clin Immunol 2015. [Epub ahead of print].

89. Wang L, Yin J, Fadel R, et al. House dust mite sublingual immunotherapy is safe and appears to be effective in moderate, persistent asthma. Allergy 2014;69(9): 1181–8.

90. Bergmann KC, Demoly P, Worm M, et al. Efficacy and safety of sublingual tablets of house dust mite allergen extracts in adults with allergic rhinitis. J Allergy Clin Immunol 2014;133(6):1608–14.e6.

91. Nony E, Bouley J, Le Mignon M, et al. Development and evaluation of a sublingual tablet based on recombinant bet v 1 in birch pollen-allergic patients. Allergy 2015;70(7):795–804.

92. Pitsios C, Demoly P, Bilo MB, et al. Clinical contraindications to allergen immunotherapy: an EAACI position paper. Allergy 2015;70(8):897–909.

93. Maloney J, Durham S, Skoner D, et al. Safety of sublingual immunotherapy Timothy grass tablet in subjects with allergic rhinitis with or without conjunctivitis and history of asthma. Allergy 2015;70(3):302–9.

94. Jutel M, Akdis CA. Novel immunotherapy vaccine development. Curr Opin Allergy Clin Immunol 2014;14(6):557–63.

95. de Azevedo MS, Innocentin S, Dorella FA, et al. Immunotherapy of allergic diseases using probiotics or recombinant probiotics. J Appl Microbiol 2013;115(2): 319–33.

96. Fili L, Cardilicchia E, Maggi E, et al. Perspectives in vaccine adjuvants for allergen-specific immunotherapy. Immunol Lett 2014;161(2):207–10.

97. Frischmeyer-Guerrerio PA, Keet CA, Guerrerio AL, et al. Modulation of dendritic cell innate and adaptive immune functions by oral and sublingual immunotherapy. Clin Immunol 2014;155(1):47–59.

98. Casale TB, Stokes JR. Immunotherapy: what lies beyond. J Allergy Clin Immunol 2014;133(3):612–9 [quiz: 620].

99. Baris S, Kiykim A, Ozen A, et al. Vitamin D as an adjunct to subcutaneous allergen immunotherapy in asthmatic children sensitized to house dust mite. Allergy 2014;69(2):246–53.

100. Rolinck-Werninghaus C, Hamelmann E, Keil T, et al. The co-seasonal application of anti-IgE after preseasonal specific immunotherapy decreases ocular and nasal symptom scores and rescue medication use in grass pollen allergic children. Allergy 2004;59(9):973–9.

101. Karlsson TR, Shakeel M, Supriya M, et al. Septoplasty with concomitant inferior turbinate reduction reduces the need for revision procedure. Rhinology 2015; 53(1):59–65.

102. Karatas A, Salviz M, Dikmen B, et al. The effects of different radiofrequency energy magnitudes on mucociliary clearance in cases of turbinate hypertrophy. Rhinology 2015;53(2):171–5.

103. Hegazy HM, ElBadawey MR, Behery A. Inferior turbinate reduction; coblation versus microdebrider—a prospective, randomised study. Rhinology 2014; 52(4):306–14.

104. Larrabee YC, Kacker A. Which inferior turbinate reduction technique best decreases nasal obstruction? Laryngoscope 2014;124(4):814–5.

105. Neri G, Mastronardi V, Traini T, et al. Respecting nasal mucosa during turbinate surgery: end of the dogma? Rhinology 2013;51(4):368–75.

106. Simmen D, Sommer F, Briner HR, et al. The effect of "pyriform turbinoplasty" on nasal airflow using a virtual model. Rhinology 2015;53(3):242–8.

107. Golding-Wood PH. Observations on petrosal and vidian neurectomy in chronic vasomotor rhinitis. J Laryngol Otol 1961;75:232–47.

108. Halderman A, Sindwani R. Surgical management of vasomotor rhinitis: a systematic review. Am J Rhinol Allergy 2015;29(2):128–34.

109. Robinson SR, Wormald PJ. Endoscopic vidian neurectomy. Am J Rhinol 2006; 20(2):197–202.

110. Lee JC, Kao CH, Hsu CH, et al. Endoscopic transsphenoidal vidian neurectomy. Eur Arch Otorhinolaryngol 2011;268(6):851–6.

111. Guo H, Liu MP. Mechanism of traditional Chinese medicine in the treatment of allergic rhinitis. Chin Med J 2013;126(4):756–60.

112. Jang TY, Kim YH, Shin SH. Long-term effectiveness and safety of endoscopic vidian neurectomy for the treatment of intractable rhinitis. Clin Exp Otorhinolaryngol 2010;3(4):212–6.

113. al-Samarrae SM. Treatment of 'vasomotor rhinitis' by the local application of silver nitrate. J Laryngol Otol 1991;105(4):285–7.

114. Bhargava KB, Shirali GN, Abhyankar US, et al. Treatment of allergic and vasomotor rhinitis by the local application of different concentrations of silver nitrate. J Laryngol Otol 1992;106(8):699–701.

115. Erhan E, Kulahli I, Kandemir O, et al. Comparison of topical silver nitrate and flunisolide treatment in patients with idiopathic non-allergic rhinitis. Tokai J Exp Clin Med 1996;21(2):103–11.

116. Jose J, Coatesworth AP. Inferior turbinate surgery for nasal obstruction in allergic rhinitis after failed medical treatment. Cochrane Database Syst Rev 2010;(12):CD005235.

117. McDonald JL, Cripps AW, Smith PK, et al. The anti-inflammatory effects of acupuncture and their relevance to allergic rhinitis: a narrative review and proposed model. Evid Based Complement Alternat Med 2013;2013:591796.

118. Feng S, Han M, Fan Y, et al. Acupuncture for the treatment of allergic rhinitis: a systematic review and meta-analysis. Am J Rhinol Allergy 2015;29(1):57–62.

119. Xue CC, Zhang AL, Zhang CS, et al. Acupuncture for seasonal allergic rhinitis: a randomized controlled trial. Ann Allergy Asthma Immunol 2015;115(4): 317–24.e1.

120. Fleckenstein J, Raab C, Gleditsch J, et al. Impact of acupuncture on vasomotor rhinitis: a randomized placebo-controlled pilot study. J Altern Complement Med 2009;15(4):391–8.

121. Chen S, Guo S, Wang J, et al. Effectiveness of moxibustion for allergic rhinitis: protocol for a systematic review. BMJ Open 2015;5(5):e006570.

122. Xue CC, Zhang CS, Yang AW, et al. Semi-self-administered ear acupressure for persistent allergic rhinitis: a randomised sham-controlled trial. Ann Allergy Asthma Immunol 2011;106(2):168–70.

123. Zhang CS, Xia J, Zhang AL, et al. Ear acupressure for perennial allergic rhinitis: a multicenter randomized controlled trial. Am J Rhinol Allergy 2014;28(4): e152–7.

124. Koreck AI, Csoma Z, Bodai L, et al. Rhinophototherapy: a new therapeutic tool for the management of allergic rhinitis. J Allergy Clin Immunol 2005;115(3): 541–7.

125. Koreck A, Szechenyi A, Morocz M, et al. Effects of intranasal phototherapy on nasal mucosa in patients with allergic rhinitis. J Photochem Photobiol B 2007; 89(2–3):163–9.

126. Tatar EC, Korkmaz H, Surenoglu UA, et al. Effects of rhinophototherapy on quality of life in persistant allergic rhinitis. Clin Exp Otorhinolaryngol 2013;6(2):73–7.

127. Casale TB, Romero FA, Spierings EL. Intranasal noninhaled carbon dioxide for the symptomatic treatment of seasonal allergic rhinitis. J Allergy Clin Immunol 2008;121(1):105–9.
128. Juto JE, Axelsson M. Kinetic oscillation stimulation as treatment of non-allergic rhinitis: an RCT study. Acta Otolaryngol 2014;134(5):506–12.
129. Cantone E, Marino A, Ferranti I, et al. Nonallergic rhinitis in the elderly: a reliable and safe therapeutic approach. ORL J Otorhinolaryngol Relat Spec 2015;77(3): 117–22.
130. Passariello A, Di Costanzo M, Terrin G, et al. Crenotherapy modulates the expression of proinflammatory cytokines and immunoregulatory peptides in nasal secretions of children with chronic rhinosinusitis. Am J Rhinol Allergy 2012;26(1):e15–9.
131. Cantone E, Marino A, Ferranti I, et al. Nasal cytological assessment after crenotherapy in the treatment of chronic rhinosinusitis in the elderly. Int J Immunopathol Pharmacol 2014;27(4):683–7.
132. Cantone E, Maione N, Di Rubbo V, et al. Olfactory performance after Crenotherapy in chronic rhinosinusitis in the elderly. Laryngoscope 2015;125(7):1529–34.
133. Miraglia Del Giudice M, Decimo F, Maiello N, et al. Effectiveness of ischia thermal water nasal aerosol in children with seasonal allergic rhinitis: a randomized and controlled study. Int J Immunopathol Pharmacol 2011;24(4):1103–9.

Moving?

Make sure your subscription moves with you!

To notify us of your new address, find your **Clinics Account Number** (located on your mailing label above your name), and contact customer service at:

Email: journalscustomerservice-usa@elsevier.com

800-654-2452 (subscribers in the U.S. & Canada)
314-447-8871 (subscribers outside of the U.S. & Canada)

Fax number: 314-447-8029

Elsevier Health Sciences Division
Subscription Customer Service
3251 Riverport Lane
Maryland Heights, MO 63043

*To ensure uninterrupted delivery of your subscription, please notify us at least 4 weeks in advance of move.